NUTRIPOINTS

CAN WORK FOR YOU TOO!

"I am hooked on the Nutripoints Program!
Thank you for your inspiration to start a
healthful, safe and permanent eating plan."

Riva Rosenfeld
North York, Ontario

"I have enjoyed your book and keep it with me
at all times. I have lost 50 pounds and finally
feel I am getting a balanced diet. I teach 6th
grade and use your information in class."

Ron Roberson
Inman, South Carolina

Continued

"I've been on your Nutripoints Program for about three weeks and I'm surprised at the extra energy it has developed; I'm 73. *Nutripoints* has become a daily reference work in our home."

James L. Jones
Allen Park, Michigan

"It is fascinating, positive and addictive. So several of us are about to get compulsive about counting Nutripoints. Thank you, and thank you."

Ellen M. Davis, et al.
The Winston School
Dallas, Texas

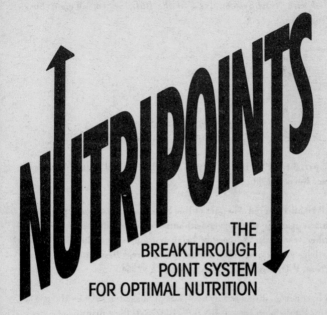

NUTRIPOINTS

THE
BREAKTHROUGH
POINT SYSTEM
FOR OPTIMAL NUTRITION

DR. ROY E. VARTABEDIAN
KATHY MATTHEWS

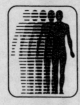

Designs For Wellness Press
P.O. Box 1450, Loma Linda, CA 92354

A hardcover edition of this book was published in 1990 by Harper & Row Publishers, Inc., ISBN 0-06-106275-9. First printing of paperback edition published in 1991 by HarperCollins*Publishers*, ISBN 0-06-109917-1.

Chart on page 146 from *Diet for a Small Planet*, © 1982 by Frances Moore Lappé. Reprinted by permission of Frances Moore Lappé and her agents, Raines & Raines, 71 Park Avenue, New York, N.Y.

First printing: March 1991
Second printing: June 1994
Third printing: January 1996

Printed in the United States of America

Designs For Wellness and logo are trademarks of Vartabedian & Associates and Dr. Roy E. Vartabedian.

TO MY GRANDMA, LOUISE VARTABEDIAN

It was my Grandma Louise's energy, positive attitude, and zest for living, combined with her compelling interest in foods that were "poisons" or "wonder foods," that inspired me to undertake nutrition and health science as my life's work. Grandma Louise lived well into her eighties. My wish is that you may benefit from the culmination of my grandmother's inspiration —Nutripoints —and that by following its principles you may enjoy as full and long a life as she did.

CONTENTS

Foreword   xiii

Acknowledgments   xv

PART I: **INTRODUCTION**   1

A Word from Kathy Matthews   3

"Update Overload" and the
    Confused Consumer   5

The Nutripoints Revolution   9

Future Foods   16

Nutripoint Numbers   18

    Nutripoint Values

    Nutripoint Quotas

    Nutripoint Balance

    Nutripoint Recovery

Nutripoints in the Real World   26

Why Nutripoints Could Be *Your*
    Nutritional Breakthrough   31

PART II: **THE SCIENCE OF OPTIMAL
NUTRITION**   37

Scared Smart   39

Beyond Calories   41

ix

Putting the Nutrients Back in
Nutrition   45
The Advantage of Natural Nutrition   50
How to Take a Vitamin   55
Is Our Food Really Safe?   59
Is Our Food Really Nutritious?   61

**PART III: THE NUTRIPOINT BUILDING
           BLOCKS**   63
The Nutripoint Formula   65
Answers to Questions About the
Nutripoint Formula   72
Essentials and Excessives   75
    The Essentials
    The Excessives

PART IV: NUTRIPOINTS AT WORK   109
Your Current Nutripoint Status   112
Keeping a Food Diary   112
Upgrading Your Diet   126
Nutrigroup Trends   130
Personalizing the Nutripoint
Program   137
The Vegetarian Option   142
Nutripoint Recovery   149
Shopping for Nutripoints   150
    Prepare to Shop
    Time Your Shopping Trips
    Shop Wisely
Eating Out   153
The Perfect Match: Boosting Your
Nutrition   158
Answers to Common Questions
About Nutripoints   159

PART V: SPECIAL LISTS   185
             Top-Ten Nutripoint Foods   187
             Nutripoint Shopping Lists   189
             A Nutrient Bang for the Buck   200

PART VI: NUTRIPOINT MENUS AND
             RECIPES   203
             Nutripoint Menus   209
             Nutripoint Recipes   225
                 Modifying Your Favorite Recipes

PART VII: NUTRIPOINT LISTS   279
             Nutrigroup Ratings   285
                 Vegetable Group
                 Fruit Group
                 Grain Group
                 Legume/Nut/Seed Group
                 Milk/Dairy Group
                 Meat/Fish/Poultry Group
             Other Groups   370
                 Fat/Oil Group
                 Sugar Group
                 Alcohol Group
                 Condiment Group
                 Miscellaneous Group
             Alphabetical Ratings   384

POSTSCRIPT   547
             An Invitation   550

REFERENCES   551

INDEX   553

ADDITIONAL NUTRIPOINT RATINGS   583

FOREWORD

Nutrition in the 1990s will be more sophisticated and more scientific than ever before. No longer will we guess at whether we are getting optimal nutrition; we will measure it accurately.

In 1968 I developed a simple and easy-to-follow point system for exercise called "aerobic" points. It revolutionized our concept of exercise. Now, at last, the same thing has been done for nutrition. A simple and easy-to-follow point system has been developed that I predict will permanently change the way we look at foods and nutrition.

After painstaking research and development using the Cooper Clinic Nutrition Database at the Aerobics Center, among others, Dr. Roy Vartabedian has formulated the Nutripoint rating system. Nutripoints, based on nutrient density, precisely quantifies the quality of 3,000 common foods by carefully comparing each food, nutrient by nutrient, to RDA standards. In addition, the system adjusts for cholesterol, sodium, total and saturated fat, sugar, caffeine, and alcohol in each food. The result is *one number* that, taking into account all these factors, tells you the bottom-line nutritional value of the food. I believe that Nutripoints will promote a major change in the American diet and will be an enormous help to everyone interested in avoiding "life-style" diseases, particularly heart disease and cancer.

A balanced program for total well-being must make nutrition its cornerstone. Nutripoints simplifies the complexities of nutrition with a point system that helps you compare foods and track your progress. The system has been used with tremendous success at the In-Residence Programs at the Aerobics Center, and I'm convinced that, coupled with an effective exercise program, it can help you achieve a healthier, happier life.

Kenneth H. Cooper, M.D.

ACKNOWLEDGMENTS

I owe a debt of gratitude to Dr. Kenneth Cooper for his assistance in making this book possible. Dr. Cooper's application of a point system to exercise in his landmark book, *Aerobics*, inspired me to apply this simple, practical concept to nutrition. In addition, his support in allowing me to devote time and energy to this book while directing the In-Residence Programs at the Aerobics Center made the project possible. By introducing me to his agent, Herbert M. Katz, he made this book a reality.

I am deeply indebted to Herb Katz. In addition to undertaking the standard responsibilities as the agent for *Nutripoints*, Herb acted as the "godfather" of the book from its inception, becoming its first champion and promoter as well as a thoughtful and discerning reader. His guidance throughout the publishing process has been invaluable.

Bill Shinker of Harper & Row has been a galvanizing force. His marketing vision and energetic commitment to *Nutripoints* have from the beginning made my association with his company an exciting experience.

Larry Ashmead, my editor at Harper & Row, has provided the enthusiasm that has kept *Nutripoints* on course right from the beginning. His immediate appreciation of the book's concept and his unflagging support have been greatly appreciated.

Margaret Wimberger, Eamon Dolan, and Anne McCoy, of

the editorial staff of Harper & Row, have been meticulous readers and have contributed greatly to the ultimate cohesion of the book.

I would also like to thank Karen Mender, Linda Michaels, Brenda Segel, Steve Magnuson, and Martin Weaver, all of Harper & Row, for their support, hard work, and dedication to this book.

My thanks to Mike Smith and Suzan Lewis, founders of Constructive Solutions, for their hard work. All the mathematical formulations and computations for *Nutripoints* were completed efficiently and accurately through their efforts, contributing to the book's scientific validity.

Kathleen Duran, R.D., Assistant Director, In-Residence Programs, supplied many of the menus and recipes for *Nutripoints*, culling them from the recipes she developed at the In-Residence Programs. She also acted as my nutritional consultant.

Ava Bursau, M.S., Associate Director, In-Residence Programs, is my able associate who helped keep things running smoothly in the In-Residence Programs and allowed me to focus on the book.

Susan Hill, my data-processing specialist, performed the herculean task of plugging 50,000 pieces of information into the computer in order to analyze the more than 3,000 foods found in *Nutripoints*.

Linda Zeiner and Susan Wampler, my executive secretary, worked on the major project of alphabetizing the food lists. Susan also helped compile the recipe section.

Scott Dyer of Tom Thumb Food Stores allowed me to obtain information on brand-name foods at his facilities in North Dallas.

I am grateful to all the manufacturers who sent information on their products, allowing us to make complete and accurate analyses of their ingredients.

Nutripoints guidelines and recommendations were developed for the average healthy adult free from disease or major risk factors. Physical variations from individual to individual may necessitate modifications of the book's suggestions. As always, common sense must be used when following a certain program or regime, and extremes must be avoided. Before starting any nutrition or exercise program, you should consult a physician who will supervise your overall program. None of the information presented here should supersede your physician's or dietitian's advice. If you experience any adverse health effects while on the *Nutripoints* program, check with your physician or dietitian.

NUTRIPOINTS

PART I

INTRODUCTION

A WORD FROM KATHY MATTHEWS

THE WORDS *REVOLUTIONARY* AND *BREAKTHROUGH* ARE SO COM-
monplace these days that when something that truly earns
these descriptions comes along we're left tongue-tied. *How do
you describe a nutritional system that replaces counting calories,
worrying over fats, sugar, and sodium, calculating cholesterol,
and figuring out RDAs—a system that does all this, and more,
with a single number that tells you all you need to know to
maintain a healthy diet?*

Revolutionary, it certainly is.

A breakthrough, unquestionably.

In the same week that I met Dr. Vartabedian, creator of
Nutripoints, I received a frantic phone call from a friend. I've
known Carol since college and we've been through the diet
wars together. About twenty pounds overweight, she had just
decided to go on a simple, safe, low-calorie diet—one of those
popular diets I'm sure you've heard of. She had also just
visited her doctor who, because of her family medical history,
had warned her that she must make a serious effort to get
plenty of calcium in her diet. He also warned her to avoid
cholesterol-rich foods, such as whole milk and other dairy
products. He said that the diet she planned to use was a good
one but that she should be careful not to skimp on the recommended protein: adequate protein was essential if she wanted
to lose weight safely and permanently.

Carol is a motivated and intelligent bank vice president.
She is quite sophisticated in her knowledge of nutrition, but
her head was spinning. "Kathy," she said on the phone, "this
isn't getting easier, it's getting harder. I want to lose weight
but I don't want to have to become a professional dietitian.
You've written two books on nutrition that were best-sellers.
What can I eat?"

I promised to help Carol but I knew that it would be a

complicated and relatively tedious task. She needed high-quality protein that was low in fat and cholesterol and probably a lot of green vegetables, some of which would help her obtain her calcium requirement. Would a broiled, skinless breast of chicken be a better choice than a broiled veal chop? And what about the days when Carol had no time to cook; were there any frozen, prepared meals that were really good, nutritionally speaking? Was it really possible to get in a full day's nutrition—all the vitamins and minerals as well as adequate protein and carbohydrates—on a low-fat, low-calorie diet? When you came right down to it, what *were* the best foods to eat? Carol's words rang in my ears and I realized that despite, or perhaps because of, the constant flood of nutritional information, finding your way through the food maze just isn't getting any easier.

Then I met Dr. Vartabedian, a nutritional pioneer who has assimilated a great deal of contradictory data, and who has gone a step beyond anyone in his field. Dr. Vartabedian had already helped nearly a thousand patients grappling with the same problems faced by my friend Carol, and who, like Carol, are intelligent, self-motivated readers of dozens of books and articles that have put them on a nutritional seesaw, trying to balance the benefits and disadvantages inherent in any given food. For example:

• This food is high in calcium but also high in fat.
• This food is low in fat but high in sodium.
• This food is high in protein but also high in cholesterol.
• This food is low in cholesterol but high in saturated, or "bad," fat.
• This food is low in calories but not very nutritious.

When I recited the litany of seemingly contradictory nutritional recommendations that confuse us all, Dr. Vartabedian acknowledged the confusion as the inspiration for Nutripoints. The following pages contain Dr. Vartabedian's explanation of the Nutripoint concept and how it works.

"UPDATE OVERLOAD" AND THE CONFUSED CONSUMER

I think it is wonderful that nutritional updates have become fixtures in the news. Unfortunately, in my experience as a nutritionist who has seen thousands of patients over the course of a career, the result of all this information is confusion. If a research finding doesn't help you in the kitchen or at the dining table, where it really counts, it can't do you any good.

When I was a student of nutrition, all my questions about the body and the foods that fuel it were readily answered by my distinguished professors. Nutrition on the molecular level, while complicated, is relatively straightforward. It was only when I began my practice that things became almost intolerably confusing, a confusion reflected in the case histories that follow:

• Mary had read in a women's magazine that if she didn't eat enough protein while trying to diet, she would lose muscle rather than fat and so regain any lost weight very quickly. But how much was enough protein? And didn't protein come mainly from meat and have a lot of fat? How could she find protein that didn't have a lot of calories?

• Roberta ate out at restaurants all the time. She knew the principles of good nutrition (avoid fried foods and creamy sauces, and so on), but what were the best, and most healthful, foods on a typical restaurant menu? Was fresh grilled tuna better or worse than baked flounder? What about a small, very lean baked pork chop compared to a few slices of lean baked ham?

• James had suffered two heart attacks and was on a low-cholesterol diet, but he frequently had to eat at restaurants and just didn't know which foods, particularly meats, were low in cholesterol. He used to think that shrimp was OK, but now he wasn't sure. Everything he read about "good" and "bad" cholesterol confused him even more.

• Ted called himself a "businessman/athlete." He jogged every morning and was in training for a local triathlon competition. He knew he needed to eat well, but he resorted to fast food all the time because he didn't like to cook. Was he getting enough of the right types of foods? Was a Celentano Chicken Primavera entree that he could cook quickly in the microwave a good nutritional choice? How would it compare with, say, a Mrs. Paul's Light and Natural Flounder Fillet?

• Barbara had three kids who were very picky eaters. She knew that it was important for them to get proper nutrition in their growing years, but their eating habits were so erratic she had no confidence that she was having any success. If they loved peanut butter and jelly sandwiches, was that better or worse than a tuna sandwich? She avoided buying breakfast cereals with a lot of sugar, but aside from that, was one brand really better than another in terms of nutrition?

• Lori and her husband had retired and faced many of the nutritional problems of the elderly: they had diminished appetites and had to carefully watch cholesterol and fat intake. Because they were eating less, they had to be particularly careful to get adequate nutrition. Lori wanted to know if those substitute foods such as Egg Beaters and Molly McButter were really OK to use. And would a vitamin pill take care of them on those days when they skipped a meal?

• Phil found himself eating at fast-food restaurants at least five times a week because they were quick and convenient. But what type of nutrition was he getting from this kind of food? Was a McDonald's Quarter Pounder better or worse than a Jack in the Box Beef Fajita Pita? What were the *best* fast foods in terms of nutritional value?

These people came to me, as an expert, with their very real and pressing questions, and I found it difficult to answer them. Most of us know what foods are "good" for us; no one would argue that a carrot or an orange is not "good." And we also feel fairly comfortable pinpointing "bad" foods; fried pork rinds and fudge sauce would be picked out of any list of suspects by just about anyone. But what about all those foods in between "good" and "bad"? How do you judge them? There was no gradient scale that could measure whether an apple was better than an orange or a fried pork rind worse than a strip of fried bacon. *Were* there any dairy foods that were low in fat and high in calcium? *Were* high-fiber breakfast cereals, particularly oat bran, really good nutritional choices? *Were* some "good" vegetables better than other "good" vegetables?

These questions frustrated me as well as my patients. I realized that it was very easy to tell people what *not* to eat, but much harder to tell them what they *should* eat. Indeed, there was an entire spectrum of food values from very good to very bad, but there was no way to measure anything between those extremes. No one believed you could compare apples and oranges, and no one had tried.

There was another factor involved. Suzanne put her finger on it for me when she came to see me about getting sufficient calcium in her pregnancy diet, while avoiding too many unnecessary calories (a very common concern).

"Dr. Vartabedian," she complained, "I'm really interested in nutrition and good food. And of course"—she gestured toward her growing waistline—"never more so than now. But lately I've noticed that every time I think about food I feel anxious. Is it good for me? Good for the baby? Is it really nutritious? Does it have too much fat? Do embryos need to restrict their cholesterol intake?

"Sometimes I'm jealous of my mother, who never worried about palm oil in her crackers, and just ate what she wanted and tried not to eat too much. I read recently that stress increases your cholesterol level. If that's true, it made me wonder if we aren't all taking one step forward and two steps back: we are so worried about how to eat right that even when we *do* eat the right things, our cholesterol levels are going up anyhow from anxiety."

Suzanne's feelings about food and eating had, over a period of years, gone from blithe unconcern, except for calories, to anxiety: diet anxiety. She knew a lot about food, but she didn't know enough to put it all together.

Suzanne was an inspiration to me. Her words rang in my ears long after her healthy baby was born and I'd moved to a fascinating job at Dr. Kenneth Cooper's Aerobics Center in Dallas. The center offers the most comprehensive, state-of-the-art wellness programs available in the world, and it gave me the opportunity to work with one of the most advanced nutritional data bases available. I knew that there must be a solution to Suzanne's dilemma—diet anxiety—and I set about to find it.

Over the course of years, working with hundreds of patients, I finally refined a system that I believe answers *all* of today's perplexing nutritional questions. It's a system that not only tells you which foods are good and which are bad but also establishes a gradient scale that measures all foods. Not only does it rate all foods, it provides a simple system that gives you an optimally balanced diet, one that allows you the luxury of choice.

Nutripoints is my answer to all the patients whose questions I had so painstakingly researched. Nutripoints is the tool that will allow them, and anyone else interested in good nutrition, to find an optimum diet.

We should not be confused about food. Above all, we should not be anxious about what we eat. My hope is that Nutripoints will be a giant step toward returning us to safe, pleasurable, healthful eating.

THE NUTRIPOINTS REVOLUTION

The Nutripoints program is something very different from anything you've come across. It is an actual nutritional advance and a quantum leap in our ability to know that we are eating healthful meals. It will provide you with an entirely new approach to eating. Here are the four revolutionary features of the Nutripoint program that make it so effective and appealing:

1. Nutripoints is the only nutritional information you'll ever need.

Nutripoints assures you that you will meet or exceed all the major nutritional guidelines—including those of the American Heart Association, the American Cancer Society, the National Cancer Institute, and the American Dietetic Association—regarding daily intakes of every major nutrient, including protein, carbohydrates, fiber, vitamins, and minerals, while at the same time staying well below the allowable levels of fat, cholesterol, sugar, and sodium.

Have you ever stood in the supermarket trying to figure out what grams of fat mean in terms of calories? Have you ever wondered what it means when a packaged food provides 100 percent of your daily requirement of one vitamin and 0 percent of everything else? Have you been on diets that you later learned were damaging to your health, even though they might be effective? Do you get confused about whether 1-percent or 2-percent milk is better for you in terms of fat content? And do you know which cheeses are lowest in cholesterol?

Before Nutripoints, you would have had to do twenty-six mathematical calculations on each food you eat to have only the *basis* for the information Nutripoints gives in one number.

Now you can forget about calories, grams of fat, and milligrams of sodium—and even forget about reading labels. And you don't have to abandon hope when you go to a fast-food restaurant. Nutripoints weighs *all* the bad factors in a food against *all* the good factors, and comes up with a simple number that tells you everything you need to know to provide the human machine with the best possible fuel.

Say you're choosing among juices. Here is a small sample of the Nutripoint ratings for juices:

Juice	Nutripoints
Unsweetened grapefruit juice	11.0
Minute Maid frozen orange juice	10.0
Dole pineapple juice	5.0
Ocean Spray Cranapple juice	1.5
Lucky Leaf apple juice	1.0

A quick glance at this chart tells you that canned pineapple juice is only half as good as orange juice. And some brands of apple juice are only one-fifth as good as some brands of orange juice. The Nutripoint charts make it easy to choose a juice that you and your family like, as well as a juice that provides good nutrition. You don't even have to know the scientific basis for the Nutripoint score, namely, that those with a higher number contain more vitamin C and less sugar than the juices with a lower score.

Now let's say you're choosing a cereal. Here are the numbers for just a few:

Cereal	Nutripoints
Whole Wheat Total	64.5
Kellogg's Product 19	56.0
Nabisco 100% Bran Cereal	31.0
Quaker Oat Squares	17.0
Kellogg's Special K	14.0
Kellogg's Fruit Loops	13.0
Post Cocoa Pebbles	7.5
Quaker 100% Natural cereal	1.0

The general trend with cereals is that the more sugar and processing that come into play and the original whole food, if any, is adulterated, the lower the level of nutrition. Consequently, cereals scoring high on the scale contain more bran or whole grain as well as less sugar (and possibly more added vitamins) than the others. Once again, if you're concerned with good nutrition, you need only look for the high numbers to find the best choices.

Whether you're choosing between broccoli or brussels sprouts, snapper or salmon, cheddar or goat cheese, or even Mars Bars or Milky Ways and Chicken McNuggets or Big Macs, *Nutripoints* is your good-food bible.

2. Nutripoints is the first positive approach to nutrition that eliminates rigid adhesion to menus and meal plans, because the balance is "built in."

Any diet in the past has had to rely on various meal plans that sometimes got pretty complicated. That's because there was no other way to ensure that people would get the right balance of foods. You can't just eat low-calorie foods and be well nourished: you need to eat from a broad spectrum of foods. The best diets were well constructed: someone figured out how much fat, protein, complex carbohydrates, and so forth were in each food and in each meal and made sure that these amounts were adequate. But you had to follow a very specific daily menu plan or a complicated system of "substitutions" in order to maintain a nutritional balance. Nutripoints makes that rigid approach history because it provides a *comprehensive system* that allows you to create your own meal plans. By following the recommendations concerning numbers of servings from the six Nutrigroups, you'll be guaranteed an optimum diet—one of your own choosing.

Though you'll find menus for those who need and/or want them, the Nutripoint program is totally flexible. Once you're familiar with Nutripoints, you need only focus on the foods you like and the foods that are readily available to you to create meals that give you the best possible nutritional value. You won't be shopping for fish to broil on a day that you're really in a mood for pasta. I've even provided some lists of the best nutritional values, in terms of your food budget, which will help you achieve an optimum diet on limited funds.

Once you're familiar with Nutripoints, you'll find it will become an instinctive way of eating. Best of all, you'll find that simply by choosing your foods from the top of the Nutripoint charts, and getting the recommended servings from every Nutrigroup, you'll be getting at least 100 percent of the RDA (Recommended Daily Allowance) for every vitamin and mineral, as well as the optimum amount of fiber, protein, carbohydrates, and fat. You'll also be limiting your total fat, saturated fat, cholesterol, sugar, sodium, caffeine, and alcohol intake.

Hundreds of Nutripoint converts agree that it's the best remedy for diet anxiety.

3. Nutripoints not only lets you know what's bad, it separates the best from the merely good.

Most foods have some bad things in them as well as some good. But how much bad and how much good? How do you evaluate this difference? Dairy foods seem to be particularly confusing today because of a very real concern about calcium. People know they need to get adequate calcium, but the foods that are very high in calcium, such as milk and cheese, are also very high in fat. Nutripoints eliminates the confusion. The higher the Nutripoint score, the lower in fat *and* the higher in calcium is the rated food. *Evaluating the critical differences in foods is what Nutripoints is all about.*

Here's an illustration of how processing lowers the Nutripoint score of a particular food.

Food	Nutripoints
Potato, baked	8.5
Potatoes au gratin	2.5
Weight Watchers baked potato with broccoli and cheese	1.5
Mashed potatoes, home recipe	1.0
Ore-Ida Golden Crinkles French fries	0.5
Betty Crocker instant mashed potatoes	−0.5
Pringle's potato chips with sour cream and onion	−1.5

You can readily see that the more a food is processed and adulterated, the more salt and fatty substances are added, and the more the original vitamin and mineral content is tampered with, the lower its Nutripoints.

Do you like yogurt? Do you think it's good for you? Here are the facts:

Yogurt	*Nutripoints*
Dannon nonfat light yogurt, all flavors	10.5
Dannon nonfat yogurt, plain	9.0
Weight Watchers Nonfat Ultimate yogurt, all flavors	8.0
Dannon low-fat yogurt, plain	5.5
Weight Watchers nonfat yogurt, peach	4.5
Yoplait nonfat light yogurt, all flavors	4.0
whole milk yogurt, plain	2.5
Yoplait low-fat strawberry yogurt	−0.5
Yoplait banana custard style	−1.0

As the fat and the sugar go up, the Nutripoints go down. Your choice might be an excellent serving of nonfat yogurt (with fresh fruit added to boost your Nutripoint score) or a yogurt that not only does you little nutritional good but actually has a negative effect on your daily nutritional status.

There are factors other than processing, factors in the food itself, that affect its Nutripoint score. Indeed, if you're someone who pays attention to good nutrition and tries to eat well, you will no doubt find that *Nutripoints is the first system to come along that tells you something you don't already know.* Here's an example. If you thought that simple steamed shrimp was a great diet food (low in calories but high in protein), you'll be interested to learn that fifteen medium shrimp earn only 0.5 Nutripoints, while half a can of low-sodium tuna in water is worth 8 Nutripoints, a far greater nutritional value. If you've been starving yourself on occasion, thinking that a lunch of a few shrimp and some lettuce is a virtuous choice, you will be delighted to learn that you're really better off with a tuna sandwich made with yogurt and vegetables on whole wheat bread. You'll be more full, you'll be better nourished, and if losing weight is your goal, you'll be better served in the long run.

Most of us know we should cut down on fat. But knowing such things isn't much help when it comes to shopping and eating. Nutripoints to the rescue: For example, did you know that Fleischmann's Egg Beaters (17.5 Nutripoints) is a terrific dairy food and a nutritionally sound substitute for scrambled eggs, which weigh in at −13.5 Nutripoints for one egg? And that Laughing Cow reduced-calorie cheese (2.5 Nutripoints) is a great substitute for cream cheese (−5 Nutripoints) when you want something to spread on a bagel?

Many people have abandoned canned fruit, thinking only fresh was of any merit, but it turns out that a half cup of canned mandarin orange slices without sugar has a Nutripoint value of 15.5, while a *fresh* pear earns only 4.5 Nutripoints. Mandarin oranges simply have more nutrition—more vitamin C and more fiber—than a fresh pear.

What about a soup for a quick lunch? Campbell's Chicken Noodle at −1.5 Nutripoints isn't the great nutritional bargain we might have expected, but Campbell's Chunky Beef at 4 Nutripoints is a good alternative. And what about those evenings when you don't have a minute to spare? Celentano Frozen Chicken Primavera (6 Nutripoints) or Chung King Frozen Beef Teriyaki (5 Nutripoints) are both quick, nutritious meals. But the Budget Gourmet Frozen Slim Chicken au Gratin (2 Nutripoints) or the Weight Watchers frozen Stuffed Sole with Newburg Sauce (1.5 Nutripoints) don't score as well.

If you're like most of my patients, just a glance at the Nutripoints food lists will be both a revelation for you and a revolution for your future diet.

4. Nutripoints allows for recovery from "being bad."

We've become so chained to the "calories per day" or "fat per day" notion of nutrition that it's a relief to substitute the Nutripoints concept, which deals with *real* nutrition in the real world. The fact is, in terms of nutrition, a day is a very short time frame. For example, your body stores vitamin A for weeks. With the Nutripoints program you no longer have to think about a twenty-four-hour make-it-or-break-it eating pattern: you can spread things out over the course of a few days. Although, for the sake of convenience, you'll still be aiming for a daily total of 100 points, you can be flexible enough to go over or under on any given day and make up for the lack within another day or two.

Because Nutripoints gives you a way of *measuring* the values of the foods you eat, it gives you an opportunity to get back on track if you fall behind.

Nutripoints is such a simple "numbers game" with negative and positive numbers that if you have a really bad day in which you eat the wrong foods—a day with a negative total of Nutripoints—you can still wind up with an excellent nutritional week.

This expansion of the basic diet time frame removes one of the most persistent and discouraging psychological barriers to effective dieting—the old "I've blown it today, so I might as well forget it" rationale.

FUTURE FOODS

You're probably aware that the foods you eat are very different from those eaten by your grandparents. What determines how "food styles" change? Agricultural trends, food storage, and distribution methods all have some effect, but a big determinant is simple fashion. It's no longer fashionable, for example, for a woman or man to display wealth with girth. It made cultural sense, once upon a time, to achieve status with the evidence of rich and lavish meals. The lean and hungry peasant would look with longing at the tubby lord. Today that trend is fully reversed: for years now people have believed that you can never be too thin or too rich.

In addition to fashion, there are practical reasons for a constantly changing and diverse national diet. A farmer, faced with a day of work from sunrise to sunset, is going to have nutritional needs that differ substantially from those of a stockbroker or a bank teller. The latter simply don't need the greater amounts of fuel required by a body that's doing hard labor.

The great nutritional challenge we face today can be simply stated. Our optimum diet has two principles that seem diametrically opposed: we need to get high levels of nutrients (to keep our bodies functioning well while helping them to fight the effects of disease, aging, and pollution), and we need to achieve this in fewer and fewer calories (to avoid excess weight that affects our appearance and our health).

These needs force us to scrutinize our foods in a new way. If we want to achieve optimum health and longevity we have to think about *nutrients per calorie.*

Nutrients per calorie is the basic cost/benefit analysis we have to keep in mind when we choose foods. It's analogous to our efforts to get the most value per dollar when buying a product. Because we are usually limiting our calorie intake, every calorie has to count in terms of overall nutritional value. Here's an example: there is ample vitamin C in half an avocado, but it will "cost" 160 calories, while a cup of grapefruit juice has nine times the vitamin C of the avocado at a "cost" of only 95 calories.

This concept of nutrients per calorie explains why junk foods are *junk:* they provide virtually no nutrition and a lot of calories. Take, for example, a typical fast-food lunch: a Big Mac with a large order of fries and a Coke. This meal gives you only 30 to 50 percent of major nutrients at a cost of 1,064 calories. For many people that's the *total* number of calories they should have in a day, and they wouldn't have gotten *half* their necessary nutrients. With Nutripoints, you can get over 100 percent of any RDA, along with optimum amounts of fiber, protein, and complex carbohydrates, with the *same* number of calories.

You must remember, also, that it costs vitamins and minerals to burn up calories. If you're not getting adequate nutrients along with the calories you're burning up, the body's stores of vitamins and minerals must be called upon to make up for the lack in the food itself. This is the not uncommon predicament that can lead to clinical or subclinical deficiencies and less-than-optimal function of various body processes.

A high nutrient-per-calorie ratio is the basic principle of every healthful diet. *Nutripoints* rates every food on the basis of this critical nutrient-per-calorie ratio. Moreover, because *Nutripoints* rates just about every conceivable food, it allows you to create your own diet, one that suits your tastes and your life-style.

NUTRIPOINT NUMBERS

Nutripoints is a very simple way of dealing with something very complex. It is a number system for rating foods.

The Nutripoint program has four important principles:

Nutripoint Values

Each food has a given Nutripoint value. It is amazingly simple: the higher the Nutripoint score of a given food, the higher it is in "good" components (including all the important vitamins and minerals, and fiber and protein), and the lower it is in "bad" components (including calories, cholesterol, total fat, saturated fat, sodium, sugar, caffeine, and alcohol). Just about every food imaginable, including basic foods, processed foods, fast foods, and even "health" foods, has been evaluated and assigned a number.

Some foods fall in a "not recommended" level and some foods are so low in Nutripoints that they have negative Nutripoint values—such as Mars Bars at −3.5 Nutripoints. Nutripoint values are provided for *all* types of foods, even poor nutritional choices. This is the way in which Nutripoints differs from typical diets. *All foods are evaluated in terms of Nutripoints.* This allows you to compare the bad with the good as well as the good with the best.

A glance at the Nutripoints for various foods is an eye-opener. For instance, we all know the old adage about an apple a day, but did you know that cantaloupe is a far better choice? In the fruit Nutrigroup, although both are "good" for you, one-quarter cantaloupe has 29 Nutripoints whereas an apple has only 4.5. The cantaloupe has fewer calories (50 versus 80) and more iron, fifty times the vitamin A, ten times the vitamin C, more folacin, thiamine, and riboflavin, and more of virtually every other nutrient than the apple. Spinach (75 Nutripoints) is a much better vegetable than plain iceberg lettuce (18 Nutripoints), even though both are low in calories.

Many people are surprised to learn that some cuts of lean beef are better choices than some types of fish. For example, lean round steak (4 Nutripoints) is a better choice than baked flounder (3.5 Nutripoints). Many people wouldn't guess that three ounces of lean, baked ham (5 Nutripoints) is a better choice than a three-ounce, lean, broiled hamburger (3 Nutripoints). Broccoli (38.5 Nutripoints) is a terrific nutritional value compared to a baked potato (8.5 Nutripoints).

As I mentioned, there are negative Nutripoints, and there's also a cut-off point below which foods are not recommended. The numbers are interesting just as a basis of comparison between foods, but you also need them to figure out your daily Nutripoint scores.

Nutripoint Quotas
The numbers assigned to foods have to be put into a workable context: what do they really add up to? You can't just eat a few servings of spinach a day and get a lot of Nutripoints and consider yourself well nourished. There has to be a balance of different types of foods over a period of time.

The Nutripoint program recommends that you get 100 Nutripoints per day, which will give you approximately 100 percent of the RDAs. Not only will you get the necessary amounts of eighteen important nutrients, you will at the same time limit the calories, sugar, cholesterol, total fat, saturated fat, sodium, caffeine, and alcohol in your diet—in one easy step helping to prevent and control heart disease, hypertension, diabetes, obesity, osteoporosis, cancer, and other life-style diseases.

Here's how Patrick, a salesman, rated on a typical day before he began the Nutripoint program:

Patrick's Diet

Food	Nutripoints
Breakfast	
2 fried eggs	−25.0
3 strips fried bacon	− 1.0
1 cup coffee	− 3.5
1 Danish	− 2.5
Lunch	
McDonald's Big Mac	− 2.0
French fries	− 2.0
Coke	− 6.0
Dinner	
3 pieces fried chicken	0.0
½ cup mashed potatoes	2.0
with gravy	0.0
Salad	33.0
with dressing	− 2.5
Total:	− 9.5

You can readily see that −9.5 Nutripoints is a very poor score for a day if the goal is 100 points. It means that Patrick is probably eating far too much fat, sodium, and calories, and is not getting nearly enough fiber and nutrients. A daily diet with a Nutripoint total in this range could spell the beginning of future health problems, as well as minor immediate symptoms. Patrick probably would complain of headaches, general sluggishness, digestive problems, inability to concentrate, and afternoon fatigue.

Of course, 100 Nutripoints is just a basic goal: you may fall below it on some days and exceed it by a wide margin on others. The following chart shows you how to assess a daily Nutripoint score:

Daily Nutripoint Scores
25	— Very poor
50	— Poor
75	— Fair
100	**— Good**
150	**— Excellent**
200+	**— Superior**

Nutripoint Balance

In order for the Nutripoint program to work, your diet must be balanced. You can't eat a cup of turnip greens (79 Nutripoints), some asparagus (44 Nutripoints), some raw radishes (29 Nutripoints), and some cucumber (20 Nutripoints) for a total of 172 Nutripoints, and call it a day. You have to choose from various food groups to be sure that you cover all the nutritional bases.

There are six basic Nutrigroups. To achieve a Nutripoint balance, you must achieve a Nutripoint goal for each group, and *you must do it within the recommended number of servings.* The serving quota is a limiting device: you want to score the highest possible number of Nutripoints, but you can't do it by simply eating enormous quantities of foods.

By following the Nutripoint program of Nutrigroups, you are assured you will meet or surpass recommendations of the

American Heart Association, the American Cancer Society, the National Cancer Institute, and the American Dietetic Association.

The following is a simple breakdown of the food group system:

Daily Nutripoint Recommendations

Servings	Nutrigroup	Nutripoints
4	Vegetables	55
3	Fruits	15
2	Grains	10
1	Legumes	5
2	Milk/dairy	10
1	Meat/poultry/fish	5
Total:		100

What does the chart mean to you on a daily basis? You are going to be making sure that you get four vegetable servings daily. Many vegetables are very high in Nutripoints, and I think you'll find it quite easy to get 55 points per day. For example, you might have a tossed salad (33 Nutripoints) at lunch, broccoli (38.5 Nutripoints) and a baked potato (8.5 Nutripoints) at dinner, and a glass of V-8 juice (24.5 Nutripoints) as a snack. This would give you four vegetable servings for a total of 105.5 Nutripoints—well above the 55 Nutripoints you're supposed to get from the vegetable group.

Of course, now and again you might have a day in which you don't do very well. Maybe you'll have a chef's salad (−1.5 Nutripoints), some French fries (1 Nutripoint), some cooked zucchini (15 Nutripoints) and some Fritos (Fritos are in the vegetable group because their principal ingredient is corn), worth −1.5 Nutripoints. Your total score on that day would be 13 Nutripoints from four servings in the vegetable Nutrigroup. You can boost your score with excellent choices from the other groups, and you can boost your long-term score with Nutripoint recovery.

Nutripoint Recovery

What does it really mean if you get more or fewer than 100 Nutripoints daily? It's an opportunity to see your nutritional status in terms of more than just one day.

Most diets are limited to a one-day pattern that, for many dieters, means walking a nutritional tightrope—if you break down and have some barbecued chicken wings at a cocktail party, you fall off the diet. This is enormously discouraging. Even if the diet tells you to view the lapse as a mistake, and to move on from there, you're never given a *method* that allows you to incorporate the mistake into the diet plan.

Nutripoints is the first nutritional system that gives you a method for recovery. Nutripoints, which is really a leap beyond dieting, gives you the flexibility to recover from a lapse. You no longer have to despair about a bad day.

While you're shooting for 100 Nutripoints per day, the program allows you to quantify the values of the foods you're eating and thereby make up for a bad day within the next day or two. If you have a business dinner that includes a high-fat Mexican meal that plunges your Nutripoints to a negative number, you can boost your scores back up to optimum levels with some high Nutripoint scores during the next few days. So if your Mexican-debacle day totals 32 Nutripoints, you can go for the gold for the next two days, trying to get well in excess of your recommended daily 100 points.

The important point is that because Nutripoints gives you a way of *measuring* the value of your nutritional intake, it also gives you a method of recovering from losses. You cannot "bank" Nutripoints: you can't prepare for a binge on Wednesday by getting high scores on Monday and Tuesday. After all, you're fooling no one but yourself if you try to use Nutripoints in that way. But you don't have to feel defeated by a day's low score.

Let's face it: not all our lapses are forced. What about when you're just dying for an ice cream cone? Or what if high-altitude amnesia forces you to eat the honey-roasted peanuts on the plane? With the Nutripoint program you have a method of atonement. You need only be sure to make up for those negative points within a couple of days.

The following record shows how Patrick improved his weekly Nutripoint score to recover from his dismal day recorded earlier:

Patrick's Improved Diet

Food	Nutripoints
Breakfast	
⅓ cup All Bran cereal	27.0
1 cup skim milk	9.5
¼ cantaloupe	29.0
With ¼ cup blueberries	3.5
With 2 oz. plain, nonfat yogurt	2.0
Lunch	
Tuna salad sandwich:	
½ cup tuna (Getting into the Nutripoint spirit, he mixed tuna with yogurt and shredded carrots and scallions to boost his score.)	15.0
2 slices whole grain bread	6.0
Fresh fruit salad	13.0
Dinner	
3 oz. chicken breast, baked, no skin	4.0
1 cup navy bean soup	13.5
Spinach salad:	
1 cup spinach	37.5
½ tomato	15.0
½ cup sliced carrots, onion, celery	15.0
1 tsp. low-cal. salad dressing	−1.0
1 cup strawberry smoothie	13.0
Total:	202.0

Patrick managed to redeem himself nicely from his −4 Nutripoint day with a total on his good day of 202 Nutripoints.

The following is a breakdown of how some of the nutrients
worked out for Patrick's good and bad days:

	Bad Day	Good Day	Ideal
Calories	3,087	1,049	1,000–2,000
% fat calories	57	15	20–30
% carb. calories	23	50	50–70
Tsp. sugar	10	3	0
Grams fiber	7	29	25–35
Mg. sodium	4,845	2,565	fewer than 3,000
Mg. caffeine	223	0	fewer than 200

While both Patrick's sample days provided virtually all the
essential nutrients (except fiber on the bad day), on the good
day he achieved this with one-third the calories while limiting
all negative factors, such as fat, sugar, and sodium. This
illustrates the concept of "nutrition per calorie": what makes
Patrick's bad day so bad is that he got bad nutritional value
per calorie. No one can afford to do that today.

I want to emphasize that Nutripoints does not encourage
or even allow for regular diet lapses. It just doesn't make
nutritional sense to try to eat well most of the time but, say,
twice a week, have a small binge. The Nutripoints program
assumes that you're serious about good nutrition. It simply
recognizes that there will be occasions when you'll eat something that isn't of good nutritional value. There's no sense in
pretending this doesn't happen, and so Nutripoints takes it
into consideration and figures it into the system.

Patients have found the recovery feature of Nutripoints
very reassuring. Many studies have shown that "restrained
eaters," who are severely limited in the type or amount of
food they can eat, will eventually binge or relapse. Nutripoints provides powerful psychological motivation because it

allows you to make up for lapses. It's also far more realistic to assume that people will have good and bad days: Nutripoints gives you a framework that takes real life into consideration.

The extraordinary benefit of Nutripoints is that if you've adopted the nutritional goals of the Nutripoint program you will probably be better nourished than you've ever been in your life, even if you have a bad day.

NUTRIPOINTS IN THE REAL WORLD

It's one thing to come up with the best all-round system for evaluating foods, but the best and most sophisticated charts in the world won't help people if they don't, or can't, use them. Nutripoints' track record for changing people's lives is convincing evidence that it's a system that's easy to live with no matter what your life-style.

The story of Joni, a Nutripoint convert who came to the program reluctantly, follows. I want to tell you about Joni because, while some patients have experienced more dramatic changes in their overall health profile, Joni illustrates two key elements of the Nutripoint program:

1. It's incredibly easy to live with.
2. It's valuable even for people who think that their diet is already nutritionally sound.

Joni is a 42-year-old manager of a corporate health plan for a large national company based in New York. Her job gives her reason and opportunity to keep up with the latest medical advances and theories, but she's also personally interested. When it came time for her company to make an arrangement with a corporate health center to do complete physicals on its employees, Joni became a "guinea pig" so that she could get a good understanding of the services offered by the center.

Though Joni hadn't had a complete physical in a few years, she had no complaints that she considered serious, or even worthy of mention. She often had a headache in the afternoon, and she was usually exhausted after work but thought that these symptoms had more to do with her demanding schedule than anything else. Although she counseled employees to get regular exercise, Joni herself was sedentary except for an occasional tennis game in the summer. She knew that she should lose about ten or fifteen pounds, but she thought her diet was pretty good except for regular business lunches when she found it impossible to eat lightly. All in all, Joni thought she was healthy, and she didn't expect any surprises from her physical.

When the printout from the health center arrived, Joni was shocked. Her cholesterol level was 228, her blood pressure was slightly elevated, her fifteen pounds of overweight was confirmed, and her treadmill time, which measured her aerobic endurance level, was terrible. Worse, her family history of osteoporosis indicated that she'd have to dramatically increase her calcium intake but, because of her high cholesterol level and her overweight, be especially careful to avoid fat. She also had a family history of breast cancer, and the latest evidence showed that a reduction in her fat intake would be imperative if she wanted to improve her chances of avoiding this disease.

Because of her work in the health field, Joni had heard about the Cooper Aerobics Center and she enrolled in our four-day Aerobics Wellness Weekend. When she arrived, she told me that the results of her physical had really overwhelmed her; it was the first time she'd felt really "mortal," as she put it. She was also confused. Though she knew what her dietary goals should be, she didn't know how to achieve them. She hated the idea of a typical diet because she really didn't believe she'd be able to stick with one. She felt she needed a "crash course" on nutrition to get her on track. Joni was very frank when she told me that she didn't expect to change her life; she just wanted to pick my brains to learn what she should be eating, and then go about things her own way. She warned me not to expect her to stay with any eating program once she was back on her home turf.

I began by giving Joni a brief explanation of the Nutripoints program. She was fascinated by the numbers and eager to see how they'd apply to her own life. I asked Joni to chart a typical day's eating. She felt she was on solid ground here. She was convinced that her diet was excellent. The following record is what she came up with:

Breakfast	*Nutripoints*
1 oat bran muffin (no butter)	3.0
Coffee	− 3.5
Cream	− 1.5
Snack	
1 container blueberry yogurt	1.0
Lunch	
Pasta primavera	3.0
Bread	2.5
Butter	− 4.0
1 glass wine	−13.0
Salad	33.5
Italian dressing	− 2.5
Dinner	
Weight Watchers frozen sweet and sour chicken	1.5
Yoplait frozen peach yogurt	− 2.0
2 glasses wine	−26.0
Total:	− 8.0

Joni said that on some days she ate much more than usual, and on others less, but that this was a fairly typical meal pattern. She thought it was pretty good—after all, she didn't eat much meat or any eggs, and she tried to avoid sweets. The fact is, Joni's total daily Nutripoint score was −8! Even if you forget about the wine she drank, which dramatically lowered her score, you're left with a score of 31. This is a dismal score, particularly when you consider that Joni thought of herself as someone well versed in nutrition.

It's shocking when you become familiar with Nutripoints and when your sense of what constitutes good nutrition changes, but Joni's diet was typical of someone who knows a fair amount about nutrition in the 1980s. She knew to avoid certain fats and sweets, but she had no notion about the *positive* elements missing in her diet. She was also eating a lot of *hidden* fats and sweets. Joni was really short-changing herself, and her body was beginning to show the symptoms.

Because Joni was so resistant to a "diet," I decided to ease her into the Nutripoint program. I told her we'd stick with her typical eating pattern but that we'd *upgrade* it with Nutripoints. The following table shows Joni's typical day on Nutripoints:

Breakfast	Nutripoints
Kellogg's corn flakes	18.0
Skim milk	9.5
¼ cantaloupe	29.0
Decaffeinated coffee	−0.5
with skim milk	2.5

Snack	
Plain, nonfat yogurt	9.0
Frozen strawberries	8.0

Lunch	
Lentil soup	8.0
Pasta with marinara sauce	1.0
Bread (no butter)	3.0
Tossed salad	33.0
"Lite" Italian dressing	−0.5
Fresh fruit salad	13.0

Dinner	
Celentano frozen Chicken Primavera	6.0
Green Giant frozen broccoli, cauliflower, carrots	33.0
Frozfruit Chunky Strawberry	1.0
Total:	173.0

Joni couldn't believe that she was eating nearly the exact same things she'd been eating before, and yet improving her diet by about 175 percent. A few simple tricks improved her Nutripoint score dramatically. For example, she found that it was no trouble to toss some frozen berries in a cup of nonfat yogurt in the morning before she left for work. The berries helped keep the yogurt cold and by the time she was ready for her snack, they were defrosted. She says the "fruit added" yogurt now tastes sickeningly sweet to her. After three days at the center eating similar meals that I had devised for her on the basis of her own preferences, Joni was a convert.

After two months on Nutripoints, Joni called me to tell me the results of her latest physical. She'd gone back to the corporate health center to get an update, and she was delighted with the news: her cholesterol level was 186, down 18 percent; her weight was down twelve pounds; and her blood pressure was completely normal.

Joni was quick to tell me that she didn't stick religiously to the program. Every now and again she slipped, but not because she wanted to. It was always because she found herself in a situation—usually a social one, such as a dinner party—in which it was nearly impossible to stick with her new patterns. For example, her worst day included a dinner party at the home of a business associate. She had a glass of red wine (−14 Nutripoints), a crabmeat appetizer with hollandaise sauce (−3.5 Nutripoints), chicken Kiev (0 Nutripoints), a salad with blue cheese dressing (19 Nutripoints), and carrot cake with cream cheese frosting (−2.5 Nutripoints). Even though Joni tried to only sample some of the dishes she thought were the worst Nutripoint values, she still found herself with a score of −4.5 Nutripoints for that meal. As she said, "The cook spent an enormous amount of time and trouble to plunge me into negative Nutripoints!" On the day of that dinner, Joni's Nutripoints came to 53. But she was only more resolved to make up for the loss and go for the top of the list for the rest of the week.

WHY NUTRIPOINTS COULD BE *YOUR* NUTRITIONAL BREAKTHROUGH

One morning, not too long ago, the phone rang in my office. It was Richard, a computer analyst who had visited the Aerobics Center two months previously with his wife. Richard had made the visit for his wife's sake, but he had no real interest in participating. As Richard was extremely overweight, but also reluctant to try any kind of diet, I was surprised to hear from him. By the time he left the Aerobics Center I believed that he had a psychological problem that was preventing him from making an effort.

"Dr. Vartabedian," Richard said, "I have a confession to make. When I got home from the Aerobics Center, I was upset. I guess I really believed that if I paid the money to be there, it would *have* to help me. Yes, I was there for my wife's sake, but I also wondered if the visit could really help me too. I almost had a chip on my shoulder about it.

"I guess because I didn't have any success, I'm ashamed to say that I made fun of the food charts my wife was using. She was making real progress and I guess I just couldn't take it. Well, a week after I got home I found myself standing at the refrigerator eating raw chocolate-chip cookie dough, right out of the roll, by the spoonful. By the time I had finished half the roll, I felt awful—dizzy and light-headed. I went to lie down, and as I was stretched out on the couch I thought, really thought, about what I had done. I was so disgusted with myself I wasn't sure which was making me sicker, the cookie dough or my own behavior. I decided to give Nutripoints a try. I knew I couldn't change overnight, but I remembered enough about what you'd said about Nutripoints to know that I could do it at my own pace. And I wanted to thank you because as of today I've lost twenty-one pounds. I also wanted to tell you that it's the only thing that's ever worked for me. The only reason that it's worked is because it's really easy. I have a long way to go, but for the first time in my life I know I'm going to make it."

I'm telling Richard's story because he illustrates what I think is the most important feature of Nutripoints: it's easy. Although many people want to improve their lives, without major motivation it's just too hard. I believe that's because diet and exercise programs are just too difficult. They're not fun: they're grim and they make you feel like a penitent. They demand major changes, that you give up patterns and habits acquired over a lifetime. Most people never experience the pleasure of a body enjoying optimum nutrition, or anything near it.

If you want to improve your nutrition but are discouraged by difficult diets with complicated menus, the Nutripoint program will change your life. One of my goals in developing Nutripoints was to find something that *everyone*—even people who would never follow a typical diet—would find accessible.

Here are the features that I think will make the difference for you. First, you'll find that it's the simplest and most positive approach to nutrition you've ever encountered. If you like, you can ease into it: just use the charts to improve the quality of everything you eat. Focus on the positive, and you'll soon find yourself avoiding the negative. I've seen many people ease into the system this way with great success. Maria is an example. She came to our thirteen-day Aerobics Program for Total Well-Being at the Aerobics Center with her husband, who was showing early signs of heart disease. She was there only to offer moral support; she exercised regularly and, though she would have liked to lose a few pounds, she didn't want to diet. As she now says, "Once I realized that I could lose a bit of weight and dramatically improve the quality of my diet simply by doing some informed compari-sons of foods and eliminating a few foods that tipped the balance the wrong way, I couldn't *help* but do it. My nutri-tional status was not great. I was eating bad stuff, and I guess without realizing it I was on a gradual decline. You just don't stop and see what you're doing to yourself day to day.

"I never would have thought about making a change with-out Nutripoints. It never occurred to me before Nutripoints just why typical reducing or health-oriented diets turned me off. They all seemed to be complicated or offer a gimmick that

I couldn't really believe in. But Nutripoints is not really a diet; it's a *tool* based on real science that allows you to go as far as you want to improve your nutrition. My husband has certainly changed his life and dramatically improved his health—his cholesterol is already down 46 points—but I always felt convinced that would happen if he made major changes in his diet. The real surprise is me. I never would have believed that I'd jump on the Nutripoint bandwagon and, given the fact that I didn't think I needed any improvement, I'm amazed at the changes I see in me and my husband. I've lost those few extra pounds, and the general improvement in the way both my husband and I feel is really wonderful. We've got more energy, we're more calm. We feel just great."

There's a second, bonus benefit to Nutripoints: you won't have to wait years to enjoy its effects. The following are the average changes experienced by participants in the thirteen-day Aerobics Program for Total Well-Being:

Weight	8 lbs., or 4% decrease
Cholesterol	14% decrease
Cholesterol/HDL ratio*	16% decrease
Glucose	10% decrease
Triglycerides	40% decrease
Treadmill time (fitness level)	19% increase
Blood pressure	6% decrease

These patients are working on exercise and stress reduction in addition to nutrition. But if you undertake the Nutripoints program with any measure of seriousness, and you work on stress reduction and exercise too, there's no reason why you

*Cholesterol levels can be measured in two ways: total cholesterol measures all types found in the blood whereas high-density cholesterol (HDL) refers to good, protective cholesterol only. The higher the HDL is in relation to total cholesterol, the better. Therefore the lower the ratio (cholesterol/HDL), the better.

can't experience similar improvements. From a short-term point of view, you'll probably experience freedom from digestive problems, sluggishness, inability to concentrate, frequent headaches, and irritability. And in mid-afternoon, when many people start to fade, you'll find that you have the energy and stamina to keep going.

PART II

THE SCIENCE OF OPTIMAL NUTRITION

SCARED SMART

FOR A MOMENT, FORGET PILLS, FORGET EXERCISE, FORGET RELAXA-tion techniques. The fact is, the single most important step you can take today to improve your overall sense of well-being and your long-term health is to improve your nutrition. Exercise works the body; food *makes* the body. There are trillions of cells in your body, and each one is made up of, and nourished by, the food you eat. You simply can't function at your best, as we'll see, if you don't eat the best foods. Of course, exercise, stress-reduction techniques, and all sensible efforts at better health make sense, but if you don't improve your nutrition, your other efforts will be virtually pointless.

Does it really matter that you keep your fat, cholesterol, and sodium levels down? That you make a point of getting all the vitamins and minerals your body needs? I'm so used to dealing with the educated demands of my patients at the Aerobics Center that I sometimes forget that anyone today needs convincing.

The people who come to me for help with their diets are highly motivated. In many cases, *motivated* is a euphemism for *terrified.* Some of my patients are actually staring death in the face. They've suffered a heart attack, maybe two. I think of these people as "scared smart." They have decided they want to live, and they're prepared to do anything it takes to make that possible. The Nutripoint program is an enormous relief to them. It's an eating program that can help them to literally save their own lives. In addition, it is easy to incorporate into their life-styles, and it allows them to devise their own eating program: many of these people believed that they would have to live on a terribly restricted, boring diet for the rest of their lives.

I hope that most of the rest of us—the lucky ones who haven't been forced to change their diets through personal illness—have moved out of the Dark Ages of nutrition, where we believed we could eat whatever we wanted and trust to luck or good genes to get us through. It just doesn't work that way. It really *is* up to you.

Cholesterol was the red flag that alerted millions of Americans to the fact that diet really does matter—that what we're eating every day is going to make a difference in how we feel both today and tomorrow. But cholesterol is only part of the story. Today, largely because of their diets, over 50 percent of Americans are at risk for heart disease, diabetes, hypertension, and cancer. The American Cancer Society recently announced that they expected one million Americans to hear a cancer diagnosis in 1989—the first time the projection has reached that mark. In addition to more than one million new cancer cases, the society projected over half a million cancer deaths for 1989. Thirty-five percent of cancers—only one of the leading causes of death—are diet related. Former U.S. Surgeon General Koop recently said that the unhealthy eating habits of as many as 1.5 million Americans may have contributed to their deaths in 1987.

It's no news that the American diet can be dangerous to your health. In 1977 George McGovern headed a congressional committee that investigated the long-term effects of what Americans eat. The McGovern committee studied the relationship between the average diet and the nation's major killers—heart disease, cancers of the colon and breast, stroke, high blood pressure, obesity, diabetes, arteriosclerosis, and cirrhosis of the liver. They estimated that if Americans modified their rich diets, there would be an 80-percent drop in the number of obese people, a 25-percent drop in deaths from heart disease, a 50-percent drop in deaths from diabetes, and a 1-percent annual increase in longevity.

It seems that every day there's a new study that demonstrates the dangers of fats and cholesterol, and the importance of fiber and various nutrients, such as calcium, in the diet. A recent study reported in the *New York Times* confirmed yet again the dangers for women of a high-calorie, high-fat diet. This study, which was the largest survey done to date, overwhelmingly demonstrated that women who ate the most fats, saturated fats, and animal protein had a three times greater chance of getting breast cancer than those whose intake of these substances was lowest. Moreover, it showed that a high-calorie diet made women almost twice as likely to develop breast cancer.

A diet high in fat, cholesterol, and calories has been definitively linked to the major life-style diseases. The answer couldn't be more obvious: if you want to avoid the major killing and debilitating diseases, improve your diet.

BEYOND CALORIES

How *do* you improve your diet? Well, you try to cut fat and cholesterol, and probably calories. But how do you actually go about doing this? The first thing you do is to discard your old notions about how to judge foods. If you're like most people, the calorie is the only food measure that you're really familiar with. It's time to forget calories and move on to Nutripoints.

To understand just how revolutionary Nutripoints are, you need only take a look at what has existed in the past to help people choose among foods.

We are all calorie nuts. We have some notion from high school that we have to have variety (something about choosing from various food groups), but counting calories has been the most common system for comparing foods. Most people who pay attention to what they eat are trying to lose weight. They look for foods that are low in calories. But we now know that calories are just one measure of the value of various foods. A diet extremely low in calories can also be a diet that is nutritionally unsound—even absolutely dangerous, as we've seen from some fad diets. A diet extremely low in calories is not necessarily a diet that will promote permanent weight loss.

RDAs (Recommended Dietary Allowances) provide some measure of food value. These figures were arrived at by the Food and Nutrition Board, a committee of the National Academy of Sciences–National Research Council. RDAs are supposed to be the "levels of intake of essential nutrients considered, in the judgment of the Food and Nutrition Board on the basis of available scientific knowledge, to be adequate to meet the known nutritional needs of practically all healthy persons."

RDAs are assigned to all foods, but unprocessed foods don't provide the handy labels that would help you determine whether a white or a sweet potato is a better choice in terms of your nutritional needs. RDAs are concerned with vitamins and minerals, but ignore critical analyses of the fat, carbohydrate, and protein contents of foods. So, while a useful beginning, it's difficult to translate RDAs into a healthful diet.

In 1973 the FDA (Food and Drug Administration) adopted its basic nutritional labeling regulations. Making use of RDAs, this was a step forward in helping people determine the nutritive value of foods. Three kinds of foods must be labeled: those that make any kind of nutritional claim, such as "high in fiber," those that are fortified with nutrients, and those that are specifically intended for children under age four. Manufacturers of other types of foods are free to voluntarily include nutritional labeling. Foods that are so labeled list the percentage of the RDA of each nutrient the food contains. Nutritional labeling is very useful in comparing the relative nutritional value of two similar foods.

While nutritional labeling is an advance for consumers, it's of limited value. Although in 1975 it was believed that roughly 85 percent of all manufacturers would be using nutritional labeling soon, by 1985 less than half of packaged foods were labeled. Moreover, some labels are almost deceptive. For example, a manufacturer must list ingredients in descending order of amounts, but sugar can be listed in various forms, such as sugar, dextrose, corn syrup, honey, molasses, and so on. If you're not sophisticated about reading labels, you can wind up buying a product that has far more sugar than a cursory glance would reveal.

Another major drawback of nutritional labeling is that it tends to highlight the vitamin/mineral content of foods while downplaying the importance of fat, carbohydrates, protein, and fiber. These major nutrients are usually listed as amounts (for example, a frozen dinner might have 8 grams of fat) rather than as percentages. This makes it more difficult for the consumer to tell how nutritious the food is. Most people simply don't know the significance of nutrients in terms of grams: is 8 grams of fat a lot or a little?

While labels might list the amounts of certain nutrients, this information still doesn't tell you what you need to know: how much is good? If you know the amount of fat, protein, fiber, or complex carbohydrates in a certain food, can you tell if it's a good choice in terms of the ideal, or in terms of what you've already eaten today? Most people just don't know if a food with 10 percent complex carbohydrates is a good choice. Finally, it is enormously time-consuming to stand in a supermarket and compare labels to check varying percentages of nutrients.

Nutritional labeling is great as far as it goes, but it doesn't offer any help with the foods we should be eating the most of: whole, unprocessed foods. You can check a label to see if Count Chocula cereal has more sugar than Fruity Pebbles, but there are no handy labels to help you determine whether an apple versus a banana, or a pork chop versus a veal chop, is a better choice in terms of your nutritional needs.

The fact is, nutritional labeling and RDAs are a useful

beginning, but for most people they are simply raw data in a form too complicated to be of much use. It's good to know that a product contains 15 percent of your daily requirement of protein, but where do you go from there? Is that an acceptable amount? Is it a good contribution to your daily protein intake? And how does it compare to other, similar products?

It's almost as if food labeling is only an intriguing set of puzzle pieces that the average consumer is unable to put together in any useful way. (Now that the FDA has proposed a rule that will allow companies to make health claims in their food labels, consumers can even be misled: a soup high in fiber would be able to claim that the fiber in the soup helps reduce the risk of cancer, without mentioning that its high sodium content contributes to hypertension.)

Unfortunately, and despite the enormous interest in nutrition today, the experts can't be of much help in determining which foods offer better nutritional value. They know that a bran muffin is better than a Twinkie . . . probably . . . unless, come to think of it, the bran muffin is commercially manufactured with palm oil and contains a lot of cholesterol.

No doctor or nutritionist can tell you which foods are best to eat because, up to now, they haven't had the "software." While the government has charts that list all of the nutrient values in thousands of foods, they're not widely available; and even if they were, most people (including doctors and nutritionists) would be overwhelmed in trying to translate this vast sea of data into any useful information. It's just too complicated. The best anyone could do up to now is to point out that some foods are better than others. Some foods low in cholesterol are high in sugar or salt. Some foods low in calories have virtually no nutritive value. Some foods that are high in protein are surprisingly high in fat. Did you know that tofu, that favorite "healthy" substitute for animal protein in many diet and vegetarian meals, is high in fat?

Nutripoints has made use of the most up-to-date information available on foods today. It has looked at nutritional labeling, RDAs, calorie and cholesterol counts, and so on, as *raw data*, which is what it really is as far as the consumer is concerned, and gone one step beyond by providing the first accurate, practical nutritional guidebook.

PUTTING THE NUTRIENTS BACK IN NUTRITION

• Anemia, from lack of iron in the diet, is the most common nutritional-deficiency disease in the country today. Symptoms include immune disorders, fatigue, learning problems in children, muscle weakness, among many others.

• Only 22 percent of Americans past the age of one meet the top recommended dietary allowances of vitamin B_6. According to the USDA, only 8 percent of women consume 100 percent of the dietary allowances of B_6. Such deficiencies have been linked to everything from asthma and PMS, to diabetes, cardiovascular disease, and cancer.

• Only 42 percent of the population consumes the recommended daily allowance of calcium. The people who need it most consume the least: 80 percent of teenage and middle-aged women consume less than half of the recommended daily allowance. Most people have heard about osteoporosis and calcium deficiency, but lack of sufficient calcium in the diet can also contribute to gum disease, high blood pressure, and even colon cancer.

These are a few facts that illustrate how many of the people in the "best-nourished nation in the world" are suffering from the first stages of malnutrition. How could this have happened? In large part it's due to our obsession with dieting, which translates into a never-ending desire to lose weight. In fact, losing weight has become such a primary focus for so many of us that we forget that *diet* refers to a system for nourishing the body rather than a means to lose weight. When was the last time a friend told you he or she was on a "diet" geared to improve consumption of all the major nutrients in order to feel better and prevent disease?

In fact, many diets today take into consideration the negative elements in American eating patterns and help you avoid excess fats, cholesterol, and sodium—although very few help you avoid all three. And most diets make you feel like you're the worst kid in second grade: the basic theme is, "don't, don't, don't; no, no, no!" Don't eat this; don't eat that; don't even think about eating all of these things!

Nutripoints goes beyond this negative approach and moves the entire idea of diet into another, positive realm. Most diets set you up for failure; there is no way you can "fail" with Nutripoints. That's because the emphasis is not on avoiding certain foods, or on eating specific foods. Rather, the emphasis is on *choice.* The Nutripoint program assumes that you are intelligent and that you are ready to improve your diet. It provides you with the information—the type of information you've never had before—that will enable you to make intelligent choices.

Most of us think of nutrition in terms of losing weight. We think if we eat foods that are low in calories, and avoid junk food, we're doing well. Unfortunately, this focus on calories has obscured the importance of adequate nutrition. The fact is, most of us are not very well nourished. We eat too much fat, too much protein, too much sugar, and we don't get enough fiber, complex carbohydrates, and certain critical nutrients in our diets.

While Americans have reduced their fat intake 12 percent since 1977, and slightly increased their complex carbohydrate intake, the improvement hasn't been enough. While we're eating 80 percent more yogurt than we were in 1983, and 43 percent more wholesome snacks (including fruits and nuts), our consumption of salty tortilla, taco, and nacho chips rose by 60 percent. We're eating less bacon, but more frankfurters and breakfast sausage. We all claim we're eating fewer sweets, but consumption of "gourmet" chocolate-chip cookies increased from fifty-five million pounds in 1985 to seventy-five million in 1987. Who's eating all this stuff?

I witnessed a typical example of how some of our misguided notions about foods have more to do with trends than with accurate information on how foods affect our bodies. I was in the supermarket watching a young man who was filling his cart. He carefully chose a bottled water, a "lite" frozen entree, a large bottle of diet soft drink, and then a huge bag of M&Ms!

While most Americans are at least aware of the shortcomings in their diets, or at least aware enough to insist that they're doing better (despite the facts that contradict them), they're still vulnerable to disease from too much fat and too little fiber.

The more surprising results of recent USDA and FDA surveys are that our diets are shortchanging us of vital vitamins and minerals. As the two top officials of the U.S. Department of Agriculture's Human Nutrition Information Service reported, "50 percent or more [of the 38,000 people surveyed] had intakes below the RDA for vitamin A, iron, calcium, magnesium, and vitamin B_6; over 30 percent of the individuals failed to meet the 70-percent RDA levels for these nutrients. Zinc and folacin are also known to be short in many diets." The report concluded that "U.S. diets do not show up well . . . when either the RDA or the [USDA's] Daily Food Guide is used as a standard." So while most of us feel fairly complacent about the nutrients we're getting from our diets, the facts tell a very different story.

The very steps we take to reduce fat (such as cutting out red meat and many dairy products) are further reducing our intake of these important nutrients.

Does it really matter if your intake of, say, iron, is low?

Most of us tend to think that a deficiency of any given nutrient is only a remote possibility. We figure that our iron intake must be OK if we don't have anemia. What most people don't appreciate is the subtle interplay of nutrients in our bodies: it doesn't take a diagnosed deficiency to make you feel tired, or make it hard for you to shake a cold. Indeed, lack of sufficient iron in your diet will begin to sap your energy and lower your physical and mental productivity long before it turns into a full-blown deficiency.

The story of Bill Walton, the basketball star, illustrates the need for adequate nutrients. When Walton was under contract with the San Diego Clippers, he had a terrible run of luck. Walton kept breaking bones, and past breaks were troubling him. His left foot had been broken twice, and didn't seem to be healing. When x-rayed, it showed evidence of osteoporosis. If he did have osteoporosis, it would explain why he'd broken so many bones: several fingers and toes, a leg, a wrist, a cheekbone, and his nose, in addition to the two breaks in his foot. But Walton drank what should have been enough milk to provide the calcium the body needs to prevent osteoporosis.

Tests on Walton's blood became an indictment of his diet: while his calcium level was high, his levels of trace elements were alarming. He had an absolute zero level of manganese, and his copper and zinc levels were one-third normal.

Walton's nutritional mistake was not his vegetarian diet, as so many people suspected, but his *unbalanced* diet. He ate mainly brown rice and vegetables supplemented with milk and, occasionally, fish. While too many people today would consider this an ideal diet—low in fat and cholesterol and high in fiber—it was destroying his body and his career. He wasn't getting the critical balance of nutrients his body needed.

When Walton supplemented his diet with the minerals he was missing, he soon recovered, his foot healed, and within six weeks he was back playing basketball.

I was fascinated by Walton's story because it's such a powerful illustration of the necessity of getting *all* the nutrients, even trace elements, if we want to perform properly. It also demonstrates how the lack of one or two nutrients can cripple the entire system. In Walton's case, calcium was unable to do its work of strengthening bones because it didn't have the minerals copper and manganese essential to the task.

Walton's diet was unusual, and his demands on his body accelerated the problems that most of us wouldn't experience so dramatically, but it's not uncommon for the average American to consume a diet that is just as unvaried and nutritionally unsound. Many people, in an effort to lose weight, go on popular diets that put their health at risk.

Many popular reducing diets are unsound, and sometimes we make them even worse by adapting them to our own desires without the requisite knowledge. Inventing our own diets, where we simply cut out foods we believe to be fattening, is another trouble area. In many cases, we wind up eating a shockingly inadequate diet that repeats one or two "low-calorie" meals virtually every day.

As I mentioned before, even people who eat a relatively good diet will unknowingly cut out essential vitamins and minerals when they reduce fat and cholesterol in their diets. Most people simply don't know how to substitute a "good" food for a "bad" one. They're not aware that the right diet can be a simple matter of intelligent substitution.

I think that the goal of *optimum nutrition* will replace concern with the calorie as we learn more about the critical role these nutrients play in ensuring our well-being.

As Paul Saltman, trace element researcher at the University of California, San Diego, says, "There is every reason to believe that millions would have more energy, and would perform at higher levels physically and mentally, if our diet were richer in certain minerals and trace metals." Nutripoints is the best method available today to help you achieve that goal.

THE ADVANTAGE OF NATURAL NUTRITION

"Why can't I just take a vitamin pill?" How many thousands of times have I heard this question? It's not surprising that people are confused on the issue of vitamin pills. The vitamin pill manufacturers spend veritable fortunes convincing us that a pill is just as good, if not better, a source of nutrition as food. And who wouldn't *want* to believe them? You don't have to shop frequently for pills. They don't take up much room. You don't have to wash or chop or stir-fry or sauté them. But the fact is, vitamin pills have virtually no real role in achieving natural nutrition.

Did you know, for example, that most of those reports you hear about that demonstrate that vitamin A or vitamin C can cure or mitigate the effects of this or that disease *do not rely on pills, but rather on food, as a source of the vitamin?* Many people hear about research that promises to help their arthritis, PMS, or whatever, and begin to dose themselves on whatever vitamin or mineral was cited as the cure. But frequently, pills had nothing to do with the reported results.

This is just one misconception about vitamins. As I'll demonstrate, there are other, even more compelling reasons for relying on *natural nutrition,* or fuel from food.

One of the cornerstones of Nutripoints is that *pills are not a substitute for food.* Let's take a look at some of the drawbacks of vitamin supplementation.

Even the best vitamins are incomplete.
    Despite what you may read or hear, vitamin supplementa-

tion is not an exact science. It's a relatively new scientific frontier: by 1913, only two vitamins had been recognized. Moreover, because we're interested in the effects of vitamins on humans, and because humans often cannot be the subjects of experiments for obvious reasons, we're limited in how much we *can* learn about the effects of vitamins on human health.

But we do know a great deal from animal experimentation. For example, guinea pigs eating a totally synthetic diet which contains all the known nutrients needed to sustain their lives will not thrive. Why? Because we're not aware of all the essential nutrients—for guinea pigs or for ourselves. Dr. Jean Mayer, one of the most highly respected authorities on nutrition, has said that "if the history of the development of our science is a dependable guide, there may be nutrients performing significant duties for us that we have not yet identified. In particular, there may be minerals functioning heroically to our benefit and all unknown to us." A vitamin pill contains the *known* micronutrients, and that's the best we can do. But no one can claim that it's complete.

Vitamin D_2, or irradiated ergosterol, for example, can be produced by irradiating yeast with ultraviolet light. Because this is a "natural" process, irradiated ergosterol can be called a "natural" vitamin. Milk and many other food products, as well as vitamin supplements, contain irradiated ergosterol. But this substance, vitamin D_2, is not the same as the D vitamin produced in the body when ultraviolet light strikes the skin. Moreover, vitamin D_2 does not supply the complex of D vitamins found in such foods as fish oils, milk fats from animals feeding on fresh greens, and liver. The fact is, the supplements we create, either naturally or otherwise, may not be exactly the same as those created by nature in foods. If the effects of these created supplements in the body are precisely the same, no one can prove it, and there's room for great skepticism on the part of the consumer.

Even the best vitamins are not perfectly balanced; some are dangerously unbalanced.

The vitamins and minerals that occur naturally in food are balanced. Nature dictates how much of a given nutrient will be present. But the contents of a vitamin pill are dictated by companies—companies that are run for profit and that sometimes pander to the public's ignorance about vitamins and how they work in the body.

It's important to remember that nutrients have to work in concert, and to take too much of one or another can be useless or even dangerous. For example, increasing zinc intake by only 3.5 milligrams per day above the RDA of 15 milligrams per day can decrease copper retention as well as interfere with calcium absorption. Large doses of folic acid can mask a vitamin B_{12} deficiency and result in serious and irreversible neurological damage. In pregnant women, large doses of folic acid can cause zinc deficiencies, which could lead to birth defects. Most people are astonished to learn that megadoses of vitamin C impair B_{12} utilization and can raise blood cholesterol.

Vitamins and minerals work in concert with one another, and we ignore this fact to our peril. Calcium, for example, is one of the most abundant minerals in the body. It's found in bone cartilage, teeth, and blood and nerve cells. We're all wary of calcium deficiencies today because of the threat of osteoporosis. But calcium supplements *can* do more harm than good. Calcium is used by the body in conjunction with magnesium. One of these minerals taken alone will have a totally different effect. For example, magnesium oxide is effective in the relief of constipation. If you take it with calcium, it will have no effect on your bowels. Too many calcium supplements, taken over a long period of time, can result in a disorder called hypercalcemia, which can eventually lead to rheumatoid arthritis. Calcium, taken in its natural form in dairy products and vegetables, eliminates the risk of such an overdose. It is the only guarantee that the body is getting the calcium it needs in concert with magnesium, and in the balance necessary for optimum functioning.

Some popular vitamin formulations completely ignore the concept of balance and can actually put you in danger. One popular brand contains a potentially toxic amount of vitamin A, minerals in insignificant amounts, and eight unrecognized nutrients. It also features a label that lists potency according to the obsolete MDR (Minimum Daily Requirement) standard, instead of the current FDA standard, the RDA (Recommended Dietary Allowance). This vitamin is also among the most expensive available.

The only way to be sure that the nutrients you ingest are properly balanced and readily absorbed by the body is to get them from food.

Vitamins can be toxic.

The body stores excess vitamin A in the liver. The fact that the liver is a storehouse for many excess vitamins is why it is also considered a valuable food (though liver has great drawbacks in nutritional terms). In any case, liver could almost be seen as one of the original megavitamins. And, like commercially produced megavitamins, it can be dangerous. For example, long ago Eskimos learned to avoid eating polar bear liver. They knew it caused death; they didn't know that it did so because of its extremely high content of vitamin A. Polar bear liver contains about one million international units (IU) in three ounces, compared to an RDA of 5,000 IU for men.

In the early sixties, approximately twenty children in New York died from vitamin A overdoses when their mothers doubled the recommended dosage of vitamin supplements. Each child took two capsules daily. This was in addition to the already generous amounts of vitamin A the children were receiving from foods in their diets.

There are also long-term dangers to the use of supplements. For example, some experts worry that consumption of large amounts of iron supplements could cause a buildup of iron in the liver, leading to serious problems in later life.

Although we've talked about the dangers of inadequate calcium intake, there's also a danger in too much calcium. As I mentioned before, due to the threat of osteoporosis, many women have begun to take calcium supplements. But very few of these women are actually aware of how much calcium they are consuming. As more and more foods are supplemented with calcium to cash in on the concern with osteoporosis, people are getting extra calcium in everything from their orange juice to their antacid tablets. This extra calcium is *in addition* to the calcium they're getting naturally in their diets from milk and other sources. Long-term high doses of calcium could have potentially harmful consequences. Moreover, calcium supplements derived from dolomite or bone meal can be contaminated with poisonous metals, such as lead.

Unfortunately, the FDA, with a few exceptions, has no authority to limit the potency of vitamin/mineral supplements. These supplements are considered foods or food additives, not drugs. While the average consumer taking an "insurance" multivitamin will not get into trouble, medically unsupervised megavitamin supplementation is a dangerous game.

Vitamin supplementation can alter your body chemistry.

There's a more subtle problem relative to vitamin/mineral supplementation. While consumers may be aware that high levels of certain nutrients can be dangerous, most are not aware that even low routine doses of vitamins can create problems by conditioning the body to *expect* higher than normal levels of certain vitamins. This is known as *systemic conditioning.* It occurs with water-soluble vitamins, and it can create withdrawal problems when the nutrient is withdrawn. There is a great deal yet to be learned about systemic conditioning in relation to nutrients, but we do know that it can affect offspring as well as the individual taking the nutrient. There have been cases of infants suffering from something called *rebound scurvy,* which causes temporary scurvylike withdrawal symptoms, because their mothers took megadoses of vitamin C while pregnant. You should certainly never take megadoses of any vitamin while pregnant. If you are currently taking megadoses of a water-soluble vitamin (including the Bs and vitamin C), be sure to cut down on your intake gradually to avoid the symptoms of withdrawal. (Megadoses of a fat-soluble vitamin, such as A, D, or E, should be ceased immediately if at toxic levels.)

You should also be aware that vitamin/mineral supplementation can alter the results of various diagnostic tests, particularly blood and urine tests. Large doses of vitamin C can give false readings for blood in stool and sugar in urine. If you take supplements, particularly in high doses, be sure to tell your doctor so that diagnostic tests can be correctly interpreted.

HOW TO TAKE A VITAMIN

Despite what I've just said, I'm not totally opposed to intelligent vitamin supplementation. If you follow Nutripoints, there is really no *need* for supplements. But some people just can't shake the belief that a vitamin will give extra insurance. To these people I recommend a single, balanced multivitamin taken every other day, or half a vitamin taken daily. Even a poor diet gets 50 to 75 percent of RDAs, and there's no need to supplement beyond this. There are some groups of people who really can benefit from a vitamin/mineral supplement: children under two years of age, and older children and elderly people who eat a limited number of foods; people on diets that contain fewer than 1,200 calories a day; pregnant women; strict vegetarians who eat no dairy products or eggs; and people with certain illnesses that seriously impair the absorption of nutrients. If you are on the lowest-calorie version of Nutripoints, you might also benefit from the half-a-vitamin-daily regime.

The following are do's and don'ts for taking vitamins:

• Do take only a vitamin that offers close to, *but no more than*, 100 percent of RDAs for all nutrients. If the levels are a *bit* higher, they're not dangerous, but they're a waste. If they're a *lot* higher (some vitamins contain 1,000 percent of the RDA for one vitamin, and 20 percent of another), they're really unbalanced and should be avoided. As you can see from the chart that follows, the best all-round brand is One-A-Day Maximum Formula. It's the one I recommend to my patients who insist on taking a vitamin.

The following list is a breakdown of various nationally available vitamins that I've listed from best to worst, beginning with my recommendations (I was astounded to find that Geritol [at the bottom of the list] is 12 percent alcohol!):

Vitamin	*Recommended*	*Comments*
One-A-Day Maximum Formula	Yes	balanced; complete; contains 100 percent of RDA; without unnecessary or unrecognized nutrients.

Vitamin	Recommended	Comments
Advanced Formula Centrum	Yes	balanced; complete; contains 100 percent of RDA; contains a few unrecognized nutrients.
Geritol Complete	No	complete; balanced, except too high in iron; contains several unnecessary, unrecognized nutrients.
Theragran-M	No	complete; unbalanced (too low in some nutrients and too high in others: 4 to 200 percent of RDA); a few unrecognized nutrients.
Myadec	No	complete; unbalanced (mostly too high in some nutrients: from 5 to 667 percent of RDA).
One-A-Day Stressgard	No	unbalanced (between 100 and 1,000 percent of RDA).
Daily Stress Natural Vitamin	No	complete; very unbalanced (17 to 3,333 percent of RDA).

Vitamin	Recommended	Comments
Stresstabs 600 +Iron	No	incomplete; unbalanced (15 to 1,000 percent of RDA).
Theragran M Stresstabs	No	incomplete; unbalanced (15 to 1,250 percent of RDA).
Allbee C-800 +Iron	No	incomplete; unbalanced (150 to 1,333 percent of RDA).
Geritol with Ferrex 50	No	incomplete; uses obsolete MDRs rather than USRDA standard; unbalanced (200 to 500 percent of MDR); contains potentially harmful levels of iron; 12 percent alcohol.

• Don't go for the highest-priced vitamin. Claims that vitamins are "natural," as opposed to "synthetic," really have no bearing on their effectiveness, and a national brand name may be no better than a much cheaper store brand.

• Do check the expiration date on any vitamins you buy. They will become ineffective over time and are best used when fresh. Store them in a cool, dark, dry place.

• Don't waste money on vitamins that contain substances for which there is no proven nutritional need. Lecithin and vitamin B$_{15}$ are two examples of such substances. Inclusion of the following in supplements only raises the price without any nutritional benefit: arsenic, cadmium, carnitine, choline, cobalt, coenzyme Q, lecithin, nickel, PABA, silicon, tin, vanadium, vitamin P, and vitamin Q.

• Unless you're under a doctor's orders, don't take vitamins that contain substances otherwise useless or dangerous. Fluoride, iodine, and phosphorus are readily available in water, salt, and protein foods. Chloride, potassium, and sodium are easily obtained from the normal diet. Molybdenum isn't a recommended mineral in supplements because its toxicity outweighs the problem of a possible deficiency. Moreover, even moderate amounts of molybdenum can cause a copper deficiency.

• Do take your vitamins with a well-balanced meal. Although there is evidence that some minerals are best absorbed on an empty stomach, the final evidence is not in, and most vitamins seem to be best absorbed when taken with foods.

IS OUR FOOD REALLY SAFE?

There is great concern today about the quality of our foods. The various additives and pesticides used to promote the growth and storage life of foods are a troubling fact of life.

I have not taken into consideration additive and pesticide use in my Nutripoint scores for a number of reasons. First, most uses of pesticides and various additives simply don't make enough of a difference in the *nutritive* value of a food. Second, their levels in any given food are simply too difficult to calibrate. Apples, for example, come from so many regions and from so many growers with varying methods of cultivation that it would be impossible to assess each in a book that covers more than 3,000 foods.

While Nutripoints cannot be your guide on how to avoid pesticides and chemicals in your food, I think it's important to be an aware and educated consumer. In 1989 there was a scare concerning the use of the chemical alar on apples. Many people stopped buying apples and apple products. But within a few weeks the *Wall Street Journal,* among others, printed lists of apple juices that had been tested and were found safe in terms of alar content. While some people were complaining about the limited number of juices they could safely give to their children, others knew that there were at least a dozen apple juice brands that were perfectly fine. The lesson is, be aware!

An excellent book that can help you make sense of the dangers of additives and pesticides is *The Goldbecks' Guide to Good Food,* by Nikki and David Goldbeck, published in paperback by New American Library. (This book is also an excellent all-round guide on how to shop for the very best foods.)

From a practical standpoint, how can you minimize the risk you take in eating certain foods? The following are some tips:

• Wash all fresh fruits and vegetables, and rinse them thoroughly.

• If foods have been waxed, peeling is more effective than washing.

• Try to buy produce that originates in this country. Imported foods may contain residues of pesticides banned here. You'll have to have the cooperation of your greengrocer or supermarket manager to learn the source of produce in your market.

• When possible, buy organically grown fruits and vegetables, or those grown under the Integrated Pest Management System, which uses alternative methods of growing and cultivation to keep chemical use at a minimum.

• Request that your supermarket carry organically grown foods. Write to corporate headquarters and express your concern about pesticide residues.

• Write federal and state government officials about your concerns regarding pesticide use. At the federal level, write the Administrator, Environmental Protection Agency, 401 M Street, SW, Washington, DC 20460; and the Commissioner, Food and Drug Administration, 5600 Fishers Lane, Rockville, MD 20857.

• To avoid risk of salmonella contamination, wash your hands thoroughly before handling poultry and eggs. Refrigerate raw and cooked poultry and eggs. Keep raw poultry and eggs away from cooked poultry and eggs. Cook eggs and poultry thoroughly. Wash surfaces that come in contact with raw poultry and eggs with warm, soapy water.

• To avoid parasites, don't eat raw seafood. Farm-raised fish and shellfish are much safer to eat raw than fish harvested in the wild.

IS OUR FOOD REALLY NUTRITIOUS?

Many people today are concerned about the actual nutritional value of foods. In fact, many of my patients have mentioned that they take vitamins, at least in part, because they don't believe that the foods they eat, even supposedly highly nutritious foods, deliver high-quality nutrients. They think this is because of the use of fertilizers, the length of time foods must travel, and the amount of time they spend on the supermarket shelves before we eat them.

Fertilizers used in commercially produced foods are not necessarily a negative in terms of good nutrition. It amuses me that the same people who are opposed to using chemical fertilizers are often devoted to vitamin/mineral supplements, which are, after all, nothing more than chemical fertilizers for the body. That aside, you should not be categorically opposed to fertilizers or chemicals, as some of them actually preserve the nutrients in foods.

What about the notion that foods are lacking in nutrients because they're grown in depleted soils? The fact is, the final agricultural product—whether apple, potato, carrot, or beet—is determined by that plant's genes, not the quality of the soil in which it grew. While the mineral content of a given food is partly determined by the soil it grew in, you can rest assured that if a vegetable reaches the marketplace, and looks, cooks, and tastes like a turnip, it's going to have all the nutrients that are normally found in a turnip.

Beyond pesticides and depleted soil, the question of storage in relation to nutrient content is a valid one. But you might be surprised to learn that the greatest loss occurs in your own kitchen. When the analyses of various foods are done to determine their nutritional content, they're not done on rare, perfect, organically grown super-foods; they're done on the very same foods you find on supermarket shelves. So when you learn that a raw sweet pepper has 140 milligrams of vitamin C, you can be confident that the sweet peppers you buy in your supermarket have very close to the same amount.

Once food gets to your kitchen, nutrition can be quickly lost through poor storage and processing. Most meats, fish, fruits, and vegetables should be promptly stored in the refrigerator. They should be carefully wrapped, and they should be washed just before eating or cooking them.

PART III

THE NUTRIPOINT
BUILDING BLOCKS

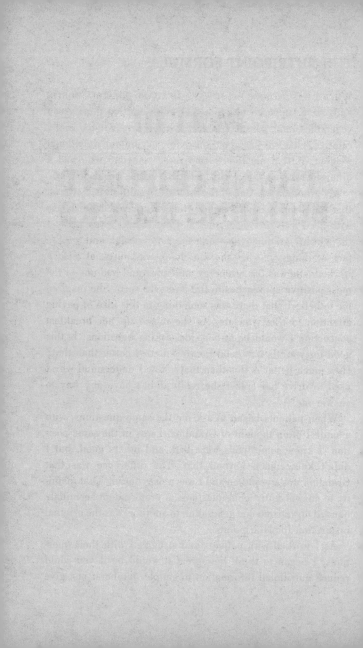

THE NUTRIPOINT FORMULA

WHEN I WAS GROWING UP, IT WAS A MEAT AND POTATOES WORLD. Kids were supposed to drink their milk and eat their green vegetables, and parents weren't supposed to eat too many calories. That was just about the extent of common nutritional wisdom. But in my family there was someone who had a different take on the world, particularly the world of food.

My grandma was one of the original "health nuts," at least that's how some people saw her when she arrived at our house with her *Prevention* magazines and her brewer's yeast. But I thought my grandma was someone very special; and, on the face of things, if what she was doing was nutty, at least it worked: she was full of energy and spirit and had one of the most positive approaches to life I've ever seen. She inspired me to believe that there was something to this idea of paying attention to what you ate. As she mixed up her breakfast concoction I would be at her side, asking questions. Is this good for you? Is that good for you? Is this better than that? How much better is this than that? Now I understand why I used to drive her crazy: she really didn't have any way to answer me.

When patients began to ask me the same questions, with a smile I often thought of Grandma. I was in the same position. I knew some foods were bad, and others good, but I didn't know much beyond that. The difference was that Grandma was a grandma and I was a *nutritionist.* That inability to answer nutritional questions, a predicament seemingly handed down from one generation to another, was the original inspiration for Nutripoints.

As I worked with patients and struggled with their questions, I began to think how great it would be if you could reduce nutritional information to simple numbers: just give each food a certain number of points for the good things it had. The major problem faced by my patients was the juggling act they faced with all the nutritional variables. They had to think about cholesterol, sodium, total fat, saturated fat, sugar, complex carbohydrates, vitamins, minerals, fiber, caffeine, and alcohol, in addition to calories. As one patient told me, "I'd have to be a walking computer to figure all this out." I knew what he meant because he'd have to be referring to labels, USDA charts, and RDAs for every food.

In 1981 I worked out a rough formula. I tested it out on a computer using USDA data on 400 foods. It seemed to work, and I was delighted, but put it aside to focus on other things. When I came to the Aerobics Center in Dallas, I revived my old idea and began to use it with patients. I assigned numbers to foods to help people choose the best ones.

The idea of a food having a number attached was a big success; patients loved it. But there was something missing. I needed a *system*—some method of helping people get a variety and a balance of foods as well as the best foods.

In 1985 I started using the basic concepts that evolved into Nutripoints: high nutrient density, low calories, and balance. All of this was done with numbers, and it was wonderfully effective. The patients at the Aerobics Center had serious health problems—such as coronary heart disease, high cholesterol, high blood pressure, obesity, and diabetes—or were engaging in poor eating habits that were contributing to a major risk for these diseases. While at the center, they had great success with my "numbers" system. There was just one problem with the early versions of Nutripoints. Patients used the numbers when they were at the clinic, but once they got home and tried to find their way without the numbers, they had difficulty sticking with their new, good eating habits.

I knew that if I wanted to help people stick with an optimum eating program, I'd have to come up with a complete system that not only rated the foods but allowed people to achieve variety and balance *within the system.* And, of course, it had to be easy—no more complicated than the simple numbers I was already working with. I could only imagine the problems the person who had never been exposed to a "wellness clinic" must be experiencing.

I began to perfect Nutripoints, working with patients in order to test its effectiveness and confirm its accessibility. It took countless hours with the computer and with data from food manufacturers and fast-food chains to come up with a program that was, first of all, accurate—more accurate than anything currently available—in rating as many foods as possible. It had to make it easy for people to get a completely balanced diet, and to do so by picking their favorite foods, or at least foods they liked, so the system had to be very flexible. Finally, it had to be easy. It had to be something that people could do at home, by themselves, and something they could stick with whether they ate at home, at restaurants, at fast-food restaurants, or at friends' houses. I'm finally satisfied that Nutripoints fulfills all of these goals.

The following pages explain how the Nutripoints formula is set up.

First, I determined the components of each food. How much of each vitamin and mineral, how much fiber, protein, complex carbohydrates, cholesterol, total fat, saturated fat, sugar, caffeine, and alcohol was in each food entry. There were eighteen *essential* elements and eight *excessive* elements in each food, the amount of which needed to be determined.

Where did the information come from? I used various

sources. The Cooper Clinic Database provided about half the information. The USDA Database was enormously helpful. I also referred to Pennington and Church's comprehensive *Nutritive Value of Foods,* as well as other nutrition books. In the case of brand-name foods and fast foods, the information came either from the manufacturer's research data or from food labels. I wrote to approximately 150 companies and received information from more than three-fourths of them. In the case of fast foods, I wrote to manufacturers and included those foods I received data on.

Once I gathered information on all the foods, I needed to analyze it in terms of what nutrients the foods contained, and how the foods compared with how much of those nutrients we need in our diets. For example, a food that has a full day's requirement of vitamin C is better than a food that has 50 percent of a day's requirement of C. The nutrient content needed to be compared with a standard.

I wanted to use a standard for each nutrient that represented the highest level of *essential* nutrients per calorie and the lowest level of *excessive* nutrients per calorie. That way I'd be able to downgrade foods that are high in nutrients but also high in calories, or, say, a food that's very high in a mineral such as calcium but also very high in fat. It was also an attempt to introduce a balance factor that limits credit for a single nutrient. If a food has 50 percent of the RDA for six nutrients, it's a better food than something that has 150 percent of the RDA for a single nutrient. A food can only get 100 percent credit for an essential (even if it has 200 percent of the RDA for a given factor), but there's no cap on how negatively the excessives can affect a Nutripoint score.

As a standard for the *essential* nutrients, I used the RDA requirements for adults, which are:

Protein (high quality)	45 g
Protein (low quality)	65 g
Vitamin A	5,000 IU
Vitamin C	60 mg
Thiamine (B_1)	1.5 mg
Riboflavin (B_2)	1.7 mg
Niacin (B_3)	20 mg
Calcium	1,000 mg
Iron	18 mg
B_6	2 mg
Folic acid	.4 mg (400 mcg)
B_{12}	6 mcg
Phosphorus	1,000 mg
Magnesium	400 mg
Zinc	15 mg
Pantothenic acid	10 mg

These levels, set by the government, are generally the highest standard for each nutrient based on the National Research Council's recommended daily allowance for various subgroups of the U.S. population. Therefore, these standards should meet, or exceed, the needs of virtually all healthy adults. As to the two kinds of protein, because we're rating each food individually, we quantified the *type* of protein, and the ratings reflect this. High-quality protein is found in animal products, and low-quality protein is found in all other foods. They're so defined because the balance of amino acids is more complete in animal protein. But in practice, you don't need to worry at all about types of protein because the balance of the Nutripoint program takes care of this for you.

Some essentials have no RDA, and therefore the following guidelines were used:

Complex carbohydrates	60 percent of total calories
Dietary fiber	35 g*
Potassium	5,625 mg†

The following standards were used as the upper limit allowable for each of the *excessive* elements in our diet:

Total fat	30 percent of total calories
Saturated fat	10 percent of total calories
Cholesterol	300 mg. per day
Sodium	3,000 mg. per day
Sugar	10 percent of total calories
Caffeine	200 mg. per day
Alcohol	½ ounce of pure alcohol per day

Once I set these standards, the computer converted these figures to a percentage of either the recommended amount (in the case of the essential nutrients), which would be a positive percentage, or the recommended limit (in the case of the excessive nutrients), which would be a negative percentage.

For example, an apple has 6 milligrams of vitamin C. So I would take 6 and divide by the RDA for vitamin C, which is 60. The resulting percentage is 10. So, for vitamin C, one of the eighteen variables, an apple scores 10 percent. The Nutripoint formula does this calculation for each one of the eighteen essentials, which include all the vitamins and minerals as well as fiber, complex carbohydrates, and protein.

Another example: an orange has 66 milligrams of vitamin C, so 66 divided by 60 (the RDA for vitamin C) equals 110 percent. An orange has 110 percent of the RDA for vitamin

*This is the upper limit of the daily recommendation of the National Cancer Institute.

†Although no RDA for potassium has been set, the National Research Council has set a "recommended safe dietary intake" of several nutrients, including potassium. This level represents the highest level within that range.

C. But the formula gives no credit beyond 100 percent for any
one of the essentials. (That's done to avoid giving too much
credit to a food that is high in only one nutrient. We don't
want a food to be at the top of the list if it has an enormous
amount of one nutrient, but not much of any other nutrients.)
Thus the percentage score for the orange in relation to vitamin C is 100 percent.

A variation of the same procedure is done for the excessives. For example, whole milk has 30 milligrams of cholesterol for an eight-ounce serving. Three hundred is the daily
limit of cholesterol, so you determine what percentage of your
daily limit is contained in that eight-ounce glass of milk.
Three hundred divided by 30 equals 10 percent. Because it's
a negative factor, this means it's a negative percentage. So
milk gets a 10-percent negative for cholesterol.

All of those percentages, negative and positive, for each
food were then added together and divided by the number of
positive factors. That percentage was then divided by the total
calories in the standard serving of that food. The result is a
fraction. The fraction was then multiplied by 100 and
rounded to the nearest half or whole number. The resulting
figure is the Nutripoint rating for that food.

I considered twenty-six factors for each of the 3,000 foods,
which translates into 78,000 info-bits that went into the rank-
ings.

One of the advantages of the Nutripoint formula is that it's
flexible. If another nutrient is discovered, or if another negative factor that affects our health is revealed, the formula can
be adjusted for this new information, and the numbers re-
crunched to come up with new, updated Nutripoint scores for
every food. It's a formula that's poised to adapt to the latest
nutritional research so that the Nutripoint score for a food
will always be the best and most complete evaluation possible.

ANSWERS TO QUESTIONS ABOUT THE NUTRIPOINT FORMULA

While I have just described the basics of how the Nutripoint formula works, I would like to answer the following common questions about it:

Are all the factors weighted equally?

In other words, does a food get as much credit for having 100 percent of the RDA of vitamin C as it does for having 100 percent of the RDA for pantothenic acid? And is having too much fat just as bad as having too much caffeine? It is obvious that some factors should be weighted, and I did so. The following are exceptions to the formula rules:

• *Dietary fiber* is weighted two times positive.

I felt that fiber is of utmost importance in the American diet, so we weighted it more positively to help steer people to foods that are rich in these factors. Weighting fiber highly also helps to lower the scores of foods that are fortified. This is done because many of them contain a lot of vitamins and minerals, but are low in fiber due to processing.

• *Cholesterol* and *alcohol* are weighted three times negatively.

I felt that cholesterol was an extremely negative factor in today's diet. By weighting it with a triple negative, I ensured that foods high in cholesterol would have lowered Nutripoint scores.

Because alcohol is negative in so many ways, I weighted it particularly negatively. It can be high in calories. It's virtually devoid of nutrients. It drains the body's stores of nutrients, particularly the B vitamins. It's a toxin. It can be psychologically harmful. For these reasons I wanted to steer people away from alcohol.

What about saturated fat? Doesn't recent research show that it's just as bad, or even worse, than eating cholesterol?

Yes, it does seem that saturated fat, which acts to elevate blood cholesterol, is a particularly negative element in the diet. The Nutripoint formula in effect weights saturated fat doubly negative because both total fat and saturated fat (a part of total fat) are given negative weights separately.

Could the formula for Nutripoints ever change?

Yes. It's possible that we'd find a more accurate way to calculate Nutripoints, especially if there's a research break-through on a new nutrient or on an element that's revealed to be particularly harmful to our health. It's important to remember, however, that whatever flaws might exist in the present system, it is consistent in its analysis, and is the best and most up-to-date system we have. Because it does the same things to all foods, and because the foods themselves will not change, it's an extraordinarily reliable guide to food value.

How did you decide what the portion size should be for each food?

The Nutripoint score is a *quality* rating. The serving size correlates with the calories in the food. In other words, the quality of the food times the calories equals Nutripoints. In order to make sure the Nutripoint value is correct, I had to be sure that the calories per serving within each group were approximately the same. I also had to be practical about amounts people typically consider to be a serving. The follow-ing lists show how the calories per serving break down in the various Nutrigroups:

Food Groups

Nutrigroup	*Calories per Serving*
Vegetable	20–60
Fruit	50–100
Grain	100–200
Legume	100–200
Milk/dairy	100–200
Meat/poultry/fish	125–250
Other Groups	
Oil	50–100
Sugar	100–200
Condiment	0–20
Alcohol	100–200

Serving sizes get smaller as the amount of calories and fat goes up. If something has, say, 100 calories, you might have a cup as a serving size, but if it's 200 calories, you might have a half cup.

Were there any surprises in the results of the Nutripoint food ratings?

Yes. For example, I was surprised at how low peanut butter rates. At .5 Nutripoints, it's low down on the legume Nutrigroup list. I thought that because it has no cholesterol and a decent amount of protein it would do better. I was also surprised at the cheeses. The fat and cholesterol in cheese really pulls it down, and many types of cheese are below the recommended level in the milk/dairy Nutrigroup. This makes it obvious that it's important to stick to the low-fat dairy foods. I was surprised at how bad eggs are. While egg whites are fine, a whole cooked egg scores —11.5—a terrible rating! It's really the cholesterol that pulls it down. Lean beef was also a surprise: it's not as bad as many people think. In fact, as you glance down the list you'll find that it's sometimes a better choice than some types of chicken. I'm sure you'll be interested to check your favorite foods in the lists and find how they score. You may be in for some surprises too.

ESSENTIALS AND EXCESSIVES

Now that you know the basics of what went into the Nutripoint formula, you might find it interesting to learn a bit more about the components of foods and how they affect your diet.

I have a somewhat *revolutionary* proposition to make: let's look at the essentials of our diet in an entirely new light. Instead of breaking things down into "sources of energy" or "percentages of daily requirements," let's be completely practical about what we need to know about food.

In fact, you don't *really* need to know anything but the numbers and Nutrigroups, but you probably have a healthy curiosity about the basic factors that go into figuring the Nutripoint numbers. So let's look at food with a fresh approach.

The factors that have been figured into the Nutripoints formula are all elements in the foods we eat. Some are good for us, but are lacking in our diets; others are good for us, but are consumed in excessive quantities; still others are bad for us, and should be avoided. I've made a practical breakdown of the elements of foods that corresponds only to what you need to know. I've divided them into two groups: *essentials* and *excessives*.

My breakdown of the essential elements in our diet is slightly unconventional. Both fat and cholesterol, for example, are indeed essential to maintain life. But, because they have become problem elements in our diets, I've moved them into the excessives category: no one in this country has to worry about getting enough fat or cholesterol in his or her diet. Calories, too, earn their place on the excessives list, even though we couldn't live without them.

My breakdown is as follows:

Essentials	Excessives
Complex carbohydrates	Total fat
Protein	Saturated fat
Dietary fiber	Calories
Vitamins*	Cholesterol
Minerals†	Sodium
	Sugar
	Caffeine
	Alcohol

The Essentials

The following are brief descriptions of the role each of these elements plays in our diets:

Complex Carbohydrates   Carbohydrates, as the name implies, are made up of carbon, hydrogen, and oxygen. Carbohydrates supply energy, in the form of blood sugar, to keep the body functioning. Carbohydrates have always seemed to me a "schizophrenic" food group: on the one hand, complex carbohydrates (those found in cereals, rice, breads, pasta, beans, nuts, and all vegetables) are really good for you. You probably eat too little of them, and one of the aims of Nutripoints is to ensure that you eat more. On the other hand, simple carbohydrates (those found in refined sugars, such as candy, cakes, puddings, soft drinks, sugar-coated cereals, and the like) are terrible for you, and you probably eat too much of them. Nutripoints has made sugar a negative factor in the Nutripoint formula and complex carbohydrates a positive fac-

* Vitamins include A, thiamin, B_2, B_3, B_6, B_{12}, C, pantothenic acid, and folacin.

† Minerals include calcium, iron, magnesium, phosphorus, potassium, and zinc.

tor so that the numbers reflect what you really need in your diet. In other words, Nutripoints weights fiber as a positive factor, and sugar as a negative factor; the system highlights the *best* carbohydrates for you.

The Nutripoint program emphasizes complex carbohydrates as a primary food. By recommending ten servings of carbohydrates daily (four of vegetables, three of fruits, two of grains, and one of legumes), it recognizes that a diet rich in complex carbohydrates can improve your energy levels and your performance, as well as help you prevent long-term disease. This emphasis on carbohydrates has replaced the old-fashioned reliance on protein as a "diet" food. Carbohydrates are low in fat, but nonetheless very satisfying. They are rich in vitamins and minerals. They "burn clean" in the body, leaving only carbon dioxide and water to be excreted (as opposed to protein, which leaves nitrogen and sulfur waste). Carbohydrates are also the major source of fuel to the brain, which relies on an optimum level of blood sugar to function properly.

Protein Along with fat and carbohydrates, protein is one of the sources of energy from food. It is essential for life. Every cell in the body contains some protein. Indeed, excluding water, half of the body's weight is protein. It's important that you get sufficient protein in your diet every day to function at an optimum level.

Most of us think of protein as the "safest" food component. We think carbohydrates are bad; we know fat is bad. But protein is something that you should eat a lot of, especially if you're on a diet. Right? Wrong! Most of us eat at least *twice* as much protein as we need. And, unlike a water-soluble vitamin, excess protein is not excreted. It's stored in the body. Because the major sources of protein we consume include meat and dairy products, which are high in fat, our high protein intake is also creating high fat, cholesterol, and calorie intakes. In short, it's making us fat. It's also putting a strain on the liver and kidneys, which are responsible for processing excess protein. Finally, excess protein consumption increases your need for calcium, and can exacerbate problems connected with a low-calcium diet.

The Nutripoints balance assures you that you're getting just the right amount of protein daily. You'll be getting high-quality protein with a balance of all the essential amino acids. But the source of some of your protein will shift: instead of getting most of your protein from meat, you'll be getting more from other sources, such as legumes. I might mention here that I've provided a vegetarian option, a Nutripoints program for those readers who prefer to omit meat entirely from their diets.

Top Tip: Protein
The best approach to giving your diet a better balance in terms of protein is to shift the major source of it from meat and dairy foods to fish, soy products (such as tofu), and dried beans and peas. There are some excellent frozen entrees that rely on tofu as their main source of protein. They're low in calories, without cholesterol, and lower in fat than meat. I highly recommend them. I've also included some delicious main course bean-based recipes, such as bean soups, which I think you'll enjoy.

Fiber   Fiber, commonly called "roughage," is a nonnutritive part of food. It has virtually no calories, and is not digested. Fiber is important in giving "bulk" to food, and in helping to move it through the intestines and colon. Lack of sufficient fiber in the diet has been linked to cancers of the colon and rectum, diverticulosis, hemorrhoids, hiatal hernia, varicose veins, and heart disease.

There are two types of fiber present in foods: soluble and insoluble. We've long been aware of insoluble fiber. It was the "rough stuff" we could depend on to promote regularity. It's insoluble because it won't dissolve in hot water. Soluble fiber, which will dissolve in hot water, has an effect on the body's metabolism of fats and sugar. Oat bran has become the most popular soluble fiber—maybe because we can put it into sweet, fatty muffins and think we're doing ourselves a nutritional favor. While it's certainly true that certain soluble fibers have a beneficial effect on blood cholesterol, fruits and vegetables, as well as beans, contain soluble fiber that's every bit as beneficial as the fiber found in oat bran.

Following the Nutripoint program will ensure that you're getting enough of both soluble and insoluble fiber. There is no need to take fiber supplements, and they can actually be dangerous if you don't take them with enough water, or if you take them to excess. Moreover, too much fiber, which is more likely to occur if you take supplements, can leach nutrients from your body as it moves food too rapidly through your digestive system. Remember: food, not pills!

The oat bran craze has recently been superseded by the rice bran craze. It seems that every few months there's a new nutritional bandwagon you can climb on. It may be megavitamins, or fiber, or tryptophan, or fish oil. As appealing as these trends can be (it's always so tempting to think that you can change and improve your life in one easy step), most of us who have seen these trends come and go recognize that they're often an exaggeration of some very complex research. The oat bran phenomenon started with some research that found that the fiber in certain foods, including beans, carrots, and oat bran, among others, was helpful in controlling cholesterol. Well, carrots and beans are not very sexy, so everyone seized on the oat bran connection. In fact, oat bran is no more effective in controlling cholesterol than a number of other fibrous foods. But who wants to eat some beans or carrots when you can have a huge, rich, sweet, fatty oat bran muffin for breakfast and feel virtuous at the same time? The fact is,

if you're serious about good nutrition, the trends are not your
best inspiration. So often they turn out to be exaggerated or
even wrong.

Nutripoints goes beyond trends in that you'll be eating the
very foods that may be discovered in the near future to be
beneficial. How can I be sure of this? Because you'll be eating
the very best, highest-quality foods. Nutripoints makes optimum nutrition an achievable goal today.

Top Tip: Fiber

Beans are an excellent source of fiber, and play too
small a role in our diets. To get the most benefit from
beans, soak them overnight and then cook them
slowly at a low temperature. If you don't soak them
and you cook them in boiling water, you'll just
toughen them and impede the availability of the fiber
and nutrients they're rich in.

Vitamins and Minerals   Adequate vitamin and mineral intake is one of the major goals of Nutripoints. The goal of the
system is to provide you with *at least* the RDA of every
essential vitamin and mineral.

Vitamins are organic substances that are essential to biochemical reactions in our bodies. Vitamins do not give us
"energy"; we rely on calories for that. They simply promote
the metabolic functions that result in energy. There are thir-
teen vitamins. Four vitamins are fat-soluble (A, D, E, and K),
and nine are water-soluble (C and the eight B-complex vitamins: thiamin, riboflavin, niacin, B_6, folic acid, B_{12}, pantothenic acid, and biotin).

Minerals are inorganic substances that, like vitamins, promote various metabolic functions in the body. The macrominerals, which are needed in relatively large amounts, include
calcium, phosphorus, magnesium, potassium, sulfur, sodium,

and chlorine. The microminerals, or trace minerals, are needed in tiny amounts. They include iron, zinc, selenium, manganese, molybdenum, copper, iodine, chromium, and fluorine. I haven't included the microminerals in the Nutripoint formula because they're not normally reported in USDA data, and getting information on amounts available in foods is difficult, if not impossible. It's also been shown that foods high in the macronutrients are also high in the micronutrients.

Here's a quick breakdown of every vitamin and mineral considered in the Nutripoint numbers, and some tips on how to guarantee your intake of that particular substance.

Vitamin A   I think of vitamin A as the "wrapper" vitamin because it's largely responsible for the health of our wrappers: our skin, hair, and mucous membranes (the linings of our mouths, stomachs, and so on). It's also involved in vision, immunity, and reproduction. Vitamin A is fat-soluble. The most exciting news about vitamin A is that researchers have recently connected a lack of vitamin A with the development of certain cancers. This is important because many of us, particularly children and adolescents, don't get nearly enough vitamin A. At the same time, there is fear among medical experts that some people, hearing of the ability of vitamin A to boost the immune system and prevent cancer, are overdosing on vitamin A. Because vitamin A is fat-soluble, and is therefore stored in the body, toxic amounts can build up and cause jaundice or liver damage. Moreover, vitamin A supplements have not been shown to help fight cancer. Beta-carotene, a precursor to vitamin A, which is found in red and yellow fruits and vegetables, is the cancer fighter, so those foods are your best sources of vitamin A. If you're getting your vitamin A in the form of beta-carotene, you won't have to worry about the dangers of overdosing.

> ## Top Tip: Vitamin A
> One of the best, quickest, and most delicious sources of vitamin A is a sweet potato. It gives you twice the RDA for vitamin A. If you've never tried a baked sweet potato, you're missing something. Just eat it hot from the oven or microwave plain, or with a bit of nonfat yogurt for a great snack or as part of a meal.

Vitamin C   Vitamin C (ascorbic acid) is one of the most well known water-soluble vitamins. It's a sort of "glue" vitamin that is important in the manufacture of collagen, which helps hold the body together. Perhaps one of the best-known roles of vitamin C is that of infection fighter.

I've learned that many people, even those who don't take any other type of vitamin, will pop a vitamin C tablet regularly, or when they feel a cold coming on. This obsession is somewhat misguided, as most of us get at least one and a half times the amount of vitamin C we need each day. At least vitamin C, because it is water-soluble, is not one of those vitamins that can readily become dangerous in high levels: the body excretes excess amounts.

> ## Top Tip: Vitamin C
> I think the best vitamin C "supplement" you can take is sweet red pepper. One-eighth of a red pepper will give you about 95 milligrams of vitamin C, or one and a half times your daily requirement. Red pepper is also very low in calories.

Vitamin B_1 (Thiamin) B_1 is known as the "energy" vitamin because one of its most important roles is in the metabolism of carbohydrates. It's also important in the functioning of nerves. It stimulates growth, helps to maintain good muscle tone, and has been shown to stabilize the appetite. Because thiamin is water-soluble, it's rarely dangerous, even when taken to excess.

Top Tip: Vitamin B$_1$

Don't add baking soda to water when you cook vegetables (as some people do to retain bright green colors). This practice depletes thiamin. Also, don't wash enriched white rice before you cook it (you can wash brown and wild rice). Don't boil any kind of rice in a lot of water until done and then drain it. Instead, measure the appropriate amount of rice and the appropriate amount of water (about twice as much water as rice), and then cook the rice until it has absorbed all the water. Throwing out water that rice has boiled in is like throwing out "vitamin soup."

Vitamin B$_2$ (Riboflavin)   Vitamin B$_2$ is necessary for carbohydrate, fat, and protein metabolism. It boosts the immune system and the formation of red blood cells. It also promotes good vision and helps keep skin, nails, and hair healthy.

Top Tip: Vitamin B$_2$

Rely on dairy products! Because so many of the sources of B$_2$ are foods low in Nutripoints, such as organ meats (which are very high in fats), low-fat or nonfat dairy foods are your best source. Keep up with the Nutripoint food groups and don't neglect your two servings of high-Nutripoint dairy foods daily. Adding some extra nonfat dry milk when you're baking (or to recipes such as meat loaf) can give you a good boost of B$_2$.

Vitamin B$_3$ (Niacin)   Vitamin B$_3$ has become a "hot" vitamin these days because of the role it plays in reducing cholesterol. In addition to this critical job, niacin is necessary for carbohydrate, fat, and protein metabolism. It helps maintain the health of your skin, tongue, and digestive and nervous systems.

The good news about niacin is that very few people have problems with deficiencies because it is so readily available from so many food sources. Just three ounces of water-packed tuna, for example, supplies about three-quarters of your daily requirement.

For reasons previously discussed concerning vitamins and their dangers, I don't recommend that you try to supplement with niacin to lower your blood cholesterol unless you're doing so under the direction of a physician. There are serious side effects connected with megadoses of niacin.

Top Tip: Vitamin B$_3$

The highest level of the RDA for niacin (for males 19 to 22 years of age) is 19 milligrams. As three ounces of tuna canned in water has 14 milligrams you can see why it is not hard to come by niacin in food. So, my suggestion on niacin is to avoid supplements. Prolonged use of megadoses can result in skin rashes, irritation of peptic ulcers, irregular heartbeat, jaundice, and promotion of gout, among other symptoms.

Vitamin B$_6$ Vitamin B$_6$ is a water-soluble vitamin that has many roles in the biochemical life of the body. It's necessary for fat, carbohydrate, and protein metabolism. It's important in the production of red blood cells and of antibodies. It helps to regulate blood glucose levels. Because vitamin B$_6$ is critical to so many functions, its lack is signaled by a wide variety of symptoms and has been connected to everything from asthma, PMS, and carpal tunnel syndrome, to diabetes, cancer, and cardiovascular disease.

So many people are so deficient in vitamin B$_6$ that the government has named it a "problem nutrient." In a recent study only 22 percent of Americans past the age of one met their recommended dietary allowances of vitamin B_6 in 1989. Because B_6 plays such an important role in so many biochemical activities in our bodies, it's important to get an adequate amount. But please don't rely on supplements. While B_6 is water-soluble, and excess amounts are largely flushed from the body, high doses (upward of 200 milligrams a day) can result in nervousness, insomnia, frequent urination, irritability, and bed wetting in children.

> ### Top Tip: Vitamin B_6
> One banana will give you over a third of your daily requirement of vitamin B_6.

Vitamin B_{12}   Vitamin B_{12} is a water-soluble vitamin that is responsible for the formation of blood cells, as well as the metabolism of carbohydrates, fats, and proteins. It's important for cell replication and helps maintain a healthy nervous system.

Because B_{12} is found in so many foods, it's rare to suffer a deficiency. The people most likely to suffer a B_{12} deficiency are strict vegetarians, and even they are not very likely to suffer a deficiency if they vary their diet.

> ### Top Tip: Vitamin B_{12}
> Stores of B_{12} can last in the body up to fifteen years. As you need only 3 micrograms daily, you really don't need to worry about a deficiency, and you can easily see why supplements of B_{12} would be superfluous for healthy people.

Pantothenic Acid   Pantothenic acid is essential for healthy skin, body growth, and the production of antibodies. It's also necessary for the conversion of fats and carbohydrates into energy. Because pantothenic acid is so readily available in foods, there's little danger of deficiency.

Top Tip: Pantothenic Acid
Because you need such small amounts, and because it's so readily available, you'll have no trouble getting adequate pantothenic acid.

Folacin Folacin aids in the metabolism of proteins, and is necessary for the growth and division of cells. Folacin is essential to your mental and emotional health.

Folacin deficiencies, particularly among women, are not uncommon. A U.S. Department of Agriculture survey revealed that many women get less than half the recommended level of folacin. If you're taking contraceptive pills, or if you've been taking aspirin because of its connection to mitigating the development of cardiovascular disease, you may need extra folacin in your diet. A number of health problems are related to folacin deficiencies, including depression, infections, cervical dysplasia in women on the pill, and cancer.

Top Tip: Folacin
To retain the most folacin in your foods, cook vegetables in the least possible amount of water or oil. Stir-frying them in the smallest possible amount of oil is the best method.

The best possible folacin boost is a spinach salad: a half cup of raw spinach gives you twice the RDA of folacin.

The emphasis on vegetables and legumes in the Nutripoint program will guarantee that you'll receive an adequate supply of folacin. Folacin is readily available in green, leafy vegetables. Those at the top of the Nutripoints list are rich in the vitamin. Even if you're among those who need extra folacin, you'll be more than adequately supplied by the Nutripoint program.

Calcium   Calcium is one of the most abundant minerals in the body, and is essential to human life. Calcium sustains the maintenance and development of bones and teeth, and is critical to blood coagulation, muscle action, heartbeat, and nerve function.

Calcium has been a "hot" mineral for a few years now, and with good reason. A government survey revealed that 68 percent of Americans are deficient in calcium. Those especially vulnerable to calcium deficiency are women: adolescent girls and middle-aged women. The deficiency shows up in later years, when these women suffer from osteoporosis—a weak bone structure that can lead to dowager's hump and easily fractured bones.

One of the reasons people have become at risk for calcium deficiency is that many of the foods that have high levels of calcium also have high levels of fat. Milk and other dairy products, which are the most common sources of calcium, are often avoided by people on a low-fat diet.

Top Tip: Calcium
A half cup of cooked broccoli or four ounces of nonfat yogurt will give you over a third of your daily requirement, while a half cup of cooked bok choy will give you well over a third. One-quarter cup of nonfat dry milk gives you over a third of your daily requirement, and it can be added to foods such as dressings, baked goods, and meat loafs to boost calcium supplies without adding many calories.

Unfortunately, many people have resorted to calcium supplements to try to increase their calcium intakes. Many people do this without being aware of what their daily intake is in the first place, so they may be getting overdoses that could be potentially dangerous. Overdoses of calcium can result in kidney stones, constipation, acid stomach, nausea, and high blood pressure. In May of 1989, the National Research Council issued a report which said that "the potential benefits of calcium intakes above the RDA . . . are not well-documented and do not justify the use of calcium supplements." I strongly recommend that you avoid calcium supplements and rely instead on the high-Nutripoint foods listed in the milk/dairy food group for the best low-fat sources of calcium. And keep in mind that weight-bearing exercise such as walking or jogging increases calcium absorption while caffeine, alcohol, and smoking decrease it.

Iron   A trace mineral essential for life, iron is the "blood mineral." It's responsible for the transport of oxygen in the body by means of the hemoglobin in red blood cells. Iron deserves attention because it is so commonly deficient in the average diet. Nearly half of the population is deficient in iron. Women are often iron deficient, particularly because of their monthly blood loss during menstruation. But young children are also commonly iron deficient.

Of all the nutrient-deficiency diseases, anemia is the most common. And if you find it hard to translate a condition such as anemia into real-life problems, you'll be amazed to learn that one study of women found that their work performance quadrupled when they increased their iron intake.

Top Tip: Iron

You can dramatically increase your iron intake by taking some vitamin C in the form of, say, orange juice with an iron-rich meal. Orange juice with breakfast, for example, can boost the absorbed iron by 200 percent. Avoid drinking coffee or tea with meals: they decrease iron absorption.

Magnesium   Magnesium is essential for every biological process. It aids in the body's use of carbohydrates, fats, and proteins, and works in conjunction with other minerals, including calcium, phosphorus, and potassium. Many of us are deficient in magnesium because of our low-calorie diets of highly processed foods. A USDA food consumption survey revealed that only 25 percent of Americans get enough magnesium. Despite deficiencies, magnesium supplements are not the answer. Magnesium is a mineral that perfectly illustrates my contention that supplements are to be avoided because they're frequently unbalanced. Because magnesium works in conjunction with calcium, for example, if you increase your magnesium intake, you must increase your calcium intake at an even ratio, and vice versa if you take calcium supplements. Very few people are aware of this relationship between minerals. If you get your minerals from foods, however, Mother Nature takes care of the balance for you.

Top Tip: Magnesium
A half cup of fresh, cooked spinach has about one-quarter of your daily magnesium requirement. Dried bran cereals such as All-Bran, Bran Buds, Bran Chex, and Bran Flakes are good sources of magnesium, with one ounce of many of them providing about one-quarter of your daily requirement.

Potassium   Potassium is the third most abundant element in the body. It works with magnesium to help regulate the heart, and with sodium to help regulate blood pressure and send nerve impulses. Fortunately, potassium is abundant in the average diet and so rarely poses the problem of deficiency. People who might be in danger of potassium deficiency include those suffering from a digestive disease, those using diuretics, and those with uncontrolled diabetes. Athletes and others who sweat profusely may find that their potassium levels are low.

Top Tip: Potassium

If you are an athlete, or if you exercise heavily in high temperatures, you should be wary of potassium depletion. Watch for weakness or fatigue over a longer than usual period. A quick recovery can be effected with a "natural potassium supplement": a glass of orange juice or a banana. Avoid potassium supplements, as overdoses pose serious risks.

Phosphorus You have a pound and a half of phosphorus in your body. Along with calcium, it's the most abundant mineral. Phosphorus, along with calcium, is responsible for the building of bones. It also plays a major role in other metabolic functions, including cell reproduction and conversion of foods to energy.

Top Tip: Phosphorus

If you frequently take antacids that contain aluminum, they can block your absorption of phosphorus. Check with your druggist to find an antacid that doesn't contain aluminum, or try to boost your phosphorus intake.

Because phosphorus is so widely available in a variety of foods (dairy products, meats, fish, grains, nuts, and beans) you rarely have to worry about a phosphorus deficiency.

Zinc Zinc is a critical trace mineral that promotes growth and healing. It aids the immune system in its efforts to prevent disease, and is important in a wide range of metabolic activities.

Marginal zinc deficiencies seem to be a common price paid for today's style of eating. Low-calorie diets are the culprits.

A USDA study revealed that only 8 percent of the surveyed groups achieved the recommended zinc levels. The typical woman eats only half the calories she would need to get sufficient zinc. Because of zinc's important role in boosting the immune system, this is a potentially dangerous nutritional situation. Zinc deficiencies also play a role in eating disorders such as anorexia nervosa and bulimia, osteoporosis, low sperm counts, gum disease, and fetal complications, including low birth weight and other disorders.

Top Tip: Zinc

One ounce of the following cereals will provide you with nearly a third of your daily zinc requirement: All-Bran, Bran Buds, 40% Bran Flakes, Nutri-Grain, and Special K. Three ounces of lean pot roast will give you half your daily zinc requirement. Three ounces of raw oysters will give you 400 percent of your daily zinc requirement.

The Excessives

The excessives are the elements in our diet that there are just too much of. As I mentioned before, most of these items are not totally bad; indeed, all of them, with the exception of caffeine and alcohol, are essential to human life. It's just that our eating patterns have emphasized these elements to our detriment. We simply can't continue to eat diets high in fat, calories, cholesterol, sodium, and sugar without paying the price in both long- and short-term symptoms and diseases.

The following are the excessives that have been figured into the Nutripoint formula:

Total fat
Saturated fat
Calories
Cholesterol
Sodium

Sugar
Caffeine
Alcohol

—

Fat Fat has become one of the biggest problems in our diet.
While fat is essential for life (as a concentrated energy source,
a carrier of fat-soluble vitamins, and a source of essential fatty
acids), too much fat is ultimately life-threatening. Most of us
are eating three to five times the amount of fat we need to
keep our bodies functioning. We really only need the equivalent of one tablespoon of fat per day. All the excess fat we're
eating is contributing to heart disease, colon and breast cancer, and obesity (which is linked to a number of other diseases).

Top Tip: Fat

I think that the "fat booby traps" are margarine and
salad dressings. Many people avoid butter because
it's high in saturated fat. Margarine is a better choice,
but margarine is still essentially fat. You can't use it
with abandon. Don't slather it on bread and sandwiches. You can eat a waffle with apple butter or
fresh fruit without missing the margarine at all. Get
out of the "fat spreading" habit. Salad dressings pose
another danger because many people find that
they're eating more salads and vegetables on the Nutripoint program. But commercial salad dressings are
loaded with fat. Even if you do virtually no cooking,
you owe it to yourself to either find a good low-fat
commercial dressing, or to try one of our Nutripoint
dressing recipes. You'll find such a dressing every bit
as flavorful as those oily ones, and far more healthful.
Make up a batch and keep it handy in your refrigerator. You can even bring a small amount with you to
a restaurant and ask for a salad without dressing so
that you can use your own.

Cutting down on fat is one of the most important things you
can do to improve your diet and thereby extend your life.

Nutripoints will make it easy for you, as fat is heavily weighted as a negative factor. By sticking to the foods that are at the high end of the Nutripoint food charts, and by being sure to limit your meat and dairy servings and portions to the Nutripoint recommendations, you'll be keeping your fat intake to 30 percent of your total calories, and your saturated fat to within 10 percent of your total calories—figures that are well within the limit set by the American Heart Association. (We break out saturated fat from the total fat because while foods with saturated fat don't contain cholesterol, they cause the body to produce cholesterol and thereby raise serum cholesterol levels.)

Calories Hi-cal, low-cal, no-cal—calories have been the dominant issue in the way most of us have approached nutrition for the past thirty years. All we want to know about calories is how to avoid them, and this obsession has given us such a distorted picture of what nutrition is all about that far too many of us are actually malnourished. A recently published book, for example, is an endless listing of the calories in every imaginable food, the premise of the book being that you can lose weight by substituting low-calorie foods for high-calorie ones. But if you binge, as you no doubt will, you can catch up by eating next to nothing until you're back to your goal. This is all pretty basic, but the implication is that you can substitute, say, a candy bar for a tuna sandwich on whole wheat and get away with it if the calories in the two foods are the same. I'm surprised that this old-fashioned approach to nutrition is still given any credence at all. The fact is, calories are just one of many factors that need to be considered in the decision as to whether a food is good or bad, nutritious or not.

Strictly speaking, calories are units of heat measurement: a calorie is the amount of energy it takes to raise the temperature of 1 gram of water 1 degree centigrade. Calories are the fuel that enable our bodies to perform their endless metabolic tasks. The average adult man burns 1,500 to 2,000 calories per day, and the average woman, 1,200 to 1,800. You need to consume about that many calories for your body to function: less and you'll force your body to call on stored energy and thereby lose weight; more and you'll store the excess calories as fat and gain weight. It's that simple.

Many of us are overweight. Some of us are overweight to the extent that it seriously affects our health. Probably *most* of us believe we are overweight by at least five or ten pounds. Many of us think that if we could only restrict our caloric intake for a while we'd get back down to what we weighed in college, or high school, or eighth grade, or whatever our personal "golden age" was. But most of us hate diets because they're boring or hard to follow, or because they make us feel sick or dizzy. In fact, I can promise you that you don't have to restrict the amount of food you eat. With the Nutripoint program you'll find that you can eat far more than you might have thought, but lose or maintain your weight (depending on your goal) by eating foods that are more nutritious and lower in calories.

Top Tip: Calories

I think the best thing you can do for yourself is to forget about calories. In the course of working with thousands of patients, I've found that the people who are the most knowledgeable about calories are also those with the most finely developed ability to "cheat" on a diet. If you can recite the number of calories in a Twinkie or Moon Pie, and think that if you skip a breakfast of equivalent calories you'll be back on track, you're only fooling yourself. *Don't worry about calories; focus instead on Nutripoints.*

Cholesterol   There is a 50-percent chance that your blood cholesterol level is higher than desirable: half of all adult

Americans have levels that are too high. There is a 25-percent chance that your blood cholesterol level is "high," meaning it's high enough to need intensive medical attention.

Although controversy continues on the precise meaning and implications of blood cholesterol levels, there is no doubt that a high level puts your life in danger. The tragedy of coronary heart disease—contributed to by high levels of blood cholesterol—certainly does that to 40 percent of its victims, the first warning sign being a fatal heart attack.

High levels of cholesterol have become the hidden time bombs in our postwar diet—a diet that's rich in fatty foods. We're now seeing the effects of a lifetime on such a diet: an increased risk of serious coronary heart disease, which is now the number one killer in this country. High cholesterol levels are the major contributor to this epidemic. Indeed, among the people of the famous Framingham, Massachusetts, study, who have been tracked now for more than forty years, only those with a cholesterol level below 150 milligrams daily have been found to be free of risk from premature death due to clogged arteries. Fortunately, the effects of a high-cholesterol diet can be mitigated and even reversed. When Nathan Pritikin completely changed his diet in middle age, as the result of serious heart disease, the results were dramatic. His autopsy revealed that his extremely low cholesterol diet had given him the unblocked, pliable arteries of a young child.

You've no doubt been reading a great deal about cholesterol for the past few years, but you may also be confused about how to translate research reports into your own "heart safe" diet. Nutripoints will eliminate this confusion because cholesterol is one of the major negative factors used in the Nutripoint analysis program. The higher the cholesterol level of a food, the lower in Nutripoints.

On the Nutripoint program, cholesterol intake is limited to 300 milligrams daily, which is in keeping with the recommendations of the American Heart Association. In addition to simply limiting cholesterol intake, Nutripoints lowers serum cholesterol levels by emphasizing fiber in the diet. This abundant fiber in the diet binds with bile acids that contain cholesterol, and thereby transports cholesterol out of the body.

The average person who follows the program will see a 14-percent reduction in two weeks, depending on how high his or her cholesterol was to begin with. (If it's very high, the reduction tends to be greater; in our live-in programs, I've seen drops of from 25 to 50 percent in people with high cholesterol. It wouldn't be unusual for someone to go from 250 to 180.)

If you are already suffering from coronary heart disease, the Nutripoint program is a safe and practical way to keep your cholesterol intake at the lowest possible level. Simply stick to the food items near the top of the list, and avoid those below the recommended level.

The following is a breakdown that you might find interesting. It identifies the worst offenders in terms of *both* cholesterol and calories. These foods show a high ratio of cholesterol to calories, and are thus double threats. Each entry has more than 1 milligram of cholesterol per calorie.

Cholesterol per Calorie

Food	Cholesterol per Calorie
Sweetbreads	10.2
Scrambled eggs	2.8
Fried eggs	2.7
Caviar	2.2
Wendy's green pepper, onion, mushroom omelet	2.2
Beef liver (fried)	2.1
Squid (boiled)	2.1

(continued)

Cholesterol per Calorie (*con't*)

Food	Cholesterol per Calorie
Carl's Jr. scrambled eggs	2.0
Paté (chicken liver, canned)	1.9
Wendy's ham, cheese, onion omelet	1.9
Omelet (ham and cheese)	1.8
Squid (raw)	1.8
Wendy's ham, cheese, mushroom omelet	1.8
Egg salad	1.7
Spinach salad (egg, bacon, ham)	1.5
Egg foo young	1.3
Wendy's Creamy Peppercorn dressing	1.3
Shrimp (steamed)	1.2
Wendy's ham and cheese omelet	1.2
Beef heart	1.1
Crabs (hard-shell, steamed)	1.0
Cheese sauce	1.0

Cholesterol is a waxy substance found only in animals. Cholesterol in food is referred to as *dietary* cholesterol, while cholesterol in our bodies is called *blood* or *serum* cholesterol. Although these substances are the same, they differ in origin: the body ingests cholesterol found in animal-based foods, and it manufactures its own cholesterol in response to consumed cholesterol. While the body needs cholesterol to function, it doesn't need to consume any. The body is capable of manufacturing enough cholesterol to fulfill all its needs. The trouble with consuming large amounts of cholesterol is that it stimulates the body to overproduce cholesterol and reduces its ability to remove dietary cholesterol from the bloodstream.

The ultimate result of excess cholesterol is clogged arteries, as the cholesterol adheres to the walls of the arteries and impairs their ability to carry oxygen through the body. Among many things, blood carries a regular supply of oxygen to the heart. Without oxygen, the heart muscle weakens, causing chest pain, heart attacks, and eventually death.

The U.S. Department of Health and Human Services makes five recommendations to help reduce your blood cholesterol levels:

1. Eat less high-fat food, especially those foods high in saturated fat.
2. Replace part of the saturated fat in your diet with unsaturated fat.
3. Eat less high-cholesterol food.
4. Choose foods high in complex carbohydrates.
5. If you are overweight, reduce your weight.

Nutripoints is a simple way to help you achieve all five of these goals.

You'll notice as you look at the food rating charts that some foods have a notation regarding cholesterol. This is because some foods, such as organ meats, while very high in nutrients, are also very high in cholesterol. If you are on a diet that severely limits your cholesterol, you should avoid such foods, even though they may be high in Nutripoints. There is a further explanation of this on page 284 just before the charts.

The FDA has defined the terms used in cholesterol labeling on foods as follows:

Cholesterol free: less than 2 milligrams per serving.

Low cholesterol: less than 20 milligrams per serving.

Cholesterol reduced: products reformulated or processed to reduce cholesterol by 75 percent or more.

The list that follows is a complete breakdown of all the sources of cholesterol in your diet. When you see any of them listed on a food label, you know the food contains cholesterol, or is a vegetable product that doesn't contain cholesterol, but is high in saturated fat, which can raise your serum cholesterol levels. (Just one gram of saturated fat is equal to eating 20 milligrams of cholesterol in its effect on your serum cholesterol levels.)

Animal fat	Hydrogenated vegetable oil*
Bacon fat	Lamb fat
Beef fat	Lard
Butter	Meat fat
Chicken fat	Palm kernel oil*
Cocoa butter*	Palm oil*
Coconut*	Pork fat
Coconut oil*	Turkey fat
Cream	Vegetable oil*
Egg and egg-yolk solids	Vegetable shortening*
Ham fat	Whole milk solids
Hardened fat or oil*	

Sodium   Sodium is a mineral that helps regulate blood pressure, and is essential for the proper functioning of the nervous system. Sodium is essential to life and, indeed, there are traces of sodium in almost everything we eat. There is more than enough sodium occurring naturally in foods to fulfill our daily requirements. The problem is, many of us consume ten to twenty-five times the amount (about one-tenth of a teaspoonful) we need.

Excess sodium can cause serious health problems, including high blood pressure, which can lead to stroke, and heart and kidney disease. Almost 20 percent of us are genetically prone to developing high blood pressure if we eat a diet that is too high in salt.

How do we avoid excess salt? Well, of course, Nutripoints has made it easy for you. Just choose foods from the top of the list and you'll be eating a diet that is naturally low in

*Contain no cholesterol, but are sources of saturated fat.

sodium. In addition, I recommend that you avoid processed foods whenever possible. The simple fact is, salt is added to so many processed foods in such large amounts that if such foods are a mainstay of your diet it's very difficult to avoid sodium. For example, a recent article in *Consumer Reports* contained the following surprising facts:

- One ounce of Kellogg's Corn Flakes has almost double the amount of sodium of an ounce of Planters Cocktail Peanuts: 260 milligrams versus 132.
- Two slices of Pepperidge Farm white bread have more sodium than a one-ounce bag of Lay's potato chips: 234 milligrams versus 191.

These two examples demonstrate that if you need to restrict your sodium intake, you'll have to do more than simply shun table salt. For one thing, sodium by itself is tasteless; it's in the form of sodium chloride that it becomes the common table salt we think of. But sodium by itself is still added to foods. Fortunately, some manufacturers are now including labeling that will help you make low-sodium choices. The following are sodium-related labeling terms as defined by the Food and Drug Administration:

Sodium free: less than 5 milligrams per serving.

Very low sodium: less than 35 milligrams per serving.

Low sodium: 140 milligrams or less per serving.

Reduced sodium: 75-percent reduction in sodium from that usually found in a product.

Unsalted, no salt added, without added salt: foods processed without salt that would ordinarily have it; e.g., "no salt added" pretzels or potato chips.

You should also be aware of other sodium-containing ingredients that could be listed on a package, including monosodium glutamate, baking soda (also identified as sodium bicarbonate), garlic salt, brine, and sodium citrate.

What of the actual amounts of sodium in a product? The Center for Science in the Public Interest recommends that if a product contains less than 135 milligrams of sodium per serving, consider it safe. If it contains more than that amount, try to find a similar product with less salt, or look for a "without added salt" version.

Because so many of my patients are concerned about sodium intake, I'm including a list of salt substitutes we use at the center. I think you'll find these suggestions very useful.

Morton Lite Salt
Morton Salt Substitute
No-Salt
Nu-Salt
McCormick's salt substitutes:
   Salt-Free Parsley Patch
   All-Purpose
   Sesame All-Purpose
   Garlic Saltless
   It's a Dilly
   Lemon Pepper
   Popcorn Blend
Mrs. Dash
Spike
Sherry (avoid "cooking sherry," as it's high in sodium)
Lemon juice
Lime juice
Garlic powder
Onion powder
Vinegar (including balsamic, rice wine, apple, red wine, raspberry, and blueberry vinegar)
Low-sodium soy sauce

Ginger
Cumin
Salsa
American Heart Association spices
Pepper
Green chili peppers
Gourmet Shop Saltless Seasonings
Low-sodium broths

Top Tip: Sodium

There are a number of ways to reduce the sodium in your diet, such as simply cutting out table salt, which you may well be familiar with. But one that I always pass on to my patients is the following: if you rinse canned tuna with tap water for one minute you will remove 80 percent of the sodium. This is an especially useful tip because tuna packed in water is so high in Nutripoints. It's also wise to rinse canned vegetables before cooking.

Sugar Sugar, along with cellulose and starch, is a principal component of carbohydrates. The body does need glucose (one of the components of sugar) to function. But sugar, as opposed to starch or complex carbohydrates, is quickly digested (there's little or no fiber to slow its absorption), and gives you an immediate burst of energy. Complex carbohydrates, on the other hand, are usually rich in fiber. They burn more slowly and give the body a more stable energy supply, as well as providing nutrients.

The drawback of sugar as a source of energy is that it contributes far too many calories in return for a very small contribution in terms of nutrients. This drawback would make sugar enough of a nutritional waste, but it's also involved in other physical problems. There's no doubt, for example, that a high sugar consumption contributes to dental caries. There is also some evidence linking excess sugar to diabetes and heart disease. Sugar is also a major culprit in causing obesity. It's so calorie-dense that it's very difficult for average people to burn off all the calories they're consuming in a day when sugar is a major component of their diet.

Despite sugar's poor nutritional value, most of us get an amazing 20 percent of our total daily calories from sugar. This means that we're eating twenty to thirty teaspoons of sugar *each day*. That's an incredible amount of sugar, and we just can't afford it in terms of weight control and in terms of the nutrients we need each day. Even if you never add sugar to any food you eat, you're still overdosing on it if you don't know how to read food labels. Did you know, for example, that some ketchups and salad dressings are about one-third sugar? Some of the mixes you use to coat meats before baking have the same percentage of sugar as a Hershey bar: 50 percent. Everything from bacon to soups, from gravy mixes to spaghetti sauces can have large amounts of hidden sugars. You probably know that some breakfast cereals have enormous amounts of sugar; indeed, a few cereals have so much sugar that it's actually the main ingredient. (And they'll still run ads claiming to be "part of a balanced breakfast"!)

Sugar is by far the most popular food additive. But if you learn its various disguises, you can avoid it. The following are the various forms of sugar you'll find listed on food labels:

Brown sugar	Turbinado sugar
Corn syrup	Caramel
Dextrose	Dextrin
Glucose	Fructose
Honey	Grape sugar
Lactose	Invert sugar
Maple sugar	Maltose
Sorghum syrup	Molasses

If you see any of these ingredients listed among the first few on a label, you know the product is high in sugar. Sometimes manufacturers will add sugar in a variety of forms. For example, you'll see corn syrup, dextrin, and molasses all listed in various places in the label. Even if they're not among the first ingredients, you can be sure that the product has plenty of sugar; if you added them all together, sugar might well be the first or second ingredient.

Of course, you don't really have to worry about reading labels because Nutripoints has done the work for you. The numbers have accounted for the amount of sugar in foods.

Finally, a word about artificial sweeteners. Patients always ask how I feel about them. The primary artificial sweetener I sanction is NutraSweet (in Equal).* It's an artificial sweetener that's a natural substance and a protein that is actually metabolized and used by the body. Saccharin (in Sweet 'n' Low) is not a nutritive substance. Because it must be excreted by the body, it has a potential, when taken in excessive amounts, to cause harm, such as cancer. Unlike NutraSweet, however, saccharin is heat stable and can be used in cooked products.

On the other hand, NutraSweet is a natural substance in an *unnatural* form (it has been processed). There may be some potential problem with it that has yet to be discovered. I therefore recommend that you limit yourself to two drinks and one food product sweetened with NutraSweet per day.

As to the question concerning NutraSweet's effect on blood sugar, I wondered if it might have an indirect effect on raising blood sugar. I used myself as a guinea pig, and here's what happened. While in a fasting state, I drank twelve ounces of Diet Pepsi (sweetened with NutraSweet), and then tested myself on a glucose meter. The Pepsi had no effect on my blood sugar. An hour later, I drank a glass of cranberry juice (which is very high in sugar), and the meter shot right up, showing an elevated blood sugar. Obviously, this isn't a scientific

*NutraSweet contains phenylalanine and should therefore be avoided by individuals with phenylketonuria.

study, but it allayed my own fears as to the effect of Nutra-Sweet on blood sugar.

Top Tip: Sugar
Satisfy your sweet tooth nature's way, with fruits that are naturally sweet. Watermelon is a good choice, and frozen grapes, while not particularly high in Nutripoints, can make a great snack.

Caffeine Caffeine is a stimulant that blocks the effects of our brain's natural tranquilizing agent, allowing the brain to temporarily move into a higher gear. It affects blood pressure and heart rate, and increases respiration. It's a diuretic as well as a vasoconstrictor and vasodilator: it allows the blood vessels of the brain to constrict, and those of the heart to dilate.

Caffeine is today's drug of choice among the vast majority of Americans. Its positive effects are undeniable: it gives a boost of energy and temporarily sharpens mental acuity; it allows you to concentrate on monotonous tasks; it's used in cold medications to counteract the sleep-inducing effects of antihistamines; and it can be useful in the treatment of certain types of headaches, as it constricts the blood vessels in the head.

But caffeine is a drug. The Department of Health, Education, and Welfare lists it, along with nicotine and heroin, as an addictive substance, and admits that if it were being introduced today, manufacturers would probably be unable to market it: caffeine would be available only by prescription.

The dangers of caffeine addiction are real. Although links between caffeine and heart disease and cancer have largely been disproven, there remains a real connection between caffeine consumption and birth defects, breast disease, digestive diseases, and anxiety. It's the more subtle effects of caffeine that are troublesome to most of us, often because we never make the link between caffeine consumption and our minor symptoms. If you suffer from insomnia, afternoon fatigue, tension headaches, and general anxiety, you might be suffering from the effects of caffeine addiction.

I suggest that you have no more than two caffeinated drinks per day, or a maximum of 200 milligrams of caffeine. I recommend you stick to decaffeinated soft drinks, coffee, and tea.

Top Tip: Caffeine

I think water-processed decaffeinated coffee or Postum (either regular or coffee flavor) makes a good substitute for regular coffee. Just be careful not to lighten your coffee substitutes with cream. Go for skim milk, or try it black.

Alcohol Alcohol is both a toxin and a drug. It's a toxin because the liver must work to detoxify it. That's why you always hear of liver damage among alcoholics; the liver is simply exhausted from its labors to detoxify a constant intake of alcohol. Alcohol is also a carbohydrate, although it's almost an "antinutrient" because it increases your need for other nutrients while contributing almost nothing of any nutritional value of its own. Alcohol is also a drug that acts as a sedative. It anesthetizes the brain beginning with the frontal lobe (reasoning section) and moving on to the speech and vision centers.

Most of us have a schizophrenic view of alcohol: we accept, and perhaps enjoy, its regular use for ourselves and among friends, but we deplore the countless lives it's ruined when abused. The problem with alcohol, of course, is control, and there can be a fine line between "regular" and "addictive" consumption of alcohol.

In addition to the seriously dangerous properties of alcohol, many people don't realize that alcohol can be destructive of nutrients. It will deplete stores of or limit the body's absorption of nutrients, including calcium, riboflavin, folic acid, iron, zinc, thiamin, folacin, and vitamins B_{12}, C, D, and A. What this means to you is that if you regularly consume alcohol with meals, say, a glass of wine with lunch and dinner, you may be counteracting the benefits of many of the nutrients you're consuming with those meals.

I think the healthiest alternative is not to drink at all. But if you wish to drink, you should take the "damage control" approach: I suggest you limit yourself to one or two drinks daily. Avoid hard liquors that are at the bottom of the Nutripoints alcohol list, and stay with wines, wine coolers, beer, and near-beer.

Top Tip: Alcohol

Why not try alcohol-free beer? Some brands have an excellent flavor and can help break a bad habit if you're accustomed to, say, having a beer when you get home from work. I also suggest that you try some of the mixed drinks without alcohol. A Virgin Mary is a good choice, as it's spicy and has a lot of flavor.

PART IV

NUTRIPOINTS
AT WORK

THIS SECTION OF THE BOOK IS DEVOTED TO EVERYTHING YOU NEED to know to use the Nutripoint program in your daily life. It will answer all your questions, from "Can I get *too many* Nutripoints?" to "What foods on a Chinese restaurant menu are the best choices?"

First, let's examine a simple breakdown of how to make the most of Nutripoints.

If you only used Nutripoints to help you choose one food over another, for example, as a guide to selecting a vegetable with a higher score (spinach at 75 Nutripoints instead of a baked potato at 8.5 Nutripoints, or a chicken salad sandwich on whole wheat at 4 Nutripoints rather than a ham and cheese sandwich on whole wheat at 1 Nutripoint), you would improve your diet. But you would not ensure that you'd get all the RDAs of the essential vitamins and minerals, or that you'd get optimum amounts of protein, carbohydrates, and fiber. And it would not ensure that you'd avoid excess calories, cholesterol, total fat, saturated fat, sodium, sugar, alcohol, and caffeine.

If you only used Nutripoints to choose one food over another, and tried to get 100 Nutripoints per day from a variety of foods, you would upgrade your diet and you would get the RDA for every vitamin and mineral. But you would not get optimum amounts of protein, carbohydrates, and fiber. And you would not be avoiding excess calories, cholesterol, total fat, saturated fat, sodium, sugar, alcohol, and caffeine.

To get the full benefit of Nutripoints, you must select foods that will give you a daily score of at least 100 Nutripoints while staying within the serving limits for each group and meeting the minimum required servings for each Nutrigroup. This is the most complete and effective use of Nutripoints. This use of the system will ensure that you get 100 percent of the Recommended Dietary Allowances; that you get optimum amounts of protein, carbohydrates, and fiber; that you avoid excess calories, cholesterol, total fat, saturated fat, sodium, sugar, alcohol, and caffeine.

YOUR CURRENT NUTRIPOINT STATUS

Before you begin using the Nutripoint program, I recommend that you take stock of your current eating habits. The best way to do this is by keeping a food diary for three days. The most immediate benefit of making a three-day food diary is that it will allow you to analyze your current diet in terms of Nutripoints. It will instantly pinpoint the weaknesses in your diet, will give you a powerful incentive to get started on Nutripoints, and will serve as encouragement when you begin to see how quickly your diet improves, and your scores go up, with just a few basic changes in your diet.

Keeping a food diary is also a helpful way to get used to using Nutripoints in your daily life: you'll become familiar with the Nutrigroups and get a handle on the highly rated foods.

KEEPING A FOOD DIARY

When patients come to the Cooper Clinic, I always ask them to make a record of what they've been eating for three typical days. You have an advantage over these patients: you can make more accurate records because you'll be doing it as it happens. (You'd be amazed at how much some of us can eat, almost unconsciously. If you tried to recall *everything* you ate two days ago, could you?)

Accuracy really counts, so please don't try to fool yourself. Remember that you don't have to show these lists to anyone if you don't want to.

I suggest that you buy a new notebook just for your Nutripoint scores. You might abandon it after a while, but in the beginning, you'll find it very helpful. You need to jot down exactly *what* you ate and in *what amounts* for each meal. It's best to record *typical* days; they don't have to be consecutive. In other words, you can record a Wednesday (skip Thursday because you were on the road and not eating typically), a Friday, and a Saturday. It's a good idea to include one weekend day as well as two weekdays. Don't forget to record snacks, beverages, and condiments. Try to make your notes as soon as possible after a meal or snack so that you can remember whether it was really three or five crackers you had.

Try to get your portion sizes as accurate as possible. Typical portion sizes would be 1 cup, 1 teaspoon, 1 tablespoon, 4 ounces, 2 slices, and so on.

The following table will help you judge portion sizes:

Typical Portion Sizes

Meat, Poultry, Fish

3 oz.	= size of palm of average woman's hand (exclude fingers)
	= amount in a sandwich
	= amount in a quarter-pound hamburger (cooked)
	= chicken breast (3 inches across)
6 oz.	= restaurant chicken breast (6 inches across)
	= common luncheon or cafeteria portion
8 oz.	= common evening restaurant portion

Cheese

1 oz.	= 1 slice on sandwich or hamburger
	= 1-inch cube or 1 wedge airplane serving
1/2 cup	= 1 scoop cottage cheese

Salads

1 cup	= dinner salad
2–4 cups	= salad bar salad

Potato

1 small	=	2½ inches long
1 medium	=	4 inches long
1 large	=	5 inches long (restaurant portion)
1 huge	=	6 inches long (meal-in-one potato)

Vegetables

½ cup = cafeteria or restaurant portion
= coleslaw or beans at a BBQ restaurant

Fats

1 tsp. margarine/butter = 1 pat
3 tsp. = 1 tbs.
1 tbs. mayonnaise = typical amount in sandwich
2 tbs. dressing = typical amount on a dinner salad
= 1 small ladle (restaurant)
= ½ large ladle (restaurant)

Beverages

1½ oz. = 1 jigger per alcoholic drink
6 oz. (¾ cup) = typical juice portion
= small glass of wine
8 oz. (1 cup) = common milk portion
12 oz. = 1 can of beer or soft drink

The following is a typical part of a daily record:

Meal	Food	Serving Size
Dinner	Chicken breast (baked, no sauce)	4 oz.
	Baked potato	1 medium
	w. margarine	2 pats
	w. cheese sauce	¼ cup
	Broccoli (steamed)	½ cup
	Apple (fresh)	1 large
	Dinner roll (no margarine)	1 small
	2-percent milk	8 oz.
Snack	Popcorn	3 cups
	Coke	12 oz.
	Chocolate candy bar w. nuts	2-oz. bar

After you have the three-day list, check each food portion
with the Nutripoint values in this book. The easiest way to
do this is to use the alphabetical listings in the back of the
book.

You're going to want to know three things for each of your
food diary entries:

1. Portion size
2. Nutripoints
3. Nutrigroup

The following is a sample Nutripoint Daily Record Sheet.
You'll notice that this table includes an "Other" column. Use
it to record points for foods in the Other Groups that you eat.
These numbers are added or subtracted from your daily total
along with the Nutrigroup totals. This record sheet will help
you figure out how to list foods so that you can readily see
how you're doing on points and portion sizes.

For a sample of how a record sheet is completed, see the
Nutripoint menus on pp. 210–224.

You'll want to check each food you consumed to learn how
many Nutripoints your serving had. The alphabetical listing
of more than 3,000 foods will probably contain any food you
might have eaten. Check it for each of the entries in your food
diary. Be sure to check the portion size listed. If you ate a cup
of something and the Nutripoints are calculated at a half cup,
you must double your Nutripoints. Conversely, if you ate a
half cup of something and the Nutripoints are calculated at
a cup, you would halve your Nutripoints for the particular
food. If you can't find a specific food listed, figure out the
components of that food and make an estimate. For example,
if you had a salad that was composed of rice, mayonnaise, and
some cut-up vegetables, check the values of each of these
ingredients and add them to arrive at a Nutripoint score for
that food.

In addition to checking your daily Nutripoint scores, you

NUTRIPOINT DAILY RECORD SHEET, DAY ____

Food Selection/Serving Size	Nutripoints							
	Veg.	Fruit	Grain	Leg.	Meat	Milk	Other	
Breakfast:								
Lunch:								
Dinner:								
Totals:								
Goals:	55	15	10	5	5	10	0	100

want to determine the balance of your diet and whether you're getting the necessary variety. So, when you check the Nutripoint score for each food, also check each food's Nutrigroup, e.g., meat/fish, grain, vegetable, and so on.

Remember that the daily Nutripoint goal is 100 points divided among the six Nutrigroups as follows:

Daily Nutripoint Recommendations

Servings	Nutrigroup	Nutripoints
4	Vegetable	55
3	Fruit	15
2	Grain	10
1	Legume	5
2	Milk/dairy	10
1	Meat/fish	5
Total:		100

Now it's time to analyze your scores. The following are the three factors you're looking at:

1. How many of the six Nutrigroups do you have points in? This will give you an idea of how varied your diet is.

2. Did you achieve the recommended number of servings for each Nutrigroup? This will show you how well balanced your diet is.

3. Did you achieve your Nutripoint goal of 100 points for the day? This will show you how nutritionally sound your diet is.

The following is a chart that suggests a simplified way to analyze your daily score. You just fill in the Nutripoints for each of the required servings of each Nutrigroup. You can then readily see if you've reached your goal for that Nutrigroup and for the day. You may well find that when you make up your food diary your scores and/or servings are way off, but this chart will at least give you a very visual way of analyzing your numbers:

Nutrigroup	Servings		Nutripoints	Goal
Vegetable	_ _ _ _	=	_____	55
Fruit	_ _ _	=	_____	15
Grain	_ _	=	_____	10
Legume	_	=	_____	5
Milk/dairy	_ _	=	_____	10
Meat/poultry/fish	_	=	_____	5
Total:				100

From the countless surveys I've done on the diet histories of patients, I've learned that there are certain patterns in the average diet. Most people find that their biggest weakness is that they don't get nearly enough variety and balance in their diet. Indeed, most people seem to choose nearly all their foods from only three out of the six Nutrigroups: meat/poultry/fish, milk/dairy, and grains. Some people do even worse and omit grains as well. Most people get few, if any, legumes, and many people fall short on fruits and vegetables.

Many people have what I think of as "miscellaneous" diets: they eat a lot of meats and dairy foods, along with a lot of miscellaneous items that don't fall into any Nutrigroup, such as sugar, fat, and condiments.

The average person gets 50 to 100 Nutripoints daily, *even when eating considerably more than the allotted number of servings.* This means that the average person is getting a poor nutritional bargain in his or her daily diet: fewer vitamins and minerals—sometimes *far* less than the RDA—at a cost of more calories than they need.

By using the Nutripoint program, you can get 100 to 200 Nutripoints daily in *significantly* fewer calories, thus enjoying a more nutrient-dense diet. And you can achieve this usually without making noticeable cuts in the *amounts* of food you eat.

The following is a sample three-day record kept by one of my patients along with a detailed nutrient analysis:

Weekday 1*

		Nutripoints	Nutrigroup
Breakfast			
(7:30 a.m.)	1 cup Kellogg's Corn Flakes	18.0	Grain
	½ cup whole milk	2.5	Milk/dairy
	1 medium banana	7.5	Fruit
	1 cup coffee	−3.5	Misc.
	Subtotal:	24.5	
Lunch			
(12:00 p.m.)	Ham sandwich	1.0	Meat
	w. mayo	−1.0	Fat
	on rye	4.5	Grain
	½ cup coleslaw	3.0	Vegetable
	1 cup potato chips	0.0	Vegetable
	12 oz. iced tea	−4.0	Misc.
	Subtotal:	3.0	
Dinner			
(7:00 p.m.)	6 oz. breaded, fried flounder fillet w. lemon	−0.5	Meat
	1 cup broccoli w. butter sauce	26.0	Vegetable
	½ cup cooked carrots w. butter	10.0	Vegetable
	1 cup coffee	−3.5	Misc.
	Subtotal:	32.0	
Snack			
(10:00 p.m.)	2 chocolate chip cookies	−4.0	Grain
	Subtotal:	−4.0	
	Daily Total:	55.5	

Nutrigroup	Points	Goal Met
Vegetable	39.0	No
Fruit	7.5	No
Grain	18.0	Yes
Legume	0.0	No
Meat	0.5	No
Milk/dairy	2.5	No
Misc.	−11.0	—
Fat	−1.0	—

*Although on this day 56 percent of the 100-point daily total was met, the goal for only one Nutrigroup was met.

WEEKDAY 1

Male, age 40 — Present Wt. (lbs.): 185 — Body Fat (%): 20
Exercise Avg.: 0 calories/day — Target Wt. (lbs.): 160 — Height (in.): 70

Nutrient Analysis

Nutrient	Present Daily Intake at 185 Lbs.		Assessment	Recommended Daily Intake at 160 Lbs.	
Calories	1,558	cal	OK	1,840	cal
Protein	71	gm	High	58	gm
Total fat	78	gm	High	41–61	gm (max.)
Polyunsat./sat. fat ratio	1.0		OK	1.0	
Cholesterol (dietary)	234	mg	OK	100–300	mg
Complex carbohydrates	143	gm	Low	230–322	gm
Sugar	10	gm	OK	0	gm
Alcohol	0.0	gm	As per Dr.	As per Dr.	
Fiber (dietary)	14	gm	Low	20–35	gm
Calcium	492	mg	Low	800	mg
Phosphorus	675	mg	OK	800	mg
Magnesium	256	mg	OK	350	mg
Sodium	2,785	mg	OK	2,000–4,000	mg
Potassium	3,045	mg	OK	3,750	mg
Zinc	6	mg	Very low	15	mg
Iron	11	mg	OK	10	mg
Vitamin A	12,354	IU	OK	5,000	IU
Thiamin (B_1)	2.3	mg	OK	1.4	mg
Riboflavin (B_2)	2.3	mg	OK	1.6	mg
Niacin (B_3)	26	mg	OK	18	mg
Pyridoxine (B_6)	2.7	mg	OK	2.2	mg
Pantothenic acid	2.8	mg	Low	5.5	mg
Folic acid	888	mcg	OK	400	mcg
Vitamin B_{12}	3.1	mcg	OK	3.0	mcg
Vitamin C	223	mg	OK	60	mg
Caffeine	473	mg	Very high	0–200	mg

Calorie Sources

Sources	Present (%)	Goal (%)
Protein	17	10–20
Fat	46	20–30
Complex carbohydrates (fruits, vegs., starches)	35	50–70
Simple carbohydrates	2	0–10
Alcohol	0	0

Weekday 2

		Nutripoints	Nutrigroup
Breakfast			
(7:30 a.m.)	1 boiled egg	−6.0	Milk/dairy
	1 blueberry muffin	0.0	Grain
	w. 1 pat butter	−2.0	Fat
	1 cup coffee	−3.5	Misc.
	Subtotal:	−11.5	
Lunch			
(12:00 p.m.)	2 pc. pepperoni pizza	−8.0	Grain
	Tossed salad	33.0	Vegetable
	w. 2 tbs. Thousand		
	Island dressing	−3.0	Fat
	Subtotal:	22.0	
Dinner			
(7:00 p.m.)	6-oz. pork chop	−2.0	Meat
	1 cup mashed potatoes	4.0	Vegetable
	w. gravy	−1.5	Fat
	½ cup green beans	12.0	Vegetable
	1 6-oz. wine	−14.0	Alcohol
	1 pc. apple pie	−8.0	Fruit
	Subtotal:	−9.5	
	Daily Total:	1.0	

Group	Points	Goal Met
Vegetable	49.0	No
Fruit	−8.0	No
Grains	−8.0	No
Legumes	0.0	No
Meat	−2.0	No
Milk/dairy	−6.0	No
Misc.	−3.5	—
Fat	−6.5	—
Alcohol	−14.0	—

WEEKDAY 2

Male, age 40	Present Wt. (lbs.): 185	Body Fat (%): 20
Exercise Avg.: 0 calories/day	Target Wt. (lbs.): 160	Height (in.): 70

Nutrient Analysis

Nutrient	Present Daily Intake at 185 Lbs.		Assessment	Recommended Daily Intake at 160 Lbs.	
Calories	2,437	cal	High	1,840	cal
Protein	88	gm	High	58	gm
Total fat	147	gm	Very high	41–61	gm (max.)
Polyunsat./sat. fat ratio	0.5		Low	1.0	
Cholesterol (dietary)	723	mg	Very high	100–300	mg
Complex carbohydrates	147	gm	Low	230–322	gm
Sugar	28	gm	OK	0	gm
Alcohol	14.8	gm	As per Dr.	As per Dr.	
Fiber (dietary)	9	gm	Very low	20–35	gm
Calcium	544	mg	OK	800	mg
Phosphorus	1,068	mg	OK	800	mg
Magnesium	196	mg	Low	350	mg
Sodium	4,403	mg	High	2,000–4,000	mg
Potassium	2,380	mg	Low	3,750	mg
Zinc	10	mg	OK	15	mg
Iron	10	mg	OK	10	mg
Vitamin A	3,072	IU	Low	5,000	IU
Thiamin (B_1)	2.2	mg	OK	1.4	mg
Riboflavin (B_2)	1.5	mg	OK	1.6	mg
Niacin (B_3)	18	mg	OK	18	mg
Pyridoxine (B_6)	1.3	mg	Low	2.2	mg
Pantothenic acid	4.3	mg	OK	5.5	mg
Folic acid	251	mcg	Low	400	mcg
Vitamin B_{12}	4.7	mcg	OK	3.0	mcg
Vitamin C	56	mg	OK	60	mg
Caffeine	175	mg	OK	0–200	mg

Calorie Sources Sources	Present (%)	Goal (%)
Protein	14	10–20
Fat	55	20–30
Complex carbohydrates (fruits, vegs., starches)	23	50–70
Simple carbohydrates	4	0–10
Alcohol	4	0

Weekend Day

		Nutripoints	*Nutrigroup*
Breakfast			
(10:00 a.m.)	2 pancakes	1.0	Grain
	w. 2 tbs. maple syrup	−5.0	Sugar
	w. 1 tsp. butter	−2.0	Fat
	2 sausages	−2.5	Meat
	8 oz. orange juice	15.0	Fruit
	1 cup coffee	−3.5	Misc.
	Subtotal:	3.0	
Lunch/Snack			
(3:00 p.m.)	Turkey sandwich	4.5	Meat
	on white bread	2.5	Grain
	w. mayo	−1.0	Fat
	w. lettuce and tomato	5.0	Vegetable
	Subtotal:	11.0	
Dinner			
(7:30 p.m.)	1 6-oz. steak	2.0	Meat
	½ cup scalloped potatoes	4.0	Vegetable
	Tossed salad	33.0	Vegetable
	w. 2 tbs. ranch dressing	−3.5	Fat
	Subtotal:	35.5	
Snack			
(9:00 p.m.)	½ cup Häagen-Dazs ice cream	−7.0	Milk/dairy
	Subtotal:	−7.0	
	Daily Total:	42.5	

Group	*Points*	*Goal Met*
Vegetable	42.0	No
Fruit	15.0	Yes
Grains	3.5	No
Legumes	0.0	No
Meat	4.0	No
Milk/dairy	−7.0	No
Misc.	−3.5	—
Fat	−6.5	—
Sugar	−5.0	—

WEEKEND DAY

Male, age 40	Present Wt. (lbs.): 185	Body Fat (%): 20
Exercise Avg.: 0 calories/day	Target Wt. (lbs.): 160	Height (in.): 70

Nutrient Analysis

Nutrient	Present Daily Intake at 185 Lbs.		Assessment	Recommended Daily Intake at 160 Lbs.	
Calories	2,430	cal	High	1,840	cal
Protein	108	gm	High	58	gm
Total fat	156	gm	Very high	41–61	gm (max.)
Polyunsat./sat. fat ratio	0.8		OK	1.0	
Cholesterol (dietary)	409	mg	Very high	100–300	mg
Complex carbohydrates	103	gm	Very low	230–322	gm
Sugar	42	gm	OK	0	gm
Alcohol	0.0	gm	As per Dr.	As per Dr.	
Fiber (dietary)	8	gm	Very low	20–35	gm
Calcium	621	mg	OK	800	mg
Phosphorus	1,169	mg	OK	800	mg
Magnesium	174	mg	Very low	350	mg
Sodium	3,034	mg	OK	2,000–4,000	mg
Potassium	2,346	mg	Low	3,750	mg
Zinc	12	mg	OK	15	mg
Iron	15	mg	OK	10	mg
Vitamin A	2,803	IU	Low	5,000	IU
Thiamin (B$_1$)	1.8	mg	OK	1.4	mg
Riboflavin (B$_2$)	1.8	mg	OK	1.6	mg
Niacin (B$_3$)	36	mg	OK	18	mg
Pyridoxine (B$_6$)	2.7	mg	OK	2.2	mg
Pantothenic acid	3.3	mg	Low	5.5	mg
Folic acid	254	mcg	Low	400	mcg
Vitamin B$_{12}$	6.4	mcg	OK	3.0	mcg
Vitamin C	47	mg	OK	60	mg
Caffeine	175	mg	OK	0–200	mg

Calorie Sources		
Sources	Present (%)	Goal (%)
Protein	17	10–20
Fat	60	20–30
Complex carbohydrates (fruits, vegs., starches)	17	50–70
Simple carbohydrates	6	0–10
Alcohol	0	0

3-DAY AVERAGE

Male, age 40	Present Wt. (lbs.): 185	Body Fat (%): 20
Exercise Avg.: 0 calories/day	Target Wt. (lbs.): 160	Height (in.): 70

Nutrient Analysis

Nutrient	Present Daily Intake at 185 Lbs.		Assessment	Recommended Daily Intake at 160 Lbs.	
Calories	2,142	cal	OK	1,840	cal
Protein	89	gm	High	58	gm
Total fat	127	gm	Very high	41–61	gm (max.)
Polyunsat./sat. fat ratio	0.7		Low	1.0	
Cholesterol (dietary)	455	mg	Very high	100–300	mg
Complex carbohydrates	131	gm	Very low	230–322	gm
Sugar	27	gm	OK	0	gm
Alcohol	4.9	gm	As per Dr.	As per Dr.	
Fiber (dietary)	11	gm	Very low	20–35	gm
Calcium	552	mg	OK	800	mg
Phosphorus	971	mg	OK	800	mg
Magnesium	209	mg	Low	350	mg
Sodium	3,407	mg	OK	2,000–4,000	mg
Potassium	2,590	mg	OK	3,750	mg
Zinc	9	mg	Low	15	mg
Iron	12	mg	OK	10	mg
Vitamin A	6,077	IU	OK	5,000	IU
Thiamin (B₁)	2.1	mg	OK	1.4	mg
Riboflavin (B₂)	1.8	mg	OK	1.6	mg
Niacin (B₃)	27	mg	OK	18	mg
Pyridoxine (B₆)	2.2	mg	OK	2.2	mg
Pantothenic acid	3.5	mg	Low	5.5	mg
Folic acid	464	mcg	OK	400	mcg
Vitamin B₁₂	4.7	mcg	OK	3.0	mcg
Vitamin C	109	mg	OK	60	mg
Caffeine	274	mg	High	0–200	mg

Calorie Sources		
Sources	Present (%)	Goal (%)
Protein	16	10–20
Fat	55	20–30
Complex carbohydrates (fruits, vegs., starches)	24	50–70
Simple carbohydrates	4	0–10
Alcohol	1	0

In addition to the food records of this particular patient, I've included a breakdown of the nutrient content of his meals. You won't need such a breakdown because the Nutripoint numbers are really a simplified version of what those numbers tell you. But I think it's interesting to see just where the weaknesses were in this patient's diet. We can see from the nutrient analysis of the three-day food report that while the total calorie intake was fine, the protein was high, the fat total was very high, the cholesterol level was very high, and the complex carbohydrate and fiber levels were very low. A few of the vitamins and minerals were low as well.

I chose this particular patient's record because it is fairly typical. It's not a terrible diet (I have seen people who earn virtually *no* Nutripoints in a three-day food record), but it shows where typical weaknesses exist. It also very quickly, in a visual way, points out where improvement can be made. Instead of looking at just numbers of calories and not really learning very much from them, you can look at the low Nutripoint numbers and see where you need to boost your scores.

Well, how did you do?

Remember that 100 daily Nutripoints is the basic goal: you may fall far below it on some days and exceed it by a wide margin on others.

UPGRADING YOUR DIET

It's time to refocus your approach to food with the help of Nutripoints. Unless your diet is truly terrible, I think you'll find this an easy shift to make. Many patients tell me that they're delighted to find that rather than being an "authoritative" diet plan that urges them to eat tons of lettuce or grapefruit, or some other food they might not like, Nutripoints leaves the choice *up to them.*

Your food diary has revealed where your diet is weak.

You're probably not eating enough different kinds of foods. Most people find that just by paying attention to balancing their diet, they improve it enormously. So you'll probably need to work on getting sufficient servings from the various Nutrigroups. But how do you choose foods *within* each group? The following are the steps you need to take:

Step 1: First, I suggest you do your own personal food survey. Go through the lists by Nutrigroups and check the foods you eat regularly. Are they high in Nutripoints? If so, great. If not, it's time to think about eliminating the foods that are low in Nutripoints, or at least those that are below the recommended level for each Nutrigroup.

Step 2: Make a list of the foods you like and eat regularly that are high in Nutripoints. This will be the basis of your new, upgraded diet. These are the foods you can rely on because you already know that you like them and that they are high in Nutripoints.

Step 3: Now you need to focus on *variety*. Go through the lists by Nutrigroups again and look for foods you like or would probably like but rarely eat. Make sure you don't neglect the Nutrigroups you're weak on. (You'll know from your food diary if, for example, you rarely eat vegetables or fruits.) Perhaps you found that you *never* eat legumes. Well, now's the time to go through that Nutrigroup list and find some legumes you like. Figure out how you're going to work them into your diet. When you first begin with Nutripoints, you may find that it's difficult to work in a serving of legumes every day. This is perfectly OK. Many people make a transitional stage in which they substitute one meat serving for one of the legume servings. (You'll want to check the menus and recipes in Part VI for some good suggestions.)

Remember that *variety* is as important as a high Nutripoint score. This pertains to choosing foods *within* a Nutrigroup as well as to choosing foods *among* Nutrigroups. Remember that each food has a unique "fingerprint" of nutrients that identifies it: it will be strong in some, weak in others. If you consistently pick only the top four vegetables, for example, you'll be missing out on the nutrients available in other vegetables you need. Keep in mind that as long as you don't go below the recommended level of foods, it's better to have a variety within a list than an extremely high score.

Step 4: An excellent way to upgrade your diet is to use Nutripoints as the basis for making *substitutions* in your diet. You would do this between foods within a single Nutrigroup. For example, say you eat a lot of pork. You might want to scan the meat/poultry/fish Nutrigroup for a food with a higher Nutripoint level. Or perhaps you like spinach and romaine lettuce equally: the next time you make a salad, include a lot of spinach and you'll be boosting your score.

Substitutions can be particularly useful when cooking. The following table offers some effective alternatives.

Cooking Substitutions

To Replace	Nutripoints	Replace With	Nutripoints
Butter	— 7.5 (per tbs.)	Safflower Oil	—2.5
		Low-cal. margarine	—2 to —1
Heavy cream	—56 (per cup)	Evaporated skim milk	19
Cream cheese	—40 (per cup)	Yogurt cheese (see page 260)	12 to 18
Eggs	—11.5 (per egg)	Egg Beaters	9 (per ¼ cup)
		Egg whites	1 (per egg)
Whole milk yogurt	2.5 (per cup)	Nonfat yogurt	9 (per cup)
Sour cream	—14 (per cup)	New Way Sour Cream (see page 271)	26 (per cup)
Sugar	—1 (per teaspoon)	Equal (NutraSweet)	0.0
Salt	0.0	salt substitutes (see page 101)	0.0
Coffee/tea	—3.0 to —3.5	Decaffeinated coffee/ tea, herb tea, or Postum	0.0 to 5.5

Step 5: Another way to upgrade your diet is to use Nutripoints to *alter your food choice.* For example, say you eat a lot of fried chicken. Why not stick with chicken if you like it, but instead of frying, try broiling? Or make your hamburgers with a leaner grade of beef. If you already eat broiled chicken, why not boost your score by taking the skin off before you broil it? If you love fruits, why not have some melon instead of your usual apple?

You can make these changes in each Nutrigroup. In the milk/dairy group you can change from regular mozzarella to low-fat mozzarella; and you can change from regular milk to 2-percent milk, from 2-percent to 1-percent milk, and then to skim milk. You can go from two eggs to one whole egg plus one egg white. Or you can switch to Egg Beaters.

Nutripoints makes it easy for you to upgrade your diet. Simply familiarize yourself with the lists. It's as easy as looking for a version of a food you like with a higher Nutripoint score.

How do you keep track of your Nutripoint scores through the day? You can continue with your food diary notebook, or you can use a sheet such as the one on page 131, which not only will help keep track of your scores but will make keeping track of your servings from the various Nutrigroups automatic. (This chart is for those who want to consume 1,000–1,200 calories per day; your chart can be personalized for your desired calorie intake, according to the guidelines on pages 137–142.)

Obviously, you might want to alter this pattern on some days. Perhaps you'll have a fruit snack instead of a fruit dessert, or perhaps you'll have a grain as a snack instead of with dinner.

A Note on Water . . .

There is one nutritional "essential" that I didn't include in the Nutripoint formula for obvious reasons: water. Your body is actually two-thirds water—forty to fifty quarts—and we can't forget that it's every bit as essential to life as food.

Most people don't give any thought to the amount of water they drink, but I think it's important to do so. You should be sure to drink six to eight 8-ounce glasses of water per day. Some people find it helpful to put six pennies in their right pocket in the morning and move one to their left pocket each time they drink a glass of water. It helps them keep track of what they're actually consuming. Following the Nutripoint guidelines for your servings of these liquids, you can substitute diet soda or juice for your water servings, but don't count caffeinated coffee or tea because they act as diuretics. If you exercise, of course, you should increase the amount of water.

NUTRIGROUP TRENDS

Many people have asked me what food types, in general, seem to be the best bets in terms of Nutripoints. It's interesting to point out that there are various trends in each Nutrigroup. If you're familiar with them, you'll be better able to choose high-Nutripoint foods, even if you don't have the charts at hand. I should mention again that you can only compare Nutripoint ratings *within* each Nutrigroup. While you *can* compare apples and oranges, you *can't* compare apples and spinach. The following are some of the major trends in the Nutrigroups.

NUTRIPOINT DAILY RECORD SHEET 1,000–1,200 CALORIES

Food Selection/Serving Size	Nutripoints							
	Veg.	Fruit	Grain	Leg.	Meat	Milk	Other	
Breakfast:								
1 Grain								
1 Milk/Dairy								
1 Fruit								
Lunch:								
1 Meat or Legume								
2 Vegetables								
1 Grain								
1 Fruit								
Dinner:								
1 Meat or Legume								
2 Vegetables								
1 Milk/Dairy								
1 Fruit								
Totals:								
Goals:	55	15	10	5	5	10	0	100

Vegetables When you're looking for the top vegetables, think light and fluffy. Green, leafy vegetables such as turnip greens, spinach, watercress, and beet greens all have terrific scores. After the leafy vegetables, which you can readily see would be both low in calories and high in nutrients, we have asparagus as well as the chunkier cruciferous vegetables, such as broccoli, cauliflower, and brussels sprouts, which are very high in vitamins A and C (the vitamins the American Cancer Society recommends you focus on as a step to reduce your risk of cancer), as well as fiber and calcium. Next, in terms of scores, we have carrots and the more watery vegetables, such as okra, tomatoes, and squash, which are also high in vitamins C and A, as well as fiber.

All the top vegetables have a tremendous ratio of nutrients per calorie, but as you continue down the list, you'll find that processing and the adding of salt and fat lower the scores of even a terrific vegetable. Keep in mind when choosing vegetables that *all* vegetables above the recommended line are really good foods and that there's no need to worry about sticking to the very top of the list for your four daily servings. As long as you are choosing from above the recommended line, you shouldn't have any trouble getting your 55 Nutripoints.

Fruit The first trend we notice in the fruits is that the tropical fruits top the charts. Cantaloupe is right at the top, along with papaya, guava, mango, and kiwi. These fruits are packed with nutrients, including vitamin C, and fiber, and are extremely low in calories for their volume. After the tropical fruits we find the citrus fruits, including the orange, mandarin orange, tangerine, and grapefruit. Then come the berries, including raspberries, blackberries, and cranberries. Most of the fruits are high in vitamins A and C and fiber, with moderately high levels of other nutrients. Again, once we get below the recommended line, the addition of sugar, salt, or fat lowers the scores. Foods such as banana cream pie (−1 Nutripoint) get about as far as you can from the basic nutritional appeal of the banana. All-American apple pie does even worse (−2 Nutripoints). Jams, jellies, and preserves hit rock bottom because virtually all nutrition, including fiber, has been processed out of them, and tons of sugar has been added. Smucker's Concord Grape Jelly (−6 Nutripoints) represents the decline of the grape to the absolute bottom of the fruit chart.

Grains At the top of the grains list you find the highly fortified cereals. There's some controversy about fortification but, in order to keep the system honest, I had to put the cereals where they fell. (Please note the caveat about fortification on page 179.) The very best cereals are those with the most balance in their fortification, as well as those that began with a quality natural food with plenty of fiber and complex carbohydrates. Whole Wheat Total is at the top of the list. As we go down the line, we'll find cereals that are less balanced in terms of fortification, or cereals with less fiber or more sugar. The top-rated natural (unfortified) cereal is wheat bran (26.5 Nutripoints), followed by wheat germ (10.5 Nutripoints) and oatmeal (4.5 Nutripoints).

A breakdown of the cereals shows that fortified whole grains top the list, followed by bran, germ, and other whole grains, and then, as you begin processing and reducing the amount of whole grain and adding sugar, salt, and fat, the scores decline. You'll find that a terrible choice for breakfast is that "health" food of the sixties and seventies—granola— in the form of Nature Valley Oats 'n Honey Granola Bar, at −2 Nutripoints.

As you move down the grain list, you find the various breads (topped by Wonder Hi-Fiber bread at 6.5 Nutripoints), rices, and pastas. Pizza makes a respectable showing and allows those who must eat at fast-food restaurants to make a

choice that will give them a grain serving as a positive contribution to their daily Nutripoint score. Pizza Hut's Hand-
Tossed Supreme Pizza, for example, weighs in at 3.5 Nutripoints for half a piece. Any good cereal for breakfast that
scores above 6.5 Nutripoints (and most do), followed by a
Pizza Hut lunch, would give you your two grain servings
above your 10 required Nutripoints for that Nutrigroup for
the day.

Legumes   Legumes are strangers to most people, though it's
time you became familiar with them. They're a good protein
alternative to meat and they're high in fiber, high in complex
carbohydrates, low in fat and cholesterol, and high in nutrients. In our legume Nutrigroup, we include not only peas and
beans but nuts and seeds. Bean sprouts top the list at 18
Nutripoints. It's easy to keep them on hand to put on sandwiches in place of lettuce, and to add to salads. Sprouting
increases the nutritional value in the bean. Peas follow
sprouted beans on the list. They're high in fiber, protein, and
complex carbohydrates, as are the next items on the list, navy
beans. Down a bit from the beans is an excellent meat substitute: the Loma Linda brand vegeburger, which is made from
soy. (These soy-based foods are processed foods, and also can
be difficult to digest. I therefore suggest that you use them
occasionally as substitutes or as convenience foods, but not
as regular components of your diet.)

   After beans, peas, and tofu come nuts. They provide protein, but they're rated lower because they're high in fat (although it's not as saturated as the fat in meat). Remember,
by the way, that there's no cholesterol in any vegetable product. As you descend the list, you find the adulterated foods,
which have been processed and have suffered the addition of
salt and sugar. Even some of the major brands of peanut
butter make a dismal showing because of the addition of salt
and sugar (Skippy at 0 Nutripoints, followed by Jif and Peter

Pan at the same score), while a healthier choice for peanut butter shows up as Health Valley No Salt Chunky peanut butter (1.5 Nutripoints).

Milk/Dairy   Because milk is an animal product, it's a good source of complete protein. It contains all the essential amino acids the body can't produce. And, of course, it's high in calcium and complex carbohydrates, as well as some of the B vitamins normally associated with beef or meat products. At the top of the milk Nutrigroup we find some interesting man-made creations, such as Egg Beaters, a fortified egg substitute that has no fat because all of the yolk has been removed. It's an especially good choice for cooking. The best natural food on the list is nonfat dry milk (12.5 Nutripoints). All of the fat and cholesterol has been removed, and what's left is protein, complex carbohydrates, and calcium. You can use nonfat dry milk in cooking: add some to meat loaf, casseroles, and other such dishes. You can, of course, also mix it with water to use in place of whole milk in baking, on cereals, and so on.

The major trend in milk foods, aside from the man-made foods, is that as the fat and cholesterol are eliminated, the Nutripoints go up. Dannon has an excellent, relatively new product in nonfat yogurt, which is just as flavorful as regular yogurt, but a much better nutritional choice because of its reduced fat. (You can always add a dash of NutraSweet [Equal] or vanilla to nonfat yogurt to give it more flavor.) With fresh fruit, yogurt makes a terrific breakfast dish, and it's great for cooking.

You can readily see how the addition of fat changes a Nutripoint score: Fleischmann's Egg Beaters are rated at 21 Nutripoints, but when they become Fleischmann's Egg Beaters with Cheez, the score plunges to 8 Nutripoints. Cheese is a problem food because of its high fat content. Formagg Cheese Substitute gets around the fat problem and weighs in at 10.5 Nutripoints. Cottage cheese is the best natural cheese choice at 5.5 Nutripoints, followed by Laughing Cow Reduced Calorie Cheese (2.5 Nutripoints).

Near the bottom of the list you find the foods that are egg, or primarily egg, with McDonald's scrambled eggs trailing the list at −19.5 Nutripoints, the second-lowest all-time low Nutripoint score (only sweetbreads, from the meat Nutrigroup, score lower, at −52).

Meat/Fish/Poultry   At the top of the meat Nutrigroup we find raw clams (13.5 Nutripoints) and raw oysters (13 Nutripoints), but the problems with contamination of shellfish make these poor choices (thus the comment on the charts, and the warning on page 284). The very lean, red meats, with their high protein and nutrient content, follow the shellfish, followed by baked and grilled fish. We're happy to see tuna in water (8 Nutripoints) rating so high, as it's such an inexpensive and readily prepared food. You'll notice that the lean beefs are right up there with the lean chicken. You don't have to eliminate red meat if you stick with the very leanest cuts. The nutrients per calorie in beef can make it a good nutritional choice. After the lean beefs we find the lean chicken and turkey choices. As with the other Nutrigroups, as you process, and add salt and fat, the Nutripoints go down. The very worst choices are fatty meats, such as bacon and the lunch meats. The organ meats above the recommended line all have a comment on them concerning cholesterol because while they're high in nutrients, and thus have relatively high Nutripoint scores, they're also very high in cholesterol, and therefore are not really good nutritional choices, especially if you're concerned about cholesterol.

Fast Foods   In general, the best choice at a fast-food restaurant is the salad bar. Following that, a stuffed potato, if not too much fat in the form of cheese or butter has been added, is a good choice. Taco Bell offers some good choices in terms

of Nutripoints. Their bean burrito with green sauce weighs in
at 4 Nutripoints, which is below your daily goal of 5 Nutripoints from the legume Nutrigroup, but is still better than a
Taco Bell Light Taco (−1.5 Nutripoints). Pizza can also be
a good nutritional choice, with Pizza Hut's Thin and Crispy
Pizza rating 2 Nutripoints. It's nearly impossible to get a good
breakfast at a fast-food restaurant, as the choices are usually
loaded with fat: butter, cheese, eggs, and sausage. Wendy's
various omelets, scoring around −10 Nutripoints, are among
the worst of all possible fast-food choices.

PERSONALIZING THE NUTRIPOINT PROGRAM

Thus far we've been talking about the basic Nutripoint program, which requires 100 Nutripoints per day. This level of
Nutripoints is geared to someone who requires 1,000–1,200
calories per day. This is the level of Nutripoints we use in the
In-Residence Programs at the Aerobics Center. We do so
because many of our patients are trying to lose some weight.
After they've finished two weeks at the clinic on this level,
we recommend that when they go home they move up to Level
2 of the program, at 1,500 calories and, in some cases, 1,800
calories. In *no* case do we recommend that anyone go below
100 Nutripoints daily because you really cannot expect to get
adequate nutrients at this level. Moreover, such a low level
of calories would have a negative effect on your metabolism.
(We don't pinpoint the calories precisely for two reasons: first,
we want to de-emphasize the importance of calories as a
measure of foods, and second, we can't specify any more
precisely without losing the element of choice that you enjoy
with Nutripoints.)

This basic level of Nutripoints we use at the clinic isn't
right for everyone. Daily nutritional needs depend on age,
sex, frame size, weight, and activity level. Obviously, a small

woman who weighs 103 pounds, and who is totally sedentary, is going to need fewer calories than a 200-pound football player in training.

In general, you may well find that you need fewer calories on Nutripoints than you might think. We've had many patients on the 1,000–1,200 regime who begin, thinking that they won't be satisfied with this number of calories. But because so much fat is eliminated from their diets, 1,000 calories turns out to be far more food than they imagined. My suggestion is to begin at a level of the system a bit lower than what you think your daily caloric needs are. If you find you're not getting enough food, move up to the next level of Nutripoints. There is an element of trial and error in choosing the right level for you. If, after being on one level for a couple of weeks, you find it's too much or too little food, adjust to the next level accordingly.

The following is a breakdown of the three levels of Nutripoints to help you figure out where you might need to personalize the system and adjust your daily total goals:

Level 1: 100 Nutripoints daily/1,000–1,200 calories

This basic level of 1,000–1,200 calories per day is adequate for those on a weight-loss program (which is why we use it at the Aerobics Center), or for a basically sedentary woman of 125 pounds or less on a weight maintenance program.

The serving recommendations are those we've already looked at:

Nutrigroup	Servings	Goal
Vegetable	4	55
Fruit	3	15
Grain	2	10
Legume/nut/seed	1	5
Milk/dairy	2	10
Meat/fish/poultry	1	5

See page 131 for the chart to use for this level.

Level 2: 150 Nutripoints Daily/1,500–1,800 calories

This level is appropriate for the following individuals: active women; inactive, heavier women; inactive to moderately active men; and men over 200 pounds who are trying to lose weight.

Nutrigroup	Servings	Goal
Vegetable	6	85
Fruit	4	20
Grain	3	15
Legume/nut/seed	2	10
Milk/dairy	2	10
Meat/fish/poultry	2	10
Total:		150

Level 3: 200 Nutripoints Daily/2,000+ calories

In this level we've increased the vegetable, fruit, and grain servings in order to increase complex carbohydrates. On Level 3, you don't have to be so particular about shooting for the top of the lists to keep calories under control; there's more margin for error when you need more calories per day. But you should still avoid any foods below the recommended level.

Nutrigroup	Servings	Goal
Vegetable	8	120
Fruit	6	30
Grain	4	20
Legume/nut/seed	2	10
Milk/dairy	2	10
Meat/fish/poultry	2	10
Total:		200

Don't be overwhelmed by the number of servings for, say, vegetables in this level of Nutripoints: you can simply in-

NUTRIPOINT DAILY RECORD SHEET 1,500–1,800 CALORIES

Food Selection/Serving Size	Nutripoints							
	Veg.	Fruit	Grain	Leg.	Meat	Milk	Other	
Breakfast:								
1 Grain								
1 Milk/Dairy								
2 Fruit								
Lunch:								
2 Meat or Legume								
3 Vegetables								
1 Grain								
1 Milk/Dairy								
1 Fruit								
Dinner:								
2 Meat or Legume								
3 Vegetables								
1 Grain								
1 Fruit								
Totals:								
Goals:	85	20	15	10	10	10	0	150

NUTRIPOINT DAILY RECORD SHEET 2,000+ CALORIES

Food Selection/Serving Size	Nutripoints							
	Veg.	Fruit	Grain	Leg.	Meat	Milk	Other	
Breakfast:								
2 Grain								
1 Milk/Dairy								
2 Fruit								
Lunch:								
2 Meat or Legume								
4 Vegetables								
1 Grain								
1 Milk/Dairy								
2 Fruit								
Dinner:								
2 Meat or Legume								
4 Vegetables								
1 Grain								
2 Fruit								
Totals:								
Goals:	120	30	20	10	10	10	0	200

crease the amounts of a serving of a single food instead of having so many different foods. For example, instead of a half cup of sliced carrots for one serving (30 Nutripoints), have a full cup for two servings (60 Nutripoints). Remember that with the fruit Nutrigroup, you can make fruit juice a serving. Many people who are on this level of Nutripoints are very active and require a fair amount of liquids throughout the day. If you are careful to have a no-sugar-added fruit juice instead of a soft drink, it will fulfill some of your fruit servings. Instead of a 7-Up (−5.5 Nutripoints), have some apple juice (2.5 Nutripoints), some orange juice (8 Nutripoints), or some orange-pineapple juice (9.5 Nutripoints).

THE VEGETARIAN OPTION

It wasn't so long ago that vegetarians were considered at best off-beat, at worst nuts. But just as people are now willing to face the fact that smoking can cause lung cancer, and that high-fat and -cholesterol diets can cause heart disease, they are also willing to entertain the notion that meat may not always be the best and only source of protein in our diets. Even groups such as the American Dietetic Association and other health organizations are saying that not only is a vegetarian diet safe (people used to worry that you couldn't get sufficient protein from it), it can also be a healthier option than a diet that includes meat.

Solely on the basis of nutritional factors, including avoidance of excessives such as cholesterol and fat, and in an effort to increase fiber, Nutripoints has already incorporated some vegetarian principles. We've decreased the number of recommended meat servings to one a day, which is fewer than most people currently eat, and we've switched the main source of protein from meat/fish/poultry to a combination of meat/fish/poultry and legumes.

The advantage of getting some of your protein from plant sources rather than solely from meat/poultry/fish is that along with protein you're getting more complex carbohydrates, more fiber, less saturated fat, and less cholesterol. As you already know, the reduction of these elements in your diet will make you less susceptible to cancer and heart disease.

In addition to avoiding the life-style diseases, there's another factor that argues in favor of shifting the emphasis from meat as the primary source of protein in your diet: by "eating low on the food chain," as vegetarians refer to this option, you lessen your chances of accumulating toxic substances. Any drug that livestock are treated with eventually winds up in their meat. A diet very high in meat is eventually introducing these toxins into your body, and no one knows what the ultimate effect of these toxins will be. In addition to toxins introduced by man in the form of drugs, animals are also more likely to harbor organisms or pathogens that can be passed to man. In general, animal diseases can be passed to us, while plant diseases cannot. When you weigh all the factors, from drug contamination to contaminants that regularly affect animals such as oysters and clams, it seems clear that you're going from increased potential for harm to decreased potential for harm when you shift your emphasis from meat to other sources of protein.

I've been a vegetarian for sixteen years, and I guess I'm living proof of what a vegetarian diet can mean in terms of health: my cholesterol runs around 140, and my recent best time on the treadmill was rated "superior." I also feel that my energy level is terrific and that my general state of health is excellent.

If you're interested in vegetarianism, you might want to consult some of the excellent books that have recently been published on the subject, including *The Vegetarian Alternative* by Vic Sussman and *The Gradual Vegetarian* by Lisa Tracy.

There are various types of vegetarians, identified as follows:

Strict vegetarian (vegan): This is the most restricted level of vegetarianism. Vegans eat no animal products, including dairy.

Lactovegetarians: These vegetarians eat milk, cheese, and other dairy products, with the exception of eggs. They also refrain from eating meat, fish, and poultry.

Ovolactovegetarians: These vegetarians eat animal protein in eggs and dairy products, but no meat, fish, or poultry.

There is a new type of vegetarian these days who doesn't eat any red meat. This isn't an official category of vegetarianism, but it's quite popular. While such people are not really vegetarians, they still represent a trend I think is good because they're avoiding a major source of fat and cholesterol, as well as any potential toxins.

The Nutripoint vegetarian option is geared to the ovolactovegetarian option because I believe it's the safest type of diet: you're totally eliminating any flesh food (meat), but you're still getting complete protein in the form of whole dairy products and low-fat cheese and yogurt. The protein level (which many people worry about) is completely adequate at 75 grams a day—clearly more than the 56 grams recommended for men and the 46 recommended for women per day.

Adequate protein has always been the controversial point of vegetarian diets, and many people have been turned off to vegetarianism by "food combining." There's something about having to worry about eating rice with beans to get certain nutrients, for example, that discourages people. They think that if they don't eat the right foods together in the precisely correct combinations, they'll wither and die. The fact is, you *do* need to pay attention to getting adequate amounts of certain foods, but this is very easy to do, and it soon becomes second nature. Most important, you don't have to combine all of these foods *in the same meal.*

The reason that animal protein is an excellent source of protein for the human body is that it contains high concentrations of essential amino acids your body needs but cannot produce on its own. Foods that are high in these essential amino acids are called "complete," or high quality. Meats are high in these amino acids because the animal has put them together from the plants it's eaten: the balance is already achieved. Meats are therefore a "complete," or high-quality, protein. To get a balance of high-quality protein without meat, you have to do the combining yourself. Some plant foods are high in one amino acid, and some are high in others: by combining them you achieve a complete protein. And, as I mentioned, you don't have to make the perfect combination at each meal; the body is far more adaptable than that. Your body has an amino acid pool that stores amino acids for future use. As long as you eat, within a period of a few days, a variety of foods that complement one another, you'll achieve the effect of high-quality protein.

Some examples of foods that in combination provide complete protein are:

Cereal w/milk	Rice w/sesame seeds
Rice/cheese casserole	Legume soup w/bread
Macaroni and cheese	Corn tortillas and beans
Cheese sandwich	Pea soup and bread
Rice/bean casserole	Lentil curry w/rice

On page 146 you'll find a graphic summary of how to achieve complete protein with combinations of foods.

You should know that a vegetarian diet is high in fiber, and

SUMMARY OF COMPLEMENTARY PROTEIN RELATIONSHIPS*

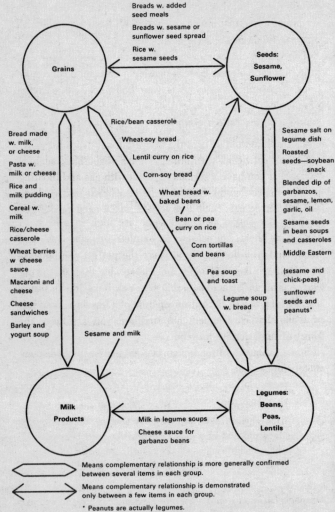

Grains

Seeds: Sesame, Sunflower

Breads w. added seed meals

Breads w. sesame or sunflower seed spread

Rice w. sesame seeds

Bread made w. milk, or cheese

Pasta w. milk or cheese

Rice and milk pudding

Cereal w. milk

Rice/cheese casserole

Wheat berries w cheese sauce

Macaroni and cheese

Cheese sandwiches

Barley and yogurt soup

Rice/bean casserole

Wheat-soy bread

Lentil curry on rice

Corn-soy bread

Wheat bread w. baked beans

Bean or pea curry on rice

Corn tortillas and beans

Pea soup and toast

Legume soup w. bread

Sesame salt on legume dish

Roasted seeds—soybean snack

Blended dip of garbanzos, sesame, lemon, garlic, oil

Sesame seeds in bean soups and casseroles

Middle Eastern

(sesame and chick-peas)

sunflower seeds and peanuts*

Sesame and milk

Milk Products

Legumes: Beans, Peas, Lentils

Milk in legume soups

Cheese sauce for garbanzo beans

Means complementary relationship is more generally confirmed between several items in each group.

Means complementary relationship is demonstrated only between a few items in each group.

* Peanuts are actually legumes.

*Adapted from Frances M. Lappé, *Diet for a Small Planet.*

you might have an adjustment period during which you'll experience excess gas. This is due to the fact that certain bacteria work to break down fiber and, in the process, give off gas. The body eventually adjusts and produces less gas, although it will still produce a bit more than when on a low-fiber diet. There are various methods to cut down on this gas.

First, be sure to cook all beans thoroughly; they're supposed to be soft, and if they're too chewy, they probably haven't been well cooked and are therefore likely to cause more gas. It often helps to soak beans in plenty of water overnight, and then discard the water and add fresh for cooking. Don't eat beans with other gaseous vegetables, such as cabbage. If you have a serious problem with gas and bloating from beans, you might want to stick to the beans that are least likely to cause gas, including lentils, black-eyed peas, lima beans, chick-peas, and white beans.

You might also notice that your body produces more frequent, and looser, bowel movements while on a high-fiber diet. This is actually good: your digestive system is getting waste out of your body as quickly as possible, and the fiber is absorbing water, which helps dilute carcinogens and excrete them. More frequent bowel movements also keep fat from sitting in the colon and causing a risk for cancer. In addition, frequent bowel movements help to flush cholesterol out of the system.

The vegetarian option for the 1,000–1,200 calorie version of Nutripoints breaks down as follows:

Nutrigroup	Servings	Goal
Vegetable	4	55
Fruit	3	15
Grain	2	10
Legume/nut/seed	2	10
Milk/dairy	2	10
Total:		100

You'll notice that this version of the vegetarian option simply substitutes one additional legume serving for the meat/poultry/fish option. If you prefer, instead of the two legume servings, you can have one legume serving and one additional milk/dairy serving.

The 1,500–1,800 calorie version is:

Nutrigroup	Servings	Goal
Vegetable	6	85
Fruit	4	20
Grain	4	20
Legume/nut/seed	3	15
Milk/dairy	2	10
Total:		150

The 2,000+ calorie vegetarian option is:

Nutrigroup	Servings	Goal
Vegetable	8	120
Fruit	6	30
Grain	4	20
Legume/nut/seed	3	15
Milk/dairy	3	15
Total:		200

As with the other higher-calorie versions of Nutripoints, you don't have to always depend on a huge number of servings from one Nutrigroup: you can sometimes simply increase the serving sizes to double the Nutripoints in a single serving. And you can get some of your vegetables, as well as fruits, in juices.

NUTRIPOINT RECOVERY

I have always found that a great limitation of a traditional "diet," which was most commonly a weight-reduction diet, was that you had to stick pretty strictly to the prescribed food choices and menus. This is not a whim of the diet-creators; in the best diets, it's done to ensure that you get an adequate balance of proteins/carbohydrates/fats, and that you get sufficient nutrients. In order for these diets to fulfill their promise of weight loss *and* adequate nutrition, they had to insist on strict compliance with the recommended menus.

What this meant in practical terms was that once you "cheated" and put butter on your toast, or ate a cookie, you were lost. You'd failed. Most people felt that following such a diet was walking a tightrope: one slip and they might as well throw in the towel. Patients had often presented their "diet histories" as a series of failed diets. Or they would lose some weight on a particular diet and then gain it all back, or gain it back with interest.

Nutripoints is different. *It puts the control back in your hands because it puts the information in your hands.* You don't have to rely on a menu plan or a list of food choices devised by someone else; you make the foods choices you like. And if you follow the system, you'll achieve your goal.

And what about those "failures"? They don't exist on Nutripoints. That's because you have the means to *quantify* your food choices yourself. This doesn't mean that you won't sometimes get fewer Nutripoints than you should, or perhaps too few or too many servings in one or more of the Nutrigroups, but when you *do* stray from the system, you can recover. This is because Nutripoints is a system of numbers. If you get fewer points on one day, you can redouble your efforts on the next day and get a higher score.

I tread lightly here because some people look upon the

recovery feature of Nutripoints as a license to binge. In other words, they think that if they get 200 Nutripoints on Tuesday, they can go wild on Wednesday and get only 10 Nutripoints and still be on top of things: the extra 100 Nutripoints on one day will help make up for the missing 90 the next. It doesn't work this way.

The basic premise of Nutripoints is that you want to improve your nutrition and your health. You know that it's not good to eat three slices of bacon and two fried eggs. Even if you eat the best diet in the world the following day, that overload of fat, cholesterol, and sodium is going to take its toll. No system can tell you that it won't. The difference with Nutripoints is that if you don't reach your goal one day, you can still recover the next by trying harder.

The way I explain this to my patients is that they don't have a license to eat a bowl of ice cream. But if they find themselves at a dinner party and the main course is cooked crab in a mayonnaise-based sauce, with broccoli in cheese sauce, and with chocolate pie for dessert, they don't have to refuse to eat. They can eat some of their meal, figure on getting a low Nutripoint score for that day, and move on the next day to choose from the tops of the Nutrigroups so that their daily "atonement" score will be particularly high. They'll be helping their bodies by making an extra effort to reduce the fat, cholesterol, and calorie intakes that were exceeded the previous day.

Because Nutripoints is a numbers system, it gives you the power to improve your overall nutritional status when circumstances have forced you into a situation that will produce a low score.

SHOPPING FOR NUTRIPOINTS

Now that you know where you stand before you embark on the Nutripoint program, I hope you're inspired to jump right

in. You can start immediately, with your next meal, if you
wish. Or you can take a day or two to familiarize yourself with
the charts and stock your kitchen with foods that are high in
Nutripoints, while you discard those that could sabotage your
score.

One patient told me after he had been on Nutripoints for
a month that the biggest change in his life was the volume
of food in his refrigerator—and it wasn't what you might
think. Before Nutripoints, he said, his refrigerator frequently
looked half empty. That's because it was filled with processed
and frozen prepared foods. After all, a box of frozen carrots
in butter sauce doesn't take up as much room as a bunch of
fresh carrots, and a frozen pot pie doesn't take up as much
room as some fresh chicken and fresh vegetables. He now
says, after Nutripoints, when he opens his refrigerator he sees
the colors of real foods instead of a lot of packages, and his
refrigerator always looks jammed.

The following are some tips on shopping that will help you
through the supermarket maze:

Prepare to Shop

1. Amazingly enough, *47 percent of all food purchases are
impulse buying*. This means that nearly half of what we buy
is just something that looks good at the moment. It may not
be a good nutritional value, or it might not even fit our
personal "food-style." Many of us go into a "supermarket
trance" the minute we hit the aisles, and begin buying for a
fantasy family. When we unload the grocery bags at home,
we too often realize that we didn't get half of what we
needed, and what we did get we don't have much use for.
The cure for this is a shopping list. Yes, it's basic, but it
works. Buy only what's on your list, and perhaps other
items that you regularly use, or that are on sale. Use the
Nutripoint "shopping lists" (see page 189) to help you find
the best nutritional bargains. If you take the time to check
these lists, you may well find that you can improve your

nutritional status just by making a few wise choices among brands.

2. Keep a list hanging in your kitchen, perhaps attached with a magnet to your refrigerator door, so that every time you notice you need something you can jot it down. Take the time to check Nutripoints for foods that could be substituted for foods that are lower in Nutripoints.

3. If you have some recipes you're going to try, be sure to check them over and add all necessary ingredients to your shopping list. It's amazing how often we never get around to preparing a certain recipe because we keep forgetting to buy that one critical ingredient.

Time Your Shopping Trips

1. Shop when your energy level is high and your temptation level low. You probably already know that you shouldn't shop when you're hungry. Don't shop when you're tired, either. One patient told me that her husband could always tell when she was exhausted: she came home from her usual after-work shopping trip with nothing but frozen entrees. If you *are* going to buy nothing but frozen entrees, at least make sure in advance that they're entrees that are high in Nutripoints.

2. If at all possible, avoid taking small children to the supermarket with you. It's terribly distracting to have to argue with a three-year-old who wants candy and sugared cereals and keep your mind on your list at the same time. If you must bring children with you, plan ahead and bring something—a small toy or healthful snack packed in a margarine tub—that will keep them occupied. One patient told me that she had her two kids help out at the market: she would instruct them to find certain items they were familiar with and praise them lavishly when they did. They enjoyed helping and were distracted from the usual supermarket temptations.

3. Frequent the biggest and best-stocked supermarket in

your area. I recommend that you look for a supermarket with the best and most extensive produce section and adopt it as your regular shopping place. The advantage of frequenting the same supermarket is that you can develop a relationship with the manager and request that they carry certain items. Some high-Nutripoint frozen dinners, for example, might not be available in your local markets, but if you request them, many managers will be happy to stock them.

Shop Wisely

1. Buy fresh fruits and vegetables in season. They're almost invariably tastier and more nutritious.

2. Never buy junk foods! If you have them in the house you'll probably eat them. Many people use guests as an excuse to buy things they ordinarily never have around. If you're having guests, prepare snacks and meals that are high in Nutripoints. They'll enjoy them as much as you, and you'll be doing them a favor by sparing them the chip and dip routine. If you must have some kind of snack food around, buy it in the smallest possible size and, if possible, in individual packages.

3. If you're buying convenience foods, make sure they're high in Nutripoints.

EATING OUT

Many of my patients ask me for tips on dining out. I wish I could evaluate all of the various restaurant preparations so that I could give you Nutripoints for each menu entry, but because of the endless variations in restaurant recipes, even for identical items, that's impossible. What this means is that a familiarity with the Nutripoint charts will help guide your food choices so that you can maintain your optimum diet. But, to some degree, without Nutripoints to guide you, you're back into the old days of watching fats and other negatives in order to eat well. The following are general tips that should help you eat well in restaurants:

• If possible, choose a restaurant in advance—a place that you know has some good Nutripoint choices on the menu. If you become a regular, many restaurants will be happy to fulfill certain requests, such as a vegetable combination dish that's not on the menu; plain, grilled fish; or meat cooked without butter. We're lucky today in that many restaurants have responded to consumer demand and become health conscious: they routinely offer grilled or baked foods, salads without dressing, vegetarian dishes, and low-fat entrees.

• Chinese, Japanese, and Indian restaurants are good choices for restaurants that tend to serve healthful foods. They use plenty of grains and vegetables, and the meat or fish portions of meals tend to be relatively small.

• If you're with a group that's ordering cocktails, stick with a carbonated soda water with a twist of lemon or lime, or perhaps a Virgin Mary or another mixed drink without alcohol. An orange juice spritzer of carbonated water and orange juice is refreshing, and is a good nutritional choice.

• If the restaurant puts bread and rolls on the table, unless others at your table object, ask them to remove the butter. It's too easy to find yourself slathering a piece of roll with butter or dabbing it on your potatoes or vegetables. You'll find that good, crusty rolls and bread really don't need butter, and the savings in terms of calories and cholesterol will be well worth it. If the restaurant doesn't serve the bread warm, you can always ask them to heat it. This brings out the natural flavors and makes it more satisfying.

• Always be sure to order salad without dressing or with dressing on the side. As we've seen, salad dressings can be a major source of fat and cholesterol if they're made with cheese or cream. Have your salad with just a bit of olive oil and vinegar, or ask if the restaurant has a low-fat or low-calorie dressing option.

• Be sure to order special dishes in advance when traveling by air. The fruit plates, vegetarian plates, and diabetic plates that most airlines serve are excellent choices, offering a delicious, fresh meal that's largely free of excess fat and sodium.

The following are tips for specific types of restaurants:

Chinese   Chinese food can be an excellent choice, as it relies on a lot of vegetables cooked quickly to retain nutrients. Stir-frying is a terrific method of cooking, and is a fixture in most Chinese restaurants. It uses very little oil, and therefore adds little fat to foods. Most Chinese vegetable and fish dishes are good choices. The only drawback to Chinese restaurants is their liberal use of MSG (which some people are allergic to), and their use of salty and/or sugary sauces. Fortunately, most Chinese restaurants are responsive to requests and quite willing to eliminate MSG, sugar, and salt from their cooking. Whole, steamed fish with sauce on the side is an excellent choice, and simple, stir-fried chicken and vegetable dishes are also good. The white or brown rice that help to round out the meal are good choices, as are the following selections: moo goo gai pan, mixed vegetables, won ton soup, and steamed dumplings. Avoid foods such as crispy fried beef, fried won tons, and any sweet and sour dishes. Yes, you can splurge on a fortune cookie. At 19 calories and very little fat, one or two won't do you too much harm.

French   French food can be difficult because of the use of sauces. If you stick with plain grilled meat or fish and simple salads, you'll be fine. Avoid anything prepared *remoulade*, because that refers to a mayonnaise sauce. Be sure to steer clear of vichysoisse and other cream-based soups, and onion soup with cheese on top. (You can ask for the onion soup without the cheese as an alternative.) Clear soups are the best choices. Stick with green salads, avoid anything that might be prepared with mayonnaise, and ask that dressing or sauce be served on the side. Bread is fine, but avoid butter, and stay away from croissants, which are loaded with butter. The best dessert bets include fresh berries, but pass up the cream.

Indian Indian restaurants provide some excellent choices because of their traditional reliance on legumes, vegetables, and yogurt-based sauces and dips. Some of the foods that are particularly good choices on an Indian menu include dal, vegetarian curries, raita, pulka (unleavened bread), basmati rice with vegetables, lentil soups, and tandoori baked chicken (which has been marinated in yogurt and roasted). Avoid puri (fried bread), samosa (fried appetizers), and any foods served with muglai (creamy curry sauce) or coconut-milk curry sauce. Be sure to avoid egg-based dishes. The biggest problem with Indian food is that many restaurants use ghee (which is clarified butter) or coconut oil (one of the few vegetable products that is a saturated fat) for cooking. Be sure to ask about this. Many restaurants will now use other oils for cooking if you so request.

Japanese Japanese restaurants can offer a good array of choices high in Nutripoints. The cuisine of Japan is low in fat, and makes good use of a variety of vegetables. Miso soup is a good choice, as it's based on soy with vegetables. Udon (noodles) served with broth and various meats and vegetables is a good main course, as are the yakitori (chicken or beef) preparations, which are meats broiled on a skewer. Be sure to avoid any fried dumplings, and any smoked or pickled foods. Tempura, which is fried, is not a good choice, and tonkatsu (fried pork) and torikatsu (fried chicken) are also to be avoided. Because of problems with seafood contamination, be very careful that the sushi you eat is from a highly reputable restaurant that serves only the freshest fish from the best sources.

Italian   We traditionally think of Italian food as being heavy, and it can be. But the fact is, southern Italian cuisine is now recognized as among the healthiest in the world. You just have to be careful to avoid northern Italian cuisine, which is rich in fat. Cioppino (seafood soup) is a good appetizer, as is minestrone soup. Steamed mussels in a red sauce can make an appetizer or a meal. Pasta with vegetable and/or tomato sauces is a good choice. Just be careful to avoid pasta selections that have cream-based sauces, or ones that are loaded with cheese. Avoid fettucini Alfredo, lasagna (except vegetable lasagna), cannelloni, and garlic bread. Plain, grilled fish or meats can be good choices.

Mexican   You have to pick and choose your way through a Mexican menu to get good nutritional value. While a dish such as chicken tostada would be a good choice, something such as a beef burrito with cheese and sour cream (heavily laden with fat and cholesterol) wouldn't. Rice, corn, and bean-based dishes can be good choices, but you must steer clear of cheese. Make sure refried beans aren't cooked in lard (which is high in saturated fat and cholesterol). Steamed corn tortillas, soft chicken tacos, black bean soup, gazpacho, and beans in a soft tortilla are all good choices. Choose the soft tacos over the crisp, as the crisp ones are fried. You can dip a plain corn tortilla in salsa, but avoid overly salted chips that are routinely served with salsa. If you can afford a dish high in fat (but low in cholesterol), you can try guacamole.

THE PERFECT MATCH: BOOSTING YOUR NUTRITION

Good nutrition depends on careful shopping, careful food storage, the best cooking techniques, and on the chemistry of the foods themselves as they work in your body. The absorption of certain nutrients can be improved when certain foods are eaten in combination; conversely, some foods inhibit the availability of nutrients when eaten with certain other foods. Alcohol, for example, impedes the body's absorption of various vitamins and minerals, including thiamin, calcium, vitamin D, folacin, and vitamin B_{12}. The following are some examples, adapted from the very informative *Jean Carper's Total Nutrition Guide*, of how you can get the best nutritional value from your foods by mixing and matching:

• Boost your iron absorption (this is particularly important for women) by adding vitamin C to any meal or food that's rich in iron. Just one glass of orange juice can boost the absorption of non-heme (nonmeat) iron by 200 to 500 percent.

• Avoid drinking tea with meals. Excess tea can help induce iron-deficiency anemia. It takes only two mugs of strong tea to reduce the amount of non-heme (nonmeat) iron you can absorb from a meal.

• White wine can boost the absorption of iron from a meal, while red wine, containing tannins, can inhibit it. This is not to encourage consuming wine, as it can destroy nutrients. It also has to be detoxified by the body. But if you must have wine, white is the better choice.

• Megadose supplements of vitamin C (one gram per meal) can impair vitamin B_{12} absorption to the point at which a deficiency can develop.

• Fruits and vegetables that are high in potassium (including spinach, beet greens, bok choy, tomatoes, beets, and cantaloupe) can help counter the effect of excess sodium in the diet. This is helpful to people who have a genetic disposition for hypertension.

• Many medications block or inhibit the absorption of various nutrients. Antibiotics, for example, can have an effect on your absorption of vitamins K and B_{12}. If you take a medication regularly, including birth control pills, check with your doctor to see if that medication has any effect on your nutritional status.

• Never add baking soda when cooking vegetables, as the alkaline solution thus created can destroy riboflavin (vitamin B_2).

ANSWERS TO COMMON QUESTIONS ABOUT NUTRIPOINTS

I've tried to cover every aspect of Nutripoints you need to know. But sometimes information is more accessible in a question-and-answer format. Also, there are certain common questions my patients ask that don't fit into neat categories. The following are the most common questions people ask about Nutripoints:

Why do I want to get more, rather than fewer, Nutripoints? Isn't this different from traditional programs that recommend you eat the least amount of calories?

For some people, adjusting to a positive goal (Nutripoints), rather than a negative one (calories), takes a bit of a psychological shift. But in the long run, as my patients tell me, it's far more appealing, and far easier to live with.

Yes, Nutripoints is different. A Nutripoint number assigned to a food is not, like a calorie, a one-dimensional number. Rather, it's an overall quality rating of the food that considers a number of factors—both positive and negative. You want to get more Nutripoints because the better a Nutripoint score, the higher the quality of a given food. The numbers are based on nutrients per calorie and the least excessives (bad elements) per calorie. The more Nutripoints you get, the more nutrition you get with the least excessives.

You might think of a Nutripoint as one point toward your vitamin quota for the day, 100 of which will give you 100 percent of the RDA, provided the points are distributed over the six Nutrigroups.

What happens if you eat too many points for the day, or for one Nutrigroup?

If you stick with the recommended number of servings for each Nutrigroup, you can't get too many Nutripoints. Anything over 100 Nutripoints for a day, or for the goal for a given Nutrigroup, is that much more nutrition you are concentrating into the food you eat. Remember that this "excess" good nutrition is fine because you are getting it in a natural form; it's nothing like taking megadoses of vitamins.

There is one problem with getting too many Nutripoints within one group. In some Nutrigroups, the only way to get super-high levels of Nutripoints, while staying within the recommended number of servings, is to pick most of your servings from the very top of the list. If you do this, it's at the expense of variety, and variety, I must stress, is very important.

Remember that each food has a "fingerprint" of nutrients that distinguishes it from other foods. If you choose all of your servings in vegetables from, say, turnip greens, you won't be diversifying your portfolio of vitamins and minerals. It would be much better to get one serving of turnip greens, and the other servings from vegetables below turnip greens that are still within the recommended area of the list.

If I eat more than 100 Nutripoints for the day, doesn't that mean that I've eaten too many calories?

Remember, the higher the Nutripoint score, the higher the density. This means the more nutrition per calorie. A high Nutripoint score means that you are getting a higher quality of food, while the number of servings you have determines the number of calories. If you get 300 Nutripoints within the recommended number of servings, you'll be within calorie limitations, and the quality of your food will be excellent.

How do you figure your score for a food item listed in the charts when you eat more or less than the serving-based points for that item? For example, if you eat an entire Arby's roast beef sandwich, but the points are only given for half a sandwich, what do you do?

Whether the points are negative or positive points, you double them if you eat double the portion listed. But don't forget that you must count that food item as *two* servings from that Nutrigroup. If you eat half the portion listed, you get half the Nutripoints, and you count that food as half a serving.

You'll notice that some foods list portion sizes that may be half of what you'd expect. For example, some of the slices of pizza are rated for half a slice. This is a tip-off that the food is calorie-dense. A large portion size is a sign that the food is a low-calorie, high-quality food, as it takes so much volume to fulfill the calorie requirement for a serving.

What happens if I eat more than the recommended number of servings per day?

There are two purposes in having a recommended number of servings per day. First, they provide the formulation within the Nutrigroups for balance between the various vitamins and minerals. Second, they provide the proper mix of carbohydrates, protein, and fats for overall daily totals. After you pick the Nutripoint level that suits you (see page 137), if you eat any more than the recommended number of servings, you will not be guaranteed your level's caloric limit.

The point I make over and over to my patients is this: when you stay within the recommended boundaries of Nutripoints, everything works. When you abandon those boundaries, you have to begin worrying about all of the old problematic factors: calories, cholesterol, sugar, fat, sodium, and so on.

If I can get my 100 Nutripoints in one serving before I fulfill the serving requirements, either for a Nutrigroup or for the day, why should I eat more food and more calories?

There are two components to an optimum diet: one is total calories, and the other is the right mix of carbohydrates, fat, and protein. Even though you get off to a good start by eating a food high in Nutripoints, you won't achieve all the requirements of your body unless you eat at least the specified number of servings per day. The goal of Nutripoints is to pick the highest-quality foods you like within each group, thus getting all of your calories, or thus limiting your calories to the right number—*at the same time* getting the proper mix of carbohydrates, protein, and fat, as well as the highest level of other nutrients, including vitamins and minerals.

What if I try to eat just foods that are high in Nutripoints, and don't bother with the serving requirements?

To get the full benefit of Nutripoints, you must consider the serving requirements along with the food scores. Think of it this way: the food scores take care of getting the best; the serving requirements take care of limiting the worst. If you pay attention just to getting foods with high scores, your nutritional status will no doubt be improved, but that's only half the picture. You still need to limit the excessives, including fat, saturated fat, cholesterol, sugar, sodium, alcohol, and caffeine. Nutripoints can assure you of achieving all these goals only if you follow the system as it was designed: high food scores in conjunction with the correct serving requirements.

I'm forced, because of business, to eat out a lot. What if I can't get in my legume serving for a day because I can't find anything appropriate on a restaurant menu?

This is a common problem, even if you don't eat out at restaurants. Many people are simply not used to buying and cooking legumes. Indeed, in the menus and recipes provided, I've assumed that you won't be able to get in the legume serving every day, and I've allowed for it by occasionally substituting a meat/poultry/fish serving.

If you miss a serving from the legume Nutrigroup, the best alternative is to substitute a serving from the meat/poultry/fish Nutrigroup. Naturally, you should try to make your substitution from the top of that Nutrigroup. You'll want to get at least a 5-Nutripoint meat/poultry/fish serving so that your total in the meat Nutrigroup for that day would be 10 rather than 5. This substitution will ensure that you're getting adequate protein for the day without too many extra calories.

What would happen if I occasionally ate a few foods from below the recommended line? What, really, is the reason for a cutoff point?

If you dip below the recommended levels on the charts, it will be more difficult to achieve the goals of the system, and it will be impossible to guarantee the results promised by Nutripoints. If you try to balance a poor choice with foods that are very high in Nutripoints, it will help you regain your balance. It's possible that the poor food choice is so high in one of the excessives that it causes you to exceed the limit for that excessive. Your other good choices are therefore limited in how much they can redeem you: they can give you optimum nutrients for that day, but they can't take away the excessive amounts of whatever excessive you've eaten.

What if I'm short in Nutripoints for one Nutrigroup, but over the goal in another: is that OK?

There's a simple answer to many questions about Nutripoints: once you abandon the program, you forfeit what it promises. I don't mean to make this sound bleak. It's just that the system has been designed to work as it's laid out. Once you begin to modify it, results can't be guaranteed. This doesn't mean that you need to abandon hope if you are short a few Nutripoints. The fact is, most people find that they're eating better on Nutripoints than they ever have in their lives, even if they don't follow the system religiously. It's impossible to say what your status would be if you were off in one Nutrigroup. If you're short by just a few points, you're probably OK. If you're short in one or two Nutrigroups every few days, you're less likely to be OK.

If you go over your Nutripoint goal for the day—say, 200 Nutripoints—how bad could it be to eat a food with a −3, which only pulls your score down a little bit?

It's difficult to appreciate at first why it's such a big deal to cut a few points off your daily score unless you understand how the numbers and servings function as *limits* as well as guidelines. If you eat a negative food when you've achieved a high Nutripoint score for the day, it means that while you've achieved all your *essential* goals, you haven't stayed within your *excessive* limits. In other words, you've probably eaten too much fat and/or cholesterol, sugar, sodium, calories. So, while you've gotten all of your vitamins and minerals, you could be harming yourself by consuming, say, too much cholesterol. You can more easily understand why this would be so just from a logical standpoint: would it make sense for someone to get a high Nutripoint score—say, 350 Nutripoints—and then eat 150 points worth of negative foods to get their final score down to 200? Of course not!

Why is there so much difference between the ratings for one Nutrigroup and another? In other words, why is the highest-rated vegetable 79 Nutripoints, while the highest dairy product gets only 23.5 Nutripoints? Does this mean we'd be better off eating just vegetables, or does it mean that a different standard was used for different Nutrigroups?

The same standard—the Nutripoint formula—was used to rate *all* foods. We can see from the ratings that, in general, vegetables offer more nutrition per calorie than milk and dairy products. So you can compare foods from Nutrigroup to Nutrigroup *in general*, but you can't finally say that because vegetables are better foods, that's all you should eat. Balance is a critical part of an optimum diet, and the only way to achieve balance is to choose foods from various Nutrigroups. The reason for this is that each Nutrigroup has its own nutrient profile, which distinguishes it from every other Nutrigroup. Although we know a great deal about the nutrients in foods, there are probably things yet to be discovered concerning micronutrients. Given this, there may be micronutrients in, say, grains, that your body requires to function. Therefore, even though a grain food has a lower score than a vegetable food, you'll be avoiding grains to your peril. The only situation in which foods from different Nutrigroups can be interchangeable is between the legume/nut/seed and meat/poultry/fish groups. This is because the basic nutrient profile critical to the human body in these groups seems to concern protein. As it's possible to get sufficient protein from plant sources, it's possible to make exchanges between these two Nutrigroups.

How can all the complex information we have about vitamins and minerals, in particular, be reduced to one number? How can you compare apples and oranges? Aren't oranges high in vitamin C while bananas are high in potassium? Can't you eat carrots because they're high in vitamin A?

While it is true that certain foods are high in specific nutrients, many of our beliefs about eating a certain food for the sake of a certain nutrient reveal more about our past inability to accurately compare foods than about the food's usefulness.

In fact, while there are about fifty nutrients, including water, that are needed daily for optimum good health, the list can be narrowed down, for practical purposes, to the ten most important, or "leader," nutrients. If you are careful to consume these leader nutrients, the other forty or so will be present in sufficient amounts to meet your nutritional needs. A study was done that demonstrated this. The study tried to discover if foods rated solely on eight vitamins and minerals (protein, vitamin A, vitamin C, niacin, riboflavin, thiamin, iron, and calcium) were valid guides to improved food choices. The foods were analyzed in various ways, and finally demonstrated that nutrient-density scores, even when based on only eight nutrients, do in fact serve as valid indicators of the overall nutritional worth of a food. They also found that high nutrient-density scores are a good measure of the nutritional complexity of a food. *Foods with the highest scores are high not just for one or two nutrients but for most nutrients.* Of the fifty foods in this study, for example, forty-three had high scores for six or more of the eight nutrients measured. Foods in the middle of the ratings had good scores for only two to five of the eight nutrients measured, and most of the bottom fifty foods failed to have a decent score for even a single nutrient.

In fact, nature, with the help of Nutripoints, has made it

easy for us: you don't have to eat two dozen foods to cover all of the major and minor nutrients, you just have to eat foods that are high in Nutripoints.

How did you arrive at the line that defines the recommended level in the lists? Why isn't it just the point at which the numbers become negative, which seems more logical?

The Nutripoint scores for foods had to take into account not only the absolute value of each individual food but how that food would fit into the pattern of balance in a daily diet. The numbers are not intended to reflect a perfect gradient; there's no point at which a food becomes taboo. My effort was, as much as possible, to eliminate the excessives and promote the essentials. It's all a question of relative values. So, as you reach the bottom of the lists, the food choices simply become comparatively poorer. If you choose too many of those poor foods, you won't meet the goals of Nutripoints. The recommended line reflects an effort to guide your choices to a point at which you can choose near the bottom of the list, *but above the recommended level,* and still achieve your Nutripoint goals.

As to why the cutoff point is not simply all negative numbers: there are some foods that are negative but that are OK to eat sometimes. Fat, for example, can be a part of your diet, but all the fats have negative numbers.

Why is it that sometimes there may be five or ten foods with the same rating? Are they all exactly the same?

When we figured out the Nutripoint scores, we carried out the numbers to the nearest one-hundredth. This means that a food might have, for example, wound up with a rating of 4.26. To avoid confusion with too many numbers (and, from a practical standpoint, because these differences are really quite minor) we rounded off these numbers. The food rated at 4.26 would have become 4.5.

If there are a number of foods listed at the same number, the order of listing reflects the small fractional differences in their ratings. They are listed in descending order. A food that appears, for example, at 4 is better than any food at 4 beneath it. Remember that these differences are so minor that, for practical purposes, foods at 4 can be considered equal.

Is a food with a score of 20 twice as good as a food with a score of 10?

Yes and no. Yes, it is twice as nutritious per calorie when adjusting for negative factors (excessives) that help determine the ratings. But no, it may not have double the nutrition. A food with a score of 10 may have nearly as much nutrition as a food with a score of 20, but the lower score may reflect the presence of negative factors that drop the rating. Hence a food with a rating of 20 is twice as good as a food with a rating of 10, *based on the criteria we have set in the Nutripoint formula.*

If a food has negative Nutripoints, does that mean it contains no nutrition?

Not necessarily. A food with negative Nutripoints may contain no nutrition plus some excessives that pull it down, or it may be extremely nutritious but be pulled down by a lot of excessives. You can't tell just by looking at the Nutripoint number. In these cases, its negative score is used to tell where it stands in comparison to other foods.

If something has 100 Nutripoints, does that mean it's a perfect food?

Not necessarily. It's possible that a food with an extremely high Nutripoint rating is high in nutrition per calorie, but it doesn't mean that it's perfectly balanced over the eighteen essentials. There really is no perfect food. Good nutrition comes from a balance that you achieve by choosing from the six Nutrigroups.

Are you absolutely positive that I'll get 100 percent of the RDA for all vitamins and minerals if I get 100 Nutripoints per day?

If you get 100 Nutripoints per day following all the guidelines of the Nutripoints program, you can be reasonably assured that you're getting 100 percent of the RDA for all of the essential vitamins and minerals. If, however, you make many of your food choices from near the bottom of the lists, it is possible that you will occasionally be slightly below 100 percent on some of the nutrients. The system has to take this very small risk if it's to allow you to make the food choices yourself. If you try to choose many of your foods from the higher portion of the list, you'll have no trouble getting 100 percent of RDAs. If you get over 100 Nutripoints, there's no doubt that you'll be reaching, and probably surpassing, the RDAs for all the essential vitamins and minerals.

Also, since your body can store nutrients for some time and can vary its ability to absorb them, it is not necessary to meet precisely all the RDAs every single day. The National Research Council that set up RDAs says, "RDA(s) are presented as *daily* allowances in order to simplify dietary calculations. Nevertheless, the various protective mechanisms of the body are such that if the recommended dietary allowance for a nutrient is not met on a particular day, a surplus consumed shortly thereafter will compensate for the inadequacy for normal individuals. In estimating dietary adequacy it would seem entirely acceptable to average intakes of nutrients over a 5–8 day period." Thus over a five- to eight-day period, a Nutripoint score of 100 each day achieved by using a variety of foods would meet the RDA standards.

Why are some foods that are high in cholesterol at the top of the list? I thought cholesterol was a negative factor and would therefore pull that food's score down.

You'll notice that there are some foods near the top of the list, particularly in the meat/poultry/fish Nutrigroup, that have a symbol identifying them as a high cholesterol food. What this means is that these foods, although high in Nutripoints, are also high in cholesterol. This occurs because these foods are extremely high in vitamins and minerals. They earned their scores honestly according to the Nutripoint formula, but their cholesterol level is nonetheless extremely high.

Most of the foods that fall into this category are organ meats, such as liver. The liver acts as a storage system in the body to store vitamins and minerals, and that's why it's so rich in nutrients. But it also produces cholesterol. About 70 to 80 percent of cholesterol is produced by the liver; the rest is gained from dietary sources. About 1,000 milligrams of cholesterol is produced by the human body each day. As animal livers also produce cholesterol, if you eat liver, you're eating a concentrated source of cholesterol. By the way, not all organ meats are rich in nutrients, and the Nutripoint charts reflect this. Sweetbreads, for example, are an organ meat, but they're not high in nutrients, and you'll find them at the very bottom of the meat/poultry/fish list.

Another reason that liver, despite its high nutritional content, may not be a good food choice is that one of the functions of the liver is to detoxify the blood. Any contaminants in the body are processed by the liver, which becomes a concentrated storage house of such toxins, which, obviously, are not a positive element in any diet.

All foods on the Nutripoints list above the recommended line that are high in cholesterol have daggers (†) next to them.

By "high in cholesterol" I mean foods that have a cholesterol per calorie ratio of 1 or above; in other words, for every calorie there is one or more milligrams of cholesterol. From a practical standpoint, this means that while these foods are high in nutrients they should be avoided, despite their high Nutripoint scores. Just one three-ounce serving of liver, for example, would have approximately 400 milligrams of cholesterol, which would put you well above the American Heart Association guidelines of 300 milligrams of cholesterol per day.

What about the fact that oxalic acid, which is a component of green, leafy vegetables, binds the calcium in greens so that it is not available and not readily absorbed by the body? Do you take this sort of thing into account in the formula?

While it's true that oxalic acid does interfere to some degree with the absorption of calcium by the body, it doesn't have as negative an effect as some people believe. Certain foods contain oxalic acid, which combines with calcium and magnesium to form insoluble compounds that are thus unavailable to the body. But most foods simply don't contain *enough* oxalic acid to bind with any significant amount of calcium or magnesium in the food. Thus, green, leafy vegetables can still be considered a good source of calcium in the diet when supplemented with a variety of low-fat dairy products.

Absorption levels could not be taken into account in the Nutripoints formula because there are simply too many variables connected with absorption that can't be quantified. In the section on food combinations (page 158), however, you'll find some helpful information on how you can boost absorption of nutrients. The section on essentials (page 76) will give you tips if you're concerned about a particular nutrient.

How does the Nutripoint program assure me that I get my citrus fruit and my green, leafy and yellow/orange vegetables every day?

The beauty of Nutripoints is that it automatically fulfills the requirements suggested by nutritionists over the years. The reason we've heard citrus fruit so highly recommended is that it's very high in vitamin C. But Nutripoints also identifies other foods that are high in C. If you choose foods from the top of the list, you'll be getting foods, citrus or not, that are most likely very high in vitamin C.

As for the green, leafy and yellow/orange vegetables, Nutripoints rates these vegetables very highly in the first place. These foods are high in vitamin A. (Green, leafy vegetables are also high in vitamin C and calcium.) The vitamin A you get from yellow/orange vegetables is in the form of beta carotene, which we've been hearing so much about recently. The body does not care whether it gets its beta carotene from green, leafy vegetables or from yellow/orange vegetables. Either one will fill the bill. Picking foods high on the Nutripoint lists will assure you that you're getting foods high in all your vitamin/mineral requirements.

Remember that it's an old-fashioned concept to assign one vitamin or one mineral to a single food. Nature has made it easy for us, as Nutripoints reveals: most foods that are generally high in one vitamin or mineral are also high in others. In other words, the good foods are usually very good, and the bad (or unnatural) ones are awful!

How does getting 100 Nutripoints assure me that I'm getting 100 percent of RDAs and limiting calories, cholesterol, sodium, sugar, caffeine, and alcohol?

The formula for Nutripoints does this by identifying foods that are simultaneously highly nutritious and low in excessives. Foods that appear below the recommended level are really the other half of the equation. If you avoid them, you'll be steering clear of foods that would put you over the limit on any one of the excessive factors. By avoiding the negative and getting the positive, you achieve your goal.

How can you say that following the program will meet, or exceed, recommendations of the American Dietetic Association, the American Heart Association, the American Cancer Society, and the National Cancer Institute?

The American Dietetic Association officially recommends the use of USRDAs for every adult. Nutripoints is designed to fulfill this requirement. The American Dietetic Association also makes the following recommendations, which are virtually identical to the USDA dietary recommendations. You'll readily see that each of these recommendations is reflected in the Nutripoint formula:

1. Eat a variety of foods.
2. Maintain a desirable weight.
3. Avoid fat, saturated fat, and cholesterol.
4. Eat foods with adequate starch and fiber.
5. Avoid too much sugar.
6. Avoid too much sodium.
7. If you drink alcohol, do so in moderation.

The American Heart Association recommends a limit of 300 milligrams of cholesterol per day and a limit of 3,000 milligrams of sodium per day. The recommended limits are part of the formulation of Nutripoints, and are the limits set in the formula.

The American Heart Association and the American Cancer Society also recommend 30 percent or less fat consumed as calories in the diet as a preventive measure against coronary heart disease and many types of cancer, particularly colon and breast cancer. Nutripoints sets 30 percent of fat as calories as the upper limit in its formulation.

The American Cancer Society recommends getting a high amount of vitamins A and C in foods, as these vitamins have been correlated with lower rates of cancer. This is one of the strengths of Nutripoints: it identifies foods highly concentrated with vitamins A and C, and thus is a cancer-prevention diet.

The National Cancer Institute recommends 25 to 35 grams of dietary fiber per day. Nutripoints sets 35 grams as the recommended amount per day in its formulation.

Picking foods from the top of the Nutripoint lists could result in a diet that betters these various guidelines.

Will the Nutripoint program help prevent cancer?

There are still many questions about the causes of cancer, but there's no doubt that there are steps you can take, in terms of nutrition, that will decrease your risks for certain types of cancer. Nutripoints will certainly lower your risk for various types of cancers, as it incorporates the basic recommendations of the American Cancer Society into the tenets of the system. These seven recommendations include:

1. Avoid obesity.
2. Cut down on total fat intake.
3. Eat more high-fiber foods.
4. Include foods rich in vitamins A and C in your daily diet.
5. Include cruciferous vegetables in your diet.
6. Eat smoked, salt-cured, and nitrite-cured foods in moderation.
7. Keep alcohol consumption moderate, if you do drink.

You'll recognize that each of these recommendations is reflected in the basic Nutripoint formula.

Does your system take into account the nutrient losses from transportation, storage, and cooking?

In general, no. It's simply impossible to account for all these factors, with the exception of cooking. You'll notice that many of the fresh foods are listed raw and cooked. This will give you an idea of how the nutrition might vary from one state to another, although sometimes the variation is simply a reflection of amounts. Raw cabbage, for example, has greater volume than cooked cabbage.

The effects of transportation and storage are too variable and can't be measured. Some of these issues are discussed on page 61.

Why did you put certain foods, such as lemons, in the condiments section when they would seem more logically placed in the fruit section?

Most of the items in the condiments group are the foods you'd expect to find there, including spices and seasonings. Other foods are listed there because they're normally eaten in such small quantities that the calorie level for a given portion would be less than 20. They couldn't logically fit into the regular fruit Nutrigroup because the serving size would have to be so large that it simply wouldn't make sense. The average number of calories for the portions in the fruit Nutrigroup are 50 to 100. For lemons to fit there, I'd have to suggest that you eat two whole lemons to count as a serving. So, one-quarter lemon at 5 or 6 calories fits logically in the condiment section. In the condiment section I've adjusted the calorie portion of the formula so that the portion sizes fit normal eating patterns.

Why do you include foods such as legumes in your system? Many people never eat them. And why is Nutripoints geared toward massive amounts of fruits and vegetables?

As Willie Sutton replied when asked why he robbed banks,
"Because that's where the money is." Legumes, fruits, and
vegetables are highly nutritious foods, and they should play
a large role in our daily diet. It's unfortunate that legumes are
unfamiliar to so many people (though I think that's changing).
Legumes are an excellent source of protein with no cholesterol, a lot of fiber, and complex carbohydrates. If we replaced
one-quarter to one-half of our meat consumption with
legumes (the Nutripoint program is designed to do this), we
would be avoiding the major causes of the most prevalent
life-style diseases, including cancer and heart disease.

As to massive amounts of fruits and vegetables, again,
that's where the nutrients are! One of the major revelations
of Nutripoints is that the best value in nutrition lies in fruits
and vegetables. That's where we get the most nutrition for the
fewest calories. The bonus of fruits and vegetables in terms
of nutrition is that these foods are also high in complex
carbohydrates and simple *bulk:* if you're dieting, they fill you
up while giving you good nutrition. This is the exact opposite
effect of junk foods, which *don't* fill you up and give you
nothing in terms of good nutrition.

**Why are some brand-name foods rated higher, and
some lower, than their corresponding basic foods?
For example, why are basic beans with pork rated 3
Nutripoints while Campbell's beans with pork is rated
2 Nutripoints?**

The ratings of basic, generic foods came from USDA data.
USDA data analyzes virtually every nutrient in a food. Manufacturers, however, analyze for basic nutrients, and their analyses can be variable and spotty. Therefore, when I plugged
information from manufacturers into the system, I had to put
a 0 for nutrients they don't provide (except cholesterol, fiber,
fat, saturated fat, and sugar—all of which, when not available, I estimated using the best available parameters). It would

be conjecture on my part to make estimates of other nutrients because they're highly variable from food to food and depend on food processing methods.

You, the reader, need to compare the numbers of brand-name foods separately from basic foods. In other words, you can't compare basic beans with pork to Campbell's beans with pork, although you can compare Campbell's beans with pork (2 Nutripoints) with Bush's beans with pork (1.5 Nutripoints) or Van Camp's vegetarian beans (3 Nutripoints).

In some cases, brand-name foods could exceed basic foods in Nutripoints because they're fortified. In most of those cases, you will see an asterisk next to the food in the chart that indicates fortification.

What about combination foods, such as lasagna, that have meat, a grain, and a vegetable in them—how did you determine which Nutrigroup to put them in?

You'll notice that I've categorized combination foods according to their major component, either by volume or calories, whichever made more sense. In the case of lasagna, it's in the grain Nutrigroup because the largest ingredient is pasta. I couldn't break down these combination foods because manufacturers provide data only for the entire dish, not the parts of the dish.

Does the Nutripoint formula take into account food additives and contaminants?

No, it doesn't. I would love to be able to do so, but there simply is no reliable, standardized way of measuring these elements in various foods. (For a fuller discussion of this subject, see page 59).

How did you gather your data?

About half my information was from the Cooper Clinic Data Base, which is based on USDA information, for which millions of dollars went into research. I feel it's the most reliable data available. In their analyses they go as far as to indicate the number of samples they tested, and the range is usually from 10 to 200. That means for some bits of information—say, the amount of vitamin A in a carrot—they might have tested 200 carrots. In most cases, they've done enough to assure accuracy, but in an occasional case I found some margin for error. For example, in a few instances I found data that was based on only one sample. This single sample disagreed with data from either a manufacturer or from another source. In those cases, I went with common sense and used my own judgment to ascertain which data made the most sense. For each food, I've looked at from one to four sources to corroborate evidence.

With brand-name foods and fast foods I've had to rely on manufacturers. In most instances, manufacturers send out samples to reliable laboratories to get their nutritional data. In most cases, these manufacturers sent me copies of the reports as they came from the labs, or they gave the name of the lab or the research company. Some manufacturers don't have their foods analyzed and have no nutritional data whatsoever. Some manufacturers based nutritional information for their products on the USDA data for basic foods and extrapolated to arrive at their own "analyses." Whenever there was doubt, inaccuracy, or contradiction, I sifted through the available evidence to come up with what I believe is the most fair and accurate interpretation of the data.

Foods are constantly changing. How can you keep up with brand names and fast foods that come out after your list was compiled?

It's true that food formulations change constantly, but I am constantly adding to the 3,000 foods, and I'd like to solicit manufacturers to send me information on their new foods, especially if they're formulating "light" or more healthful foods. We'd love to include such foods in new editions of *Nutripoints*. I'd also like to think that with the advent of Nutripoints, manufacturers will have all the more reason to create more healthful foods. If consumers know which foods are better for them, surely it's an incentive to buy, and there's nothing like consumer pressure, or the pressure of the marketplace, to convince manufacturers to create more healthful formulations of foods.

Why are supplemental foods rated higher than natural foods? For example, I noticed that most of the cereals that are fortified have much higher scores than the natural, unfortified cereals. I thought you believed in getting vitamins naturally.

Yes, I do believe in getting vitamins naturally. That's why we have an asterisk next to a food that is significantly fortified. *Significantly fortified* means that 50 percent or more of the nutrition comes from fortification. In these cases, when foods are highly fortified, we have to take a look at the basic food that existed before the fortification. For example, Whole Wheat Total is basically a good food. Everything from the whole wheat is there, including the fiber and other basic nutrients. The fortification is added to something real. But if you look at Cap'n Crunchberries, you'll see a different story. In that case, there's no real basic food at all. You simply have to use common sense. If Cap'n Crunchberries is the only thing the kids will eat, you could do worse (although I do believe it's best to avoid such foods from the beginning so that kids don't get used to having them). A helpful way to judge a cereal that's highly fortified, and therefore high in Nutripoints, is to check the ingredients list on the box: if sugar is listed near the beginning of the ingredients, you'll know that the cereal is highly sweetened and, despite the fortification, not a good nutritional bet.

Is Whole Wheat Total at 64.5 Nutripoints better than

Shredded Wheat at 5 Nutripoints? That's a toss-up. I think that Total might be considered marginally better because it does start with something good and adds vitamins to that basic food, but it's certainly not ten times better than Shredded Wheat, as the Nutripoint numbers might suggest. If you're looking at cost, it could well be that if you're following Nutripoints and thereby getting at least 100 percent of your RDA for all the vitamins and minerals, you're paying too much for Whole Wheat Total, which is charging you for vitamins you're already getting.

What about oysters and clams? I notice they're high on the list, but are they good food choices?

While it's true that oysters and clams are high on the list, you'll notice that they're marked with a double dagger (‡) indicating caution. I had to grant them their high number of Nutripoints because that's how the system worked out. They're very high in certain minerals, including calcium, iron, zinc, phosphorus, and potassium, but I don't believe they're particularly good food choices because of the problems with shellfish contamination. Pollution of our coastal waters seems to be a sad fact of contemporary life, and shellfish, as bottom feeders, are more likely than other fish to become heavily contaminated. Moreover, when we eat shellfish, we eat the entire animal, not just a gutted fillet (which has had the liver and other repositories of many harmful pollutants removed). A recent publication from the National Centers for Disease Control pointed out that while certain diseases, including typhoid fever, hepatitis A, and cholera, have long been associated with shellfish ingestion, today we're finding that certain viruses are being transmitted by consuming them. As it's simply too difficult to monitor the harvesting and distribution of shellfish, I think that your best bet is to avoid eating shellfish, particularly raw shellfish.

What if someone doesn't have problems with choles-terol, high blood pressure, or weight control, but wants to get good nutrition? Your system has a built-in bias against cholesterol, sodium, sugar, and fat—but foods that are high in these elements can also be very nutritious, right?

Nutripoints rates the food, not the eater. Foods that are highly rated are the best available for the body, based on today's scientific research. We know that excess cholesterol, sodium, sugar, and fat are not good for the body. If you're lucky enough not to have a problem with any life-style dis-eases today, that, unfortunately, doesn't mean you won't be facing them tomorrow. A prudent diet is also a *preventive* diet. All people have an "excessive threshold" that seems to allow them to consume a certain amount of food that isn't good for them, but they then reach a point at which they're trying to *reverse* a problem such as high blood pressure, overweight, or diabetes. A prudent diet, one that follows Nutripoints, is going to protect you in the future, as well as make you feel good today.

Is Nutripoints for everyone?

Nutripoints is primarily for healthy adults. It's not de-signed for anyone under age eighteen who might need addi-tional calcium and protein in his or her diet. Nutripoints is designed for people who are sedentary to moderately active, with no special medical problems that might involve diet. It's wise to check with your physician if you have any medical condition that might require special attention before you em-bark on the Nutripoints program.

Can I follow Nutripoints if I have food allergies?

If you have any particular medical condition, you should consult with your doctor before beginning Nutripoints. A doctor or nutritionist could help you adapt Nutripoints to suit your particular condition.

Is there a Nutripoint program for kids or for people with special needs, such as pregnant women and athletes?

Not right now, although we're working on such a program and hope in the future to come up with various versions of Nutripoints that will accommodate people with special needs.

How is Nutripoints used at the Aerobics Center in the In-Residence Programs?

At the Aerobics Center, Nutripoints is used primarily as a weight-loss program and as a total nutrition program for those who want to maintain their weight. In the future, we'll have a version of Nutripoints geared to weight loss for the general public; this book is geared to every healthy adult, although many people find that they lose weight using Nutripoints as it's outlined in this book, particularly if their diet was generally poor.

Why didn't someone think of Nutripoints before?

It took the happy marriage of computer technology and the latest nutritional data to produce Nutripoints. I have to assume that it wasn't done before because it never occurred to anyone that it *could* be done. Point systems that rate foods had been designed, but no one had developed a system that so exhaustively quantifies every element of a food, as well as putting that food into a total system that assures optimum nutrition. Certainly no nutrition plan has ever been offered that allows you complete freedom to choose, given only the limitations of the foods' Nutripoint scores.

Do you use the Nutripoint program yourself?

Yes, I do. I kept a diet diary for two weeks before I began using Nutripoints. Because I am a nutritionist and a vegetarian, my diet was already pretty good: low in fat and high in fiber, vitamins and minerals. But my diet survey revealed that I was getting between 150 and 200 Nutripoints daily and about 1,500 to 2,000 calories. Now, with Nutripoints, I'm getting between 200 and 300 Nutripoints daily, and I'm eating roughly the same number of calories.

Do you plan on creating a computer program to make it easier to compute daily running tallies of Nutripoints in each Nutrigroup?

Yes. We have recently developed the Diet Tracking Software for Nutripoints that you can use in your personal computer. If you're interested in this program, write to Nutripoint Research, P.O. Box 1450, Loma Linda, CA 92354 or use the handy order form at the back of this book.

PART V

SPECIAL LISTS

To make Nutripoints even more useful, we've created some special lists that highlight certain features of the system. They include:

- Top-Ten Nutripoint Foods
- Shopping Lists
- Bang-for-the-Buck Lists

TOP-TEN NUTRIPOINT FOODS

The following lists are a handy breakdown of the top ten foods in each of the Nutrigroups:

Vegetables
Turnip greens
Spinach
Bok choy
Mustard greens
Beet greens
Parsley
Broccoli
Watercress
Romaine lettuce
Dandelion greens

Fruits
Cantaloupe
Guava
Papaya
Strawberries
Black currants
Mango
Kiwi
Litchi

Mandarin oranges
Honeydew melon

Grains*
Wheat bran
Wheat germ
High-fiber Ryvita snackbread
Ralston hot, high-fiber cereal
Wasa Fiber-Plus Crispbread
Quaker Oat Bran cereal
3 Minute Brand instant oat bran cereal
Wonder Hi-Fiber bread
Health Valley vegetarian amaranth pilaf
Whole wheat bread/English muffin

Legumes
Bean sprouts
Green peas
Navy beans
Green pigeon peas
Health Valley split green pea soup
Lima beans
Black-eyed peas
Kidney beans
Loma Linda vegeburger
Lentils

Milk/Dairy
Fleischmann's Egg Beaters
Sego Diet Lite milk drink
Carnation low-fat milk, no-sugar Instant Breakfast
Carnation instant nonfat dry milk
Formagg pasteurized cheese substitute
Dannon nonfat light yogurt, all flavors
Tofutti Egg Watchers egg substitute
Scramblers egg substitute

*This list excludes fortified cereals.

Skim milk
Canned evaporated skim milk
Skim buttermilk

Meat/Fish/Poultry
Raw clams
Raw oysters
Baked venison
Canned clams
Chicken of the Sea chunk-light low-sodium tuna in water
Baked pike
Steamed/poached salmon
Baked halibut
Baked red snapper
Baked freshwater bass

NUTRIPOINT SHOPPING LISTS

Using Nutripoints well means shopping wisely. The food rating lists, both the Nutrigroup lists and the alphabetical lists, will be enormously helpful to you when you compare foods by type or by brand. But there are certain items we buy frequently, so I have provided lists comparing these by Nutripoints. This will save you searching through the lists to look for, say, the highest-rated spaghetti sauce. I think you'll find these lists enormously helpful, and I suggest that you draw up the same lists for food items you frequently buy, which I might not have included.

I have omitted from these lists items that have a dagger indicating cholesterol in the Nutrigroup and alphabetical lists, as I don't recommend you choose them. I have also omitted, for the same reason, items that fall below the recommended level for each Nutrigroup. I have also left out some generic foods because the point of these lists is to help people shop and compare, and in some cases the generic food ratings are meant more as a general reference. I've included some Nutripoint recipe foods where appropriate as a basis for comparison.

You'll also notice that I've only rated foods in the six major Nutrigroups and in the fat/oil group.

Vegetables

Frozen Vegetables	Nutripoints
Birds Eye spinach (whole leaf)	57.0
Birds Eye broccoli spears	46.0
Birds Eye cauliflower and red peppers	41.5
Pictsweet broccoli, carrots, and cauliflower	36.0
Green Giant broccoli, cauliflower, and carrots	33.0
Birds Eye baby carrots w. water chestnuts	31.0

Canned Vegetables	Nutripoints
Del Monte Early Garden spinach	35.5
Libby's mixed vegetables (natural pack)	18.5
Green Giant 50-percent Less Salt asparagus	14.5
Green Giant asparagus cuts	14.0
Green Giant mushrooms	13.0
Del Monte whole green beans	13.0
Green Giant 50-percent Less Salt green beans	8.0
Del Monte Golden Family-Style corn (no salt)	6.0
Green Giant Kitchen-Cut green beans	4.5
Green Giant whole kernel corn	2.0

Spaghetti Sauce	Nutripoints
Pritikin	9.5
Aunt Millie's meatless	4.0
Prego no-salt	4.0
Aunt Millie's w. peppers and sausage	3.5
Ragú home-style w. mushrooms	3.0

Soups	Nutripoints
Nutripoint clear spinach	23.5
Health Valley no-salt vegetable	13.0

Vegetables *(cont.)*

Health Valley vegetable	12.5
Health Valley no-salt tomato	12.0
Health Valley tomato	11.5
Health Valley chunky 5-bean vegetable	11.0
Progresso tomato w. vegetables	6.5
Pritikin vegetable	6.5
Campbell's chunky vegetable	5.0
Campbell's vegetarian vegetable	4.5
Campbell's minestrone	3.5

Fruits

Juices	*Nutripoints*
Nutripoint Sunrise Cooler	15.5
Nutripoint Strawberry Smoothie	13.0
Ocean Spray low-cal. Cranapple	12.5
Minute Maid orange juice (w. calcium)	11.0
Tropicana orange juice	11.0
Citrus Hill orange juice (w. calcium)	10.5
Ocean Spray low-cal. cranberry	10.5
Minute Maid orange juice (frozen)	10.0
Sundance orange juice sparkler	8.0
Ocean Spray grapefruit juice	8.0
Ocean Spray cranberry juice cocktail	7.0
Sundance grapefruit juice sparkler	7.0
Ocean Spray pink grapefruit juice	6.0
Welch's unsweetened grape juice (frozen)	5.5
Dole pineapple juice	5.0
Hawaiian Punch low-cal. fruit drink	4.5
Seneca apple juice (frozen)	4.5
Kiwi Island sweetened kiwi juice	4.5

Frozen Fruit	*Nutripoints*
Budget Gourmet apples glazed w. raspberry sauce	10.5
Birds Eye frozen strawberries (light syrup)	8.5
Birds Eye frozen strawberries (heavy syrup)	5.0

Fruits *(cont.)*

Dried Fruits	*Nutripoints*
Sun Maid dried apricots	8.0
Del Monte dried apricots	7.5
Sunsweet whole prunes	6.0
Sunsweet pitted bite-size prunes	5.0
Sun Maid dried peaches	5.0
Sun Maid mission figs	4.5
Sun Maid calimyrna figs	4.0
Sun Maid dried mixed fruits	3.5
Sun Maid dried fruit bits	3.5
Sun Maid zante currants	3.5
Sun Maid golden raisins	3.0

Grains

Breads	*Nutripoints*
Wonder Hi-Fiber	6.5
The Sourdough whole wheat stone-ground	6.0
Roman Oat Bran and Honey Light	5.5
Fresh Horizons wheat	5.0
Pepperidge Farm whole wheat thin	4.5
Earth Grains wheat Lite 35	4.5
Roman Meal	4.5
Country Hearth stone-ground whole wheat	4.5
Wonder 100% whole wheat	4.0
Earth Grain honey wheatberry	4.0
Oroweat Bran'nola	3.5
Thomas' Protogen Protein	3.5
Earth Grain stone-ground wheat	3.5
Home Pride 100% whole wheat	3.5
Earth Grain salt-free sandwich	3.5
Arnold original Bran'nola	3.5
Arnold honey wheatberry	3.5
Earth Grains honey wheatberry	3.5
Roman Meal honey nut and oat bran	3.5
Oatmeal Goodness oatmeal and bran	3.5
Oatmeal Goodness oatmeal and sunflower seeds	3.5

Grains *(cont.)*

Crackers	Nutripoints
High Fiber Ryvita	9.0
Wasa Crispbread (fiber plus)	7.5
Ralston Rykrisp	5.0
Wasa Golden Rye crispbread	4.0
Wasa Hearty Rye crispbread	3.5
Ryvita Dark Rye crispbread	3.0
Ralston Rykrisp seasoned	3.0

Prepared Pasta	Nutripoints
Nutripoint Angel Hair w. Sunshine Sauce	10.0
Nutripoint Fresh Pasta Salad	4.5
Green Giant Pasta Accents w. Cheddar	4.0
Green Giant Garden Gourmet Cheddar Rotini	4.0
Green Giant Pasta Accents w. Garlic	3.5
Morton spaghetti and meatballs frozen dinner	3.5

Unprepared Pasta	Nutripoints
Prince enriched macaroni and spaghetti	4.0
Buitoni Hi-Protein spinach linguine	3.5
Muellers macaroni (all types)	3.5
Prince Superoni	3.0
Buitoni linguine	3.0
Creamette Rainbow rotini	3.0
San Giorgio spaghetti	3.0
Celentano frozen cavatelli	3.0
Ronzoni spaghetti	3.0
No Yolks cholesterol-free egg noodles	3.0
Borden's Creamette spinach macaroni ribbons	3.0
San Giorgio linguine	2.5
Borden's Creamette elbow macaroni	2.5
Borden's Creamette spaghetti	2.5

Muffins	Nutripoints
Nutripoint Muffin	10.5
Whole wheat English muffin	6.0

Grains *(cont.)*

Health Valley raisin oat bran muffin	5.0
English muffin w. raisins	4.5
Roman Meal English muffin	4.5
Pepperidge Farm English muffin	4.0
Nutripoint oat bran muffin	3.5
Arnold Extra Crisp muffin	3.5
Oroweat Health Nut English muffin	3.0
Thomas' regular English muffin	2.5
Arrowhead Mills oat bran wheat-free muffin	2.5
Thomas' honey wheat English muffin	2.0

Pancakes/Waffles	*Nutripoints*
Nutripoint Whole Grain Pancake	5.5
Eggo Common Sense oat bran waffle (frozen)	3.5
Aunt Jemima Complete Buttermilk pancake mix	3.5
Aunt Jemima Original Complete pancake mix	2.5
Aunt Jemima blueberry waffles	2.0

Rice	*Nutripoints*
Wild rice (no salt)	5.5
Green Giant frozen wild rice w. sherry	4.5
Brown rice (no salt)	4.0
Spanish rice	4.0
Mahatma brown rice	3.5
Pritikin brown rice pilaf w. vegetables	3.0
White rice (no salt)	3.0
Minute Rice	2.5
Arrowhead Mills Quick brown rice	2.5
Uncle Ben's converted white rice	2.5
Mahatma long grain enriched rice	2.0
Carolina long grain enriched rice	2.0

Legumes/Nuts/Seeds

Soups	*Nutripoints*
Nutripoint French Market	17.0
Health Valley minestrone	14.0

Legumes/Nuts/Seeds *(cont.)*

Nutripoint lentil	13.5
Health Valley split pea	10.0
Health Valley lentil	8.0
Health Valley black bean	7.5
Nile Spice Foods lentil curry couscous	6.5
Hain Natural split pea	4.0
Nutripoint Hot and Sour	4.0
Progresso minestrone	4.0
Campbell's green pea	2.5
Progresso split green pea	2.5
Campbell's Chunky Old-Fashioned Beans 'n Ham	2.0

Milk/Dairy

Yogurt	*Nutripoints*
Dannon nonfat light, all flavors	10.5
Dannon plain nonfat	9.0
Weight Watchers Nonfat Ultimate, all flavors	8.0
Dannon plain low-fat	5.5
Weight Watchers nonfat peach	4.5
Yoplait nonfat light, all flavors	4.0
Dannon low-fat Fresh Flavors (all flavors)	2.0
Blue Bell frozen low-fat peaches and cream	2.0
Dannon Extra Smooth Fruit (all flavors)	2.0
Blue Bell frozen low-fat fruit (all flavors)	2.0
Borden low-fat Swiss Style Lite-Line plain	1.5
Dannon low-fat Fruit on Bottom (all flavors)	1.0
Dannon Dan'Up low-fat yogurt drink	0.5
Dannon low-fat with nuts, raisins, and fruit	0.5

Cheeses	*Nutripoints*
Formagg cheese substitute	10.5
Dry cottage cheese	5.5
Nutripoint Honey Cream Cheese	5.5
Low-fat cottage cheese (1-percent)	4.5
Wendy's imitation Parmesan	4.5
Low-fat cottage cheese (2-percent)	3.0

Milk/Dairy (cont.)

Laughing Cow reduced-calorie	2.5
Cottage cheese	1.5
Wendy's imitation cheese	1.5
Weight Watchers low-fat cottage cheese	1.5
Borden sharp cheddar flavor	1.0
Low-fat ricotta	0.5
Low-fat mozzarella	0.5
Parmesan	0.5
Kraft reduced-fat Swiss	0.5
Land O Lakes skim mozzarella	0.5
Lipton pasteurized American	0.0
Borden low-fat mozzarella	0.0

Eggs	*Nutripoints*
Nutripoint Garden Scrambled Egg Beaters	23.5
Fleischmann's Egg Beaters	17.5
Weight Watchers Tofutti egg substitute	10.0
Scramblers egg substitute	10.0
Fleischmann's Egg Beaters w. Cheez	6.0
Egg white	6.0
Nutripoint Garden Scrambled Eggs	5.5
Second Nature egg substitute	4.5

Dinner Entrees	*Nutripoints*
Celentano cannelloni Florentine	5.5
Nutripoint Five-Cheese Casserole	5.5
Celentano manicotti (frozen)	2.0
Celentano stuffed shells (frozen)	2.0
Celentano broccoli-stuffed shells (frozen)	1.5
Le Menu stuffed three-cheese shells (frozen)	1.0
Weight Watchers baked cheese ravioli (frozen)	1.0
Patio cheese enchilada dinner (frozen)	1.0
Budget Gourmet cheese manicotti w. meat sauce	0.5
Le Menu three-cheese manicotti in tomato sauce	0.5
Budget Gourmet Slim cheese ravioli	0.5
Stouffer's Lean Cuisine cheese cannelloni	0.5
Weight Watchers frozen cheese manicotti	0.0

Meat/Fish/Poultry

Seafood	Nutripoints
Nutripoint Scallop Kabob	16.5
Raw clams	13.5
Nutripoint Red Snapper Veracruz	13.5
Raw eastern oysters	13.0
Nutripoint Lettuce-Wrapped Salmon	10.5
Canned clams	8.0
Raw Pacific oysters	8.0
Chicken of the Sea chunk-light low-sodium tuna in water	8.0
Pike (baked)	7.5
Salmon (steamed)	7.5
Halibut (baked)	7.5
Red snapper (baked)	7.0
Bumble Bee tuna, chunk-light, in water	7.0
Freshwater bass (baked)	7.0

Poultry preparations	Nutripoints
Nutripoint Chicken Stir-Fry	8.5
Nutripoint Chicken Salad	6.5
Quail (no skin)	6.0
Nutripoint Cajun Chicken Breast Sandwich	5.5
McDonald's chicken salad oriental	5.0
Nutripoint Chicken Enchiladas	5.0
Nutripoint Grilled Chicken w. Mango Sauce	4.5
Light meat turkey (baked, no skin)	4.5
Chicken breast (baked, no skin)	4.0
Chicken salad sandwich on whole wheat	4.0
Nutripoint Turkey Sandwich	4.0

Beef	Nutripoints
Nutripoint Beef Asada	7.0
Nutripoint Aerobics Hamburger	5.0
Chung King frozen beef teriyaki	5.0
Lean beef round steak (broiled)	4.0
Lean beef flank steak (broiled)	4.0
Lean beef top loin (broiled)	4.0
Lean beef tenderloin fillet (broiled)	3.5

Meat/Fish/Poultry (cont.)

Lean beef chuck roast (braised)	3.5
Lean hamburger (broiled)	3.0
Beef, macaroni, and tomato sauce	3.0
Beef jerky	2.5
Lean beef rib-eye steak (broiled)	2.5
Lean porterhouse steak (broiled)	2.5
Lean T-bone steak (broiled)	2.5

Tuna*	Nutripoints
Chick/Sea chunk-light, low-sodium, in water	8.0
Bumble Bee chunk-light, in water	7.0
Bumble Bee solid white, in water	6.5
Fresh broiled tuna	6.5
Chick/Sea chunk-light, in water	6.5
Chick/Sea chunk-light, in water and oil	6.0
Star Kist solid white, in water	6.0
Chick/Sea solid white, in water	5.5
Chick/Sea chunk-white diet albacore, low-sodium, in water	5.0
Chick/Sea tonno solid light, in oil	4.0
Chick/Sea albacore solid white, in oil	4.0
Chick/Sea chunk-light, in oil	3.5

Soups	Nutripoints
Progresso Home Style chicken	5.5
Pritikin chicken w. ribbon pasta	4.5
Campbell's chunky beef	4.0
Campbell's turkey vegetable	2.5
Nile Spice Foods chicken vegetable couscous	2.0

Frozen Dinners	Nutripoints
Celentano frozen chicken primavera	6.0
Chung King beef teriyaki	5.0

*You can improve the points on almost any tuna by rinsing it in water to remove salt.

Meat/Fish/Poultry *(cont.)*

Morton sliced beef	4.0
Morton frozen turkey dinner	4.0
Healthy Choice chicken oriental	3.5
Healthy Choice chicken Parmigiana	3.5
Healthy Choice sweet and sour chicken	3.0
Healthy Choice beef sirloin tips	3.0
Dining Lite chicken a la king	3.0
Chung King beef pepper oriental	3.0
Chung King frozen imperial chicken	3.0
Gorton's frozen ocean perch fillet	2.5

Fats/Oils

Spreads	*Nutripoints*
Weight Watchers reduced-calorie no-salt margarine	−2.0
Promise margarine	−2.0
Mrs. Filbert's family spread margarine	−2.0
Hain safflower margarine	−2.5
Blue Bonnet reduced-calorie spread	−2.5
Mazola unsalted margarine	−2.5
Mazola Lite corn oil margarine	−2.5
Parkay soft diet margarine	−2.5
Kraft diet Touch of Butter spread	−2.5
Weight Watchers reduced-calorie margarine	−2.5
Fleischmann's diet margarine	−2.5

Dressings	*Nutripoints*
Nutripoint Lite Blue Cheese	8.0
Nutripoint Slim Guacamole Dip	7.5
Nutripoint Lite Ranch	3.5
Nutripoint Lite Orange Vinaigrette	2.5
Nutripoint Lite Caper Dressing	2.0
Nutripoint Lite Mayo Mix	1.5
Nutripoint Lite Vinaigrette	−1.5
Kraft Catalina French	−2.0
Kraft French	−2.5

A NUTRIENT BANG FOR THE BUCK

The lists that follow give you a way of stretching your food dollars by listing foods that are extremely high in nutrients while low in cost. We figured out the "Nutripoints per dollar" for each food and list the highest foods in each Nutrigroup here. The cost was based on the average price in local markets: some foods, particularly fruits and vegetables, may differ in cost in your area. They will, of course, be cheaper when in season.

Vegetables
Bok choy
Turnip greens
Cabbage
Parsley
Broccoli
Birds Eye whole leaf spinach
Mustard greens
Brussels sprouts
Cauliflower
Romaine lettuce
Raw spinach
Asparagus
Birds Eye broccoli, carrots, and red peppers (frozen)
Watercress
Red peppers

Fruits
Cantaloupe
Watermelon
Mandarin oranges (canned)
Orange juice
Orange
Kiwi fruit
Plums (canned, unsweetened)

Peach (fresh)
Honeydew melon
Papaya
Nectarine (fresh)
Grapefruit
Strawberries (fresh)
Casaba melon
Apricots (dry)
Apricot (fresh)
Mango
Guava

Grains
All Bran, Extra Fiber
Whole Wheat Total
Total Corn Flakes
Total Oatmeal
Product 19
Just Right
Just Right w. Fruit and Nuts
Fiber One
100% Bran
Bran Buds
Total Raisin Bran
All Bran
Kretschmer Toasted Wheat Bran
40+ Bran Flakes
Fruitful Bran
Kellogg's Corn Flakes
Post Natural Bran
Grape-Nuts
Honey Buc Wheat Crisp

Legumes/Nuts/Seeds
Split peas
Mung bean sprouts
Arrowhead Mills dry soybeans

Navy beans
Pinto beans
Garbanzo beans
Baked beans w. tomato sauce
Kidney beans
Lentils
Peas (frozen)
Black-eyed peas (canned)
Birds Eye frozen peas
Health Valley split pea soup
Tofu
Health Valley minestrone soup
Health Valley black bean soup

Milk/Dairy
Carnation instant nonfat dry milk
Evaporated skim milk
Fleischmann's Egg Beaters
Carnation Instant Breakfast (no sugar)
Nonfat yogurt
Diet Sego
Egg white
Fleischmann's Egg Beaters w. Cheez

Meat/Fish/Poultry
Chick/Sea chunk-light tuna, in spring water
Salmon
Halibut
Raw oysters
Raw clams
Red snapper
Swordfish
Flank steak
Fresh tuna

PART VI

NUTRIPOINT MENUS AND RECIPES

THIS IS THE PART OF NUTRIPOINTS THAT'S DESIGNED TO GET YOU into the kitchen. You'll find sample menus that cover fourteen days. For all the menu items that are identified by "Nutripoint"—for example, Nutripoint Grilled Cajun Chicken Breast or Nutripoint Caper Dressing—you'll find recipes in the recipe section. The page number following each dish on the menu refers to the page where the recipe appears.

The menus really serve two purposes. They're meant to be *used.* If you're the type of person who likes to have things spelled out, who likes to shop in advance and plan ahead, you'll love the menus because they'll answer all your questions about what you should be eating on Nutripoints.

The menus are also meant to serve as inspiration. You might want to mix and match various foods on different days. As long as you stick with the correct number of servings for each Nutrigroup, this is fine.

Kathleen S. Duran, R.D., the assistant director of nutrition for the Aerobics Center In-Residence Programs, developed our recipes. In developing the menus and recipes, we focused on taste, variety, and practicality. These menus and recipes are ones that we've used with great success with participants of the In-Residence Programs. As you'll see, the recipes taste great! We've received countless compliments on them from people who asked for recipe printouts to bring home. While aiming for high Nutripoint scores, we also kept in mind that a food not widely available or terribly expensive is not a good choice. We tried to use foods that are readily available in your supermarket, and we tried to make the recipes simple and easy to follow. Our goal was an eating program that would be high in Nutripoints, satisfying, tasty, and easy to live with.

As for Nutripoint scores, you can think of the two-week sample menus as a standard, optimum diet. The Nutripoint totals for each day range from 200 to 300 points for a 1,000 to 1,200 calorie diet. It's possible to get even higher scores than this, but, as I've said, we were concerned with practicality, and we wanted a meal plan that was easy and fun as well as nutritious. We analyzed the nutrients in Day 1 of the menus just to give you an idea of how the numbers might work out on a typical Nutripoint menu. You can see that they're well within the guidelines for an optimum diet.

If you need to increase your calorie level from the basic level of the menus and recipes, please refer to page 137 of Part IV for information on how to do this. The simplest way is to increase the serving sizes or to have additional portions of the suggested foods.

You may notice that we strayed from the serving recommendations in some cases, and you'll find it instructive to learn why because it may affect the way you use Nutripoints in your daily life.

We used a legume serving about half the time in place of a meat serving. We found that most people find it much easier to adapt to Nutripoints when they begin with roughly half the legumes in their diet that we ultimately recommend.

In some cases we used a grain entree with some low-fat cheese for protein instead of a meat or legume serving. On Day 6, for example, we have a grain serving (Nutripoint Spinach Lasagna) at lunch and omit a legume serving. Because the high-quality protein in the Nutripoint Red Snapper Veracruz more than satisfies our protein requirements, we went for additional complex carbohydrates in place of the legume serving. You might want to do this once or twice in the course of a two-week program. On Day 7 we skipped a grain serving because of the rice in the Nutripoint Herbed Lentils and Wild Rice casserole.

On some days we might skip a serving of vegetables if there is a good quantity of vegetables in another dish. On Day 4, for example, we skipped the vegetable at lunch because of the vegetables in the Nutripoint Chicken Stir-Fry. By making such substitutions, you'll find Nutripoints very easy to live with.

You'll notice that we used skim milk every day. You can use 1-percent or 2-percent milk if you prefer, but you should avoid whole milk entirely: it simply has too much fat.

You can mix and match recipes. For example, the Nutripoint Blackberry Freeze can be used along with the Nutripoint Banana Gladje. Some people find the Blackberry Freeze too strong on its own, but just delightful with the Banana Gladje.

I hope you'll be creative with your own combinations of Nutripoint foods. I'd welcome any recipes that you might care to share with me. I'd like to use any especially good ones, with proper credit of course, in future editions of this and other Nutripoint books. You can send them to me at Nutripoint Research, P.O. Box 1450, Loma Linda, CA 92354.

NUTRIPOINT MENUS

NUTRIPOINT 1,000–1,200 CALORIE MENU								
Day: 1	**Nutripoints**							
Food Selection/Serving Size	Veg.	Fruit	Grain	Leg.	Meat	Milk	Other	
Breakfast:								
Whole Wheat Total cereal, 1 cup			64.5					
Skim milk, 1 cup						9.5		
Cantaloupe melon, 1/4 pc.		29						
Lunch:								
Nutripoint Cajun Chicken Breast Sandwich, 3 oz.					5.5			
Tomato, 1/4 pc.	7.5							
Loose-leaf lettuce, 1 pc.	3							
Whole wheat bun, 1 pc.			6					
Nutripoint Spinach Salad, 2 cups	65							
Nutripoint Lite Zero Dressing, 2 tbs.							1	
V-8 Spicy Vegetable Juice, 6 oz.	26							
Fresh orange, 1 pc.		13.5						
No-calorie beverage								
Dinner:								
Nutripoint French Market Soup, 1 cup				17				
Nutripoint Tossed Salad, 2 cups	51.5							
Nutripoint Lite Caper Dressing, 2 tbs.							2	
Lowfat (2-percent) cottage cheese, 1/2 cup						3		
Nutripoint Fresh Fruit Platter, 1/2 cup		17						
No-calorie beverage								
Totals:	153	59.5	70.5	17	5.5	12.5	3	321
Goals:	55	15	10	5	5	10	0	100

Nutrient Analysis: Nutripoint 1,000–1,200 Calorie Menu, Day 1

Nutrient

Calories	1,214.000 cal
Protein	89.000 gm
Total fat	17.000 gm
Saturated fat	2.501 gm
Cholesterol (dietary)	99.000 mg
Complex carbohydrates	176.000 gm
Sugar	3.000 gm
Alcohol	0.098 gm
Fiber (dietary)	33.000 gm
Calcium	1,090.000 mg
Phosphorus	1,292.000 mg
Magnesium	452.000 mg
Sodium	1,988.000 mg
Potassium	4,508.000 mg
Zinc	25.000 mg
Iron	36.000 mg
Vitamin A	27,284.000 IU
Thiamin (B_1)	7.325 mg
Riboflavin (B_2)	3.717 mg
Niacin (B_3)	43.000 mg
Pyridoxine (B_6)	3.861 mg
Pantothenic acid	16.307 mg
Folic acid	1,676.000 mcg
Vitamin B_{12}	8.206 mcg
Vitamin C	429.000 mg
Caffeine	0.000 mg

Calorie Sources

Sources	Percentage
Protein	29
Fat	12
Complex carbohydrates (fruits, vegs., starches)	59
Simple carbohydrates (sugar)	0
Alcohol	0

NUTRIPOINT 1,000–1,200 CALORIE MENU								
Day: 2	**Nutripoints**							
Food Selection/Serving Size	Veg.	Fruit	Grain	Leg.	Meat	Milk	Other	
Breakfast:								
Nutripoint Fruited Cinnamon Cereal, 1 cup			5					
Skim milk, 1 cup						9.5		
Fresh blueberries, 1/2 cup		7						
Lunch:								
Nutripoint Beef Asada, 1 pc.					7			
Nutripoint Tossed Salad, 2 cups	51.5							
Nutripoint Lite Ranch Dressing, 2 tbs.							2	
Nutripoint Fresh Fruit Slices, 1 cup		23.5						
No-calorie beverage								
Dinner:								
Nutripoint Crunchy Fish, 3 oz.					6.5			
Nutripoint Vegetable Medley, 1 cup	48.5							
Nutripoint Spinach Salad, 2 cups	65							
Nutripoint Lite 16-Island Dressing, 2 tbs.							1	
Nutripoint Wild Rice Soup, 1 cup			10.5					
Skim milk, 1 cup						9.5		
Nutripoint Blackberry Freeze, 3/4 cup		8.5						
Totals:	165	39	15.5	0	13.5	19	3	255
Goals:	55	15	10	5	5	10	0	100

NUTRIPOINT 1,000–1,200 CALORIE MENU								
Day: 3	**Nutripoints**							
Food Selection/Serving Size	Veg.	Fruit	Grain	Leg.	Meat	Milk	Other	
Breakfast:								
Eggo Common Sense Oat Bran Waffles, 1½ pcs.			3.5					
Dannon Lowfat Yogurt, 1 cup						5.5		
Nutripoint Hot Peach Topping, ½ cup		7						
Lunch:								
Nutripoint Lettuce-Wrapped Salmon w/Herb Sauce, 4 oz.					10.5			
Nutripoint Salad Greens with Balsamic Vinegar, 2 cups	42							
w. mushrooms (⅓ cup)								
w. tomato (⅓ pc.)								
w. carrots (⅓ pc.)	33							
Nutripoint Fresh Pasta Salad, ½ cup			4.5					
Nutripoint Banana Gladje, ⅓ cup		6						
No-calorie beverage								
Dinner:								
Nutripoint South-of-the-Border Vegetarian Chili, ¾ cup				13				
Nutripoint Tossed Salad, 2 cups	51.5							
w. broccoli (½ cup) and cauliflower (½ cup)	41							
Nutripoint Lite Ranch Dressing, 2 tbs.							2	
Skim milk, 1 cup						9.5		
Nutripoint Rainbow Compote, ½ cup		18						
Totals:	167.5	31	8	13	10.5	15	2	247
Goals:	55	15	10	5	5	10	0	100

NUTRIPOINT 1,000–1,200 CALORIE MENU								
Day: 4	**Nutripoints**							
Food Selection/Serving Size	Veg.	Fruit	Grain	Leg.	Meat	Milk	Other	
Breakfast:								
Nutripoint Bran Muffin, 1 pc			10.5					
Nutripoint Garden Scrambled Egg or with Egg Beaters egg, 3/4 cup						5.5/ 23.5		
Fresh grapefruit, 1/2 pc.		13						
Lunch:								
Nutripoint Chicken Stir-Fry, 1 cup					8.5			
Nutripoint Tossed Salad, 2 cups	51.5							
Nutripoint Hot and Sour Soup, 1/2 cup				2				
Fresh sliced pineapple, 1/2 cup		8						
No-calorie beverage								
Dinner:								
Nutripoint Venison w. Juniper Berry Sauce, 6 oz.					6.5			
Nutripoint Spinach Salad, 2 cups	65							
Nutripoint Lite Orange Vinaigrette Dressing, 2 tbs.							2.5	
Cooked broccoli flowerettes w. Butter Buds	38.5							
Orzo pasta, 1 cup			5					
Skim milk, 1 cup						9.5		
Nutripoint Poached Pears, 1/2 pc.		4						
Totals:	155	25	15.5	2	15	15/ 33	2.5	230/ 248
Goals:	55	15	10	5	5	10	0	100

NUTRIPOINT 1,000–1,200 CALORIE MENU								
Day: 5	**Nutripoints**							
Food Selection/Serving Size	Veg.	Fruit	Grain	Leg.	Meat	Milk	Other	
Breakfast:								
Product 19 cereal, 1 cup			56					
Skim milk, 1 cup						9.5		
Banana, 1/2 pc.		7.5						
Lunch:								
Health Valley 5-Bean Minestrone Soup, 1 1/2 cups				14				
Ryvita High Fiber Crackers, 2 pcs.			2					
Wasa Fiber Plus Crackers, 2 pcs.			5					
Nutripoint Tossed Salad, 2 cups w. green peppers, alfalfa sprouts, red cabbage	51.5 28							
Nutripoint Lite Ranch Dressing, 2 tbs.							2	
Nutripoint Sunrise Cooler, 1/2 cup		15.5						
Dinner:								
Nutripoint Chicken Salad, 3/4 cup (on a bed of lettuce)					6.5			
Nutripoint Tossed Salad, 2 cups	51.5							
Nutripoint Lite Orange Vinaigrette Dressing, 2 tbs.							2.5	
Carrot sticks, 1 pc. carrot	35.5							
Plain, lowfat yogurt, 1/2 cup						3.5		
Nutripoint Fresh Fruit Platter, 1 cup		34						
Totals:	166.5	57	63	14	6.5	13	4.5	322.5
Goals:	55	15	10	5	5	10	0	100

NUTRIPOINT 1,000–1,200 CALORIE MENU								
Day: 6	**Nutripoints**							
Food Selection/Serving Size	Veg.	Fruit	Grain	Leg.	Meat	Milk	Other	
Breakfast:								
Nutripoint Whole Grain Pancakes, 4 pcs.			5.5					
Skim milk, 1 cup						9.5		
Nutripoint Hot Blueberry Topping, 1/2 cup		2.5						
or Nutripoint Hot Red Raspberry Topping, 1/2 cup		9						
Lunch:								
Nutripoint Spinach Lasagna, 1 cup			10					
Nutripoint Vegetable Medley w. Butter Buds, 1 cup	48.5							
Nutripoint Tossed Salad, 2 cups	51.5							
Nutripoint Lite Vinaigrette Dressing, 2 tbs.							-1.5	
Nutripoint Strawberry Smoothie, 1 cup		13						
Dinner:								
Nutripoint Red Snapper Veracruz, 3 oz.					13.5			
Nutripoint Spinach Salad, 2 cups	65							
Nutripoint Lite Caper Dressing, 2 tbs.							2	
Cooked peas and carrots, 1/2 cup	28							
Skim milk, 1 cup						9.5		
Peach Vitari Soft Serve, 1/2 cup		6.5						
Totals:	193	22/ 28.5	15.5	0	13.5	19	.5	263.5 /270
Goals:	55	15	10	5	5	10	0	100

NUTRIPOINT 1,000–1,200 CALORIE MENU								
Day: 7	**Nutripoints**							
Food Selection/Serving Size	Veg.	Fruit	Grain	Leg.	Meat	Milk	Other	
Breakfast:								
Whole Wheat Bagel			4					
Nutripoint Honey Cream Cheese, 1/4 cup						5.5		
Skewer of fresh fruit, 1 cup (pineapple, cantaloupe, strawberries)		52						
Lunch:								
Nutripoint Herbed Lentils and Wild Rice, 1 cup				6.5				
Baked potato	17							
Nutripoint New Way Sour Cream, 1/4 cup						6.5		
Nutripoint Tossed Salad, 1 cup Nutripoint Lite Ranch Dressing, 2 tbs.	26						2	
Cadbury Diet Chocolate Soda, 12 oz.								
Dinner:								
Nutripoint Grilled Chicken w/Mango Sauce, 4 oz.					4.5			
Nutripoint Vegetable Medley, 1 cup	48.5							
Nutripoint Tossed Salad, 1 cup Balsamic vinegar, 1 tbs.	26						0	
Fresh strawberries, 1 cup		19						
No-calorie beverage								
Totals:	117.5	71	4	6.5	4.5	12	2	217.5
Goals:	55	15	10	5	5	10	0	100

NUTRIPOINT 1,000–1,200 CALORIE MENU								
Day: 8	**Nutripoints**							
Food Selection/Serving Size	Veg.	Fruit	Grain	Leg.	Meat	Milk	Other	
Breakfast:								
40+ Bran Flakes, 2/3 cup			21					
Skim milk, 1 cup						9.5		
Fresh-squeezed orange juice, 6 oz.		11.5						
Lunch:								
Nutripoint Aerobics Burger Whole wheat bun			6		5			
Nutripoint Tossed Salad, 2 cups Nutripoint Lite Blue Cheese Dressing, 2 tbs.	51.5						4	
V-8 juice, no salt, 6 oz. (w. lemon)	28.5							
Nutripoint Fruit Salad Plate, 1 cup		28.5						
Dinner:								
Nutripoint Grilled Salmon w. Yellow Bell Pepper Sauce, 4 oz.					7			
Nutripoint Marinated Asparagus, 8 pcs.	38.5							
Nutripoint Spinach Salad, 2 cups Nutripoint Lite Orange Vinaigrette Dressing, 2 tbs.	65						2.5	
Nutripoint Key Lime Mousse, 1/2 cup						5.5		
Totals:	183.5	40	27	0	12	15	6.5	284
Goals:	55	15	10	5	5	10	0	100

NUTRIPOINT 1,000–1,200 CALORIE MENU

Day: 9	Nutripoints							
Food Selection/Serving Size	Veg.	Fruit	Grain	Leg.	Meat	Milk	Other	
Breakfast:								
Instant Total Oatmeal w. skim milk, 1/2 cup			51					
Hot Kashi cereal (pilaf), 1/4 cup			3					
Skim milk, 1 cup						9.5		
Raisins, 1/4 cup		4						
Lunch:								
Nutripoint Chicken Enchiladas, 2 pcs.					5			
Cooked frozen corn, 1/2 cup	8							
Nutripoint Tossed Salad, 2 cups w. fresh red peppers (1/2 pc.) and fresh green peppers (1/2 pc.)	51.5 20							
Nutripoint Lite Ranch Dressing, 2 tbs.							2	
Fresh fruit salad, 1/2 cup		13						
Dinner:								
Nutripoint French Bread Pizza, 1 pc.			6					
Nutripoint Coleslaw, 3/4 cup	15							
Skim milk, 1 cup						9.5		
Mandarin orange in juice, 1/2 cup		15.5						
Totals:	94.5	32.5	60	0	5	19	2	213
Goals:	55	15	10	5	5	10	0	100

NUTRIPOINT 1,000–1,200 CALORIE MENU								
Day: 10	**Nutripoints**							
Food Selection/Serving Size	Veg.	Fruit	Grain	Leg.	Meat	Milk	Other	
Breakfast:								
Just Right cereal w. fruit and nuts, 3/4 cup			36.5					
Skim milk, 1 cup						9.5		
Fresh raspberries, 1/2 cup		12.5						
Lunch:								
Nutripoint Tuna Salad, 1/2 cup					5			
Raw vegetables: Carrots (1 pc.)	35.5							
Celery (2 pcs.)	7							
Radishes (1/3 cup)	10							
Whole wheat bread, 2 pcs.			6					
Fresh apple (1/2 pc.)		2						
Orange slices (1/2 pc.)		7						
Dinner:								
Nutripoint Lentil Soup, 1 cup				13.5				
RyKrisp crackers, 2 pcs.			2					
Nutripoint Spinach Salad, 2 cups	65							
Nutripoint Lite Ranch Dressing, 2 tbs.							2	
Raw cauliflower, 1 cup	40.5							
Low-fat (2-percent) cottage cheese, 1/2 cup						3		
Fresh papaya, 1/2 pc.		20.5						
Totals:	158	29.5	44.5	13.5	5	12.5	2	265
Goals:	55	15	10	5	5	10	0	100

NUTRIPOINT 1,000–1,200 CALORIE MENU								
Day: 11	Nutripoints							
Food Selection/Serving Size	Veg.	Fruit	Grain	Leg.	Meat	Milk	Other	
Breakfast:								
Quaker Puffed Wheat, 1/2 cup			3					
Kretschmer Honey Wheat Germ, 1/4 cup			8					
Skim milk, 1 cup						9.5		
Nutripoint Fresh Fruit Slices, 1 cup		23.5						
Lunch:								
Nutripoint Jambalaya, 1 cup			7.5					
Cooked kidney beans, 1/2 cup (mix with Jambalaya)				8.5				
Nutripoint Tossed Salad, 2 cups Nutripoint Lite Vinaigrette Dressing, 2 tbs.	51.5						-1.5	
Cooked okra, 1/2 cup	31							
Sliced tomatoes, 1/4 pc.	7.5							
Sundance Apple Juice Sparkler, 6 oz.		2.5						
Dinner:								
Pan-fried bass (Pam w/olive oil) w. lemon					7			
Nutripoint Home-Style Potatoes, 1/2 cup	5.5							
Nutripoint Tossed Salad, 1 1/2 cups w. cooked green beans, 1/2 cup	45							
Nutripoint Lite Orange Vinaigrette Dressing, 2 tbs.							2.5	
Dannon low-fat yogurt w. vanilla and Equal to taste, 1 cup						5.5		
Fresh apricot pieces (added to yogurt), 3 pcs.		13.5						
Totals:	140.5	42	18.5	8.5	7	15	1	232.5
Goals:	55	15	10	5	5	10	0	100

NUTRIPOINT 1,000–1,200 CALORIE MENU								
Day: 12	**Nutripoints**							
Food Selection/Serving Size	Veg.	Fruit	Grain	Leg.	Meat	Milk	Other	
Breakfast:								
Whole wheat English muffin, 1 pc.			5.5					
Laughing Cow Reduced-Calorie Cheese, 2 pcs.						2.5		
Sliced fresh nectarine, 1 pc.		10						
Hot herb tea, 1 cup							.5	
Lunch:								
Nutripoint Marinated Hawaiian Chicken, 4 oz.					3.5			
Nutripoint Potato Salad, 1/2 cup	9							
Nutripoint Cold Mixed-Vegetable Salad, 1/2 cup	17							
Fresh mango slices, 1/2 pc.		17.5						
No-calorie beverage								
Dinner:								
Nutripoint Scallop Kabobs w. Scallop Sauce, 2 pcs.					16.5			
Wild rice pilaf, 1/2 cup			6.5					
Tomato slices, 1/2 pc.	15							
Nutripoint Spinach Salad, 2 cups Nutripoint Lite Orange Vinaigrette Dressing, 2 tbs.	65					2.5		
Skim milk, 1 cup						9.5		
Sugar Free Cherry Jell-O Gelatin (w. canned peaches), 1/2 cup		10.5						
Totals:	106	38	12	0	20	12	3	191
Goals:	55	15	10	5	5	10	0	100

NUTRIPOINT 1,000–1,200 CALORIE MENU								
Day: 13	**Nutripoints**							
Food Selection/Serving Size	Veg.	Fruit	Grain	Leg.	Meat	Milk	Other	
Breakfast:								
Nutripoint Oat Bran Muffin, 1 pc.			3.5					
Egg Beaters eggs w. Cheez, 1/2 cup						6		
Fresh kiwi slices, 1 pc.		17						
Lunch:								
Nutripoint Navy Bean Soup, 1 cup (French Market recipe w. navy beans)				17				
Nutripoint Spinach Salad, 2 cups Nutripoint Lite Vinaigrette Dressing, 2 tbs.	65						-1.5	
Honeydew and cantaloupe melon slices, 1 cup		21.5						
No-calorie beverage								
Dinner:								
Nutripoint Chicken Primavera (Tyson's Diced Chicken Meat, 3 oz., and Nutripoint Fresh Pasta Salad, 1 cup)			9		4			
Nutripoint Tossed Salad, 2 cups Nutripoint Blue Cheese Dressing, 2 tbs.	51.5						4	
Skim milk, 1 cup						9.5		
Fresh watermelon chunks, 1 cup		10.5						
Totals:	116.5	49	12.5	17	4	15.5	2.5	217
Goals:	55	15	10	5	5	10	0	100

NUTRIPOINT 1,000–1,200 CALORIE MENU								
Day: 14	**Nutripoints**							
Food Selection/Serving Size	Veg.	Fruit	Grain	Leg.	Meat	Milk	Other	
Breakfast:								
Shredded Wheat 'n Bran cereal, ²/₃ cup			6					
Skim milk, 1 cup						9.5		
Fresh peach slices, 1 pc.		11						
Lunch:								
Nutripoint Angel Hair Pasta w. Sunshine Sauce, 1¹/₂ cups			4.5					
Nutripoint Tossed Salad, 2 cups	51.5							
w. bean sprouts, 1 cup				9				
w. fresh peas, ¹/₄ cup				3.5				
w. garbanzo beans (¹/₄ cup)				2				
Nutripoint Lite Orange Vinaigrette Dressing, 2 tbs.							2.5	
Nutripoint Rainbow Compote, ¹/₂ cup		18						
w. Nutripoint Banana Mint Sauce, 2 tbs.						3		
Dinner:								
Baked sole w. lemon and Butter Buds, 6 oz.					6			
Baby brussels sprouts, ¹/₂ cup	25							
Nutripoint Spinach Salad, 2 cups	65							
Nutripoint Lite Ranch Dressing, 2 tbs.							2	
Nutripoint Bananas Flambé, ¹/₃ cup						2.5		
Totals:	141.5	29	10.5	14.5	6	15	4.5	221
Goals:	55	15	10	5	5	10	0	100

NUTRIPOINT RECIPES

List of Recipes

Soups

Lentil Soup	230
French Market Soup	231
Hot and Sour Soup	232
Wild Rice Soup	233
Clear Spinach Soup	234
Chilled Blueberry Soup	234

Sandwiches

Turkey Sandwich	234
Cajun Chicken Sandwich	235
French Bread Pizza	236
Open-Face Pita Sandwich	236

Salads

Tossed Salad	237
Spinach Salad	237
Black Bean Dip	238
Salad Greens with Balsamic Vinegar	238
Slim Guacamole Dip	239
Coleslaw	239
Tuna Salad	240
Chicken Salad	240
Potato Salad	241
Cold Mixed-Vegetable Salad	241

Vegetable Dishes

South-of-the-Border Vegetarian Chili	242
Vegetable Medley	243
Vegetable Stir-Fry	243
Marinated Asparagus	244
Seasoned Turnip Greens	244
Home-Style Potatoes	245

Seafood Dishes

Scallop Kabobs	245
Red Snapper Veracruz (with Wild Rice)	246
Lettuce-Wrapped Salmon	247
Herb Sauce	247
Jambalaya	248
Grilled Salmon with Yellow Bell Pepper Sauce	249
Crunchy Fish	250

Meat and Poultry Dishes

Aerobics Burger	250
Beef Asada	251
Chicken Enchiladas	252
Chicken Stir-Fry	253
Lemon Chicken	254
Low-Fat Fried Chicken	254

225

Pasta and Grain Dishes

Five-Cheese Casserole 228
Angel Hair Pasta with
  Sunshine Sauce 255
Spinach Lasagna 256
Herbed Lentils and Wild
  Rice 257
Fresh Pasta Salad 258

Fruit Dishes

Fresh Fruit Slices 258
Fruit Salad Plate 258
Rainbow Compote 259
Fresh Fruit Platter 259
Key Lime Mousse 260
Fruit-Yogurt Pie 260
Poached Pears 261
Bananas Flambé 262
Blackberry Freeze 262
Banana Gladje 263
Applesauce 263

Breakfast Dishes

Bran Muffins 264
Oat Bran Muffins 265
French Toast 265
Garden Scrambled
  Eggs 266
Fruited Cinnamon
  Cereal 266
Whole Grain Pancakes 266
Hot Blueberry Topping 267
Hot Peach Topping 267

Hot Red Raspberry
  Topping 268
Honey Cream Cheese 268

Dressings and Sauces

Lite Spicy Mustard
  Dressing 268
Lite Zero Salad Dressing 269
Balsamic Vinegar
  Dressing 269
Blue Cheese Salad
  Dressing 269
Lite 16-Island Dressing 270
Honey Yogurt Dressing 270
Lite Mayonnaise Mix 270
New Way Sour Cream 271
Lite Caper Dressing 271
Lite Vinaigrette Dressing 272
Lite Orange Vinaigrette
  Dressing 272
Lite Ranch Dressing 273
Juniper Berry Marinade
  and Sauce (for Venison,
  Quail, or Chicken) 274
Hawaiian Marinade for
  Chicken or Fish 275
Tomato Sauce 276
Mango Sauce 276
Scallop Sauce 277
Banana Mint Sauce 278

Fruit Drinks

Strawberry Smoothie 278
Sunrise Cooler 278

MODIFYING YOUR FAVORITE RECIPES

Many of us have favorite recipes that we continue to make, even though we know they've got too much fat in them. But they're so good! And the family loves them! And you grew up having them every week, so they bring back memories. The excuses are endless.

We'd like you to pick out four favorite recipes and try modifying them to cut the fat *down,* not *out.* We all know general tips, such as bake, don't fry; use lemon juice and herbs instead of fat for seasoning; replace high-fat dairy products with low-fat ones; choose lean cuts of meat, well trimmed. These aren't new ideas, but sometimes it's hard to translate them into practical reality. Look at the two sample recipes on pages 228 and 229 to see how we do it—then work on some of your own. The text that appears in boldface represents a modification.

———————— • Five-Cheese Casserole • ————————

½ pound **lean** ground beef* ⎱
½ pound ground turkey   ⎰ (vs. hamburger)
1 onion, chopped
15 ounces tomato sauce
¾ teaspoon each dried basil and oregano
¼ teaspoon salt
½ cup **1-percent fat cottage cheese** (vs. 4%)
2 ounces **light cream cheese** (vs. regular: saves half the
   fat)
¼ cup **light sour cream** (vs. regular: saves half the fat)
½ cup **plain lowfat yogurt** (vs. sour cream)
1 tablespoon Parmesan cheese
8 ounces noodles, cooked
½ **cup** grated **part-skim mozzarella** cheese (vs. Swiss)
¼ **cup** grated **sharp cheddar** cheese (vs. ½ cup mild
   Cheddar: sharp is more flavorful, so less can be used)

DIRECTIONS Preheat oven to 350°F. Cook meat in **non-stick skillet** until browned (no fat needed for browning). **Pour off any excess fat and rinse meat with warm water.** Add onion and cook for 5 minutes. Stir in tomato sauce and seasonings. In a separate bowl blend together cottage cheese, cream cheese, sour cream, yogurt, and Parmesan cheese. Spray a 9 × 13-inch baking dish with **no-stick vegetable oil cooking spray** (instead of regular oil). Layer the baking dish with half the noodles, half the meat sauce, and all of the cheese mixture. Repeat with the rest of the noodles and sauce. Top with mozzarella and cheddar cheeses. Bake 30 minutes.

This recipe yields six very large servings. Before making our modifications, each serving contained 470 calories and 30 grams of fat. With our changes, each serving now has 317 calories and 10 grams of fat. It's amazing what a little creativity can do. Note that we didn't "save" by cutting down the total amount of food, but by making lower-calorie substitu-

* Try adding broccoli or any other vegetable to increase portion size and decrease calories (broccoli has only 25 calories per half cup).

tions. And we didn't remove the things that make it wonderful, such as the bubbling cheese on top. Remember, healthy eating can also taste good.

SERVES: 6   SERVING SIZE: 1 heaping cup

5.5 nutripoints

―――――――――― • Bran Muffins • ――――――――――

1½ cups **Whole Wheat Total** (or any other bran cereal)
½ cup **orange juice** (vs. ½ cup apple juice), boiling
4 **egg whites** (vs. 3 eggs)
½ cup ½-percent-fat buttermilk
4 ounces **orange juice concentrate** (vs. 4 ounces apple juice concentrate)
3 tablespoons safflower oil ⎫
1 large ripe **banana**, mashed ⎬ (vs. ½ cup safflower oil)
½ cup **currants** (vs. ½ cup raisins)
2 **tablespoons** honey, brown sugar, or molasses (vs. ¾ cup)
½ teaspoon vanilla extract
1 cup **whole wheat flour** ⎫
½ cup white flour ⎬ (vs. 1½ cups white flour)
1½ teaspoons baking soda
2 teaspoons baking powder
¾ teaspoon ground cinnamon
¾ teaspoon ground nutmeg
Zest of 1 orange, chopped fine

DIRECTIONS   Preheat oven to 400°F. Combine Total in a large bowl with boiling orange juice. Let cool. Add the egg whites, milk, orange juice concentrate, oil, banana, currants, honey, and vanilla. Mix well. In a small bowl, combine flours, baking soda, baking powder, and spices. Add to wet mixture and mix very well.* Spray a 12-cup muffin tin with **nonstick spray**. Spoon batter into muffin cups. Bake for 20 minutes, or until done.

SERVES: 12   SERVING SIZE: 1 muffin   10.5 nutripoints

*Batter can be stored in refrigerator up to two weeks.

SOUPS

──────────── • Lentil Soup • ────────────

- 3 medium tomatoes, diced
- 2 cups dried lentils
- 3 medium onions, chopped
- 3 carrots, chopped
- 4 celery stalks, chopped
- 3 small potatoes, peeled and diced
- 4 sprigs parsley, chopped
- 1 can (28 oz.) tomatoes, with liquid
- 1 green pepper, chopped
- 3 cloves garlic, minced
- 2 bay leaves
- 2 tablespoons dried basil
- 1 teaspoon cayenne pepper
- 8 cups vegetable stock or chicken stock (low-sodium)
- 1 teaspoon salt
  Freshly ground black pepper

DIRECTIONS   In a large pot, combine all ingredients except the black pepper. Bring to a boil, cover, and simmer for 2 to 3 hours. Add black pepper to taste.

SERVES: 10   SERVING SIZE: 1½ cup   13.5 nutripoints

per serving

———————— • French Market Soup • ————————

¼ cup dried pinto beans
¼ cup dried lentils
¼ cup dried red beans
¼ cup dried split peas
¼ cup dried black beans
¼ cup dried black-eyed peas
¼ cup dried navy beans
¼ cup dried baby lima beans
¼ cup dried barley

DIRECTIONS   Thoroughly mix dry beans in bowl. Split into two equal portions. Use one portion for this recipe and save other portion until you make the soup again. Soak beans overnight in 1½ quarts of water. Pour out soaking water and place the beans in a large Dutch oven with 1½ quarts of fresh water. Bring to a boil, reduce heat and simmer for 3 hours, and then add:

3 stalks celery, chopped
1 15-ounce can tomato sauce
1 medium onion, chopped
2 bay leaves
1 green bell pepper, seeded and chopped
¼ teaspoon dried thyme
1 14½-ounce can tomatoes
1 clove garlic
6 ounces lean turkey ham, cut into small pieces

DIRECTIONS   Continue to cook 1 to 1½ hours. Just before serving, add black pepper to taste.

SERVES: 12   SERVING SIZE: 1 cup   17.0 nutripoints

—————————— • Hot and Sour Soup • ——————————

   4 black Chinese mushrooms (follow package directions
      for dried mushrooms), sliced
 1/4 pound boneless lean pork, cut into matchsticks
      (optional)
   1 tablespoon dry sherry
   4 cups chicken broth
   1 1/2-pound chicken breast, cut into matchsticks
 1/4 pound tofu, cut into half-inch cubes
   2 tablespoons rice wine vinegar
   1 tablespoon soy sauce
   2 tablespoons cornstarch
 1/4 cup water
1/2–3/4 teaspoon white pepper
 1/2 cup sliced bamboo shoots
   1 teaspoon sesame oil
   1 egg white, lightly beaten
   2 scallions, chopped

DIRECTIONS   Combine pork with sherry and let stand 10
minutes. Heat chicken broth to boil and add mushrooms,
pork, chicken, and bamboo shoots. Stir, reduce heat, cover,
and simmer for 5 minutes. Add tofu, vinegar, and soy sauce.
Heat covered 1 minute. Blend cornstarch with cold water.
Add to soup and cook until thickened. Add pepper and sesame oil. Slowly pour beaten egg white into soup while stirring. Sprinkle with scallions. Serve.

SERVES: 8   SERVING SIZE: 1 cup   4.0 nutripoints

———————— • Wild Rice Soup • ————————

        2 teaspoons margarine
      1/2 cup leeks, finely diced
      1/2 onion, finely diced
      1/2 cup carrots, finely diced
      1/2 cup celery, finely diced
        1 red pepper, seeded and finely diced
        1 tablespoon flour
    2 1/2 cups chicken stock
      1/3 cup wild rice
      1-2 tablespoons dry sherry
      1/8 teaspoon salt
      1/2 cup evaporated skim milk
        1 teaspoon chopped parsley

DIRECTIONS In a 2- to 3-quart saucepan, heat the margarine over medium heat. Add the leek, onion, carrots, celery, and red pepper. Cover pot and "sweat" the vegetables until translucent, about 7 minutes. Add the flour and stir well. Cook gently over low heat for approximately 3 minutes, stirring constantly. Add chicken stock gradually, making an increasingly thinner paste, until all stock has been added. Simmer 10 minutes. Add the wild rice, sherry, and salt. Simmer until rice grains have swollen and are tender, 30 to 40 minutes. Add evaporated skim milk and continue to cook on gentle heat. Garnish with parsley (you may want to add a dash more sherry just before serving).

SERVES: 8   SERVING SIZE: 1 cup   10.5 nutripoints

————————• Clear Spinach Soup •————————

    3 cans low-sodium chicken broth
    2 cups chopped fresh spinach
    1 tomato, chopped
    1 tablespoon low-calorie margarine
      Juice of 1/2 lemon
      Mrs. Dash (seasoning) and black pepper to taste

DIRECTIONS   Bring broth to a boil. Add remaining ingredients and cook until spinach barely wilts. Serve immediately.
    SERVES: 6   SERVING SIZE: 1/2 cup   23.5 nutripoints

————————• Chilled Blueberry Soup •————————

    2 cups fresh or frozen blueberries (no added sugar)
  3/4 cup apple juice
  1/2 cup orange juice
    1 drop lemon extract
      Dash of freshly grated nutmeg
      Orange slices
      Plain nonfat yogurt

DIRECTIONS   Place first 4 ingredients in a saucepan. Bring to a boil over medium heat. Reduce heat and simmer 1 to 2 minutes. Add nutmeg. Pour soup into a blender and process until smooth. Chill. Garnish with orange slices and dollops of yogurt.
    SERVES: 4   SERVING SIZE: 3/4 cup   6.0 nutripoints

SANDWICHES

————————• Turkey Sandwich •————————

    2 slices whole wheat bread
    1 teaspoon low-cal. mayonnaise
    2 teaspoons plain low-fat yogurt
    1 ounce turkey, skinless light meat
  1/4 cup alfalfa sprouts
  1/4 tomato

DIRECTIONS   Toast bread. Mix mayonnaise and yogurt in a small bowl. Spread mayonnaise mixture on toast. Assemble using remaining ingredients.

SERVES: 1   SERVING SIZE: 1 sandwich   4.0 nutripoints

————————— • Cajun Chicken Sandwich • —————————

        5 skinless, boneless chicken breasts
     10 slices whole grain bread, toasted
        2 cups coarsely shredded lettuce

MARINADE: 1/4 cup water
            1/4 cup Kikkoman teriyaki marinade
            1/4 cup red wine
       1 1/2 teaspoons dried thyme
       1 1/4 teaspoons cayenne pepper
       1 1/4 teaspoons black pepper
       1 1/4 teaspoons white pepper
          1 teaspoon garlic powder

SPREAD: 1/2 tablespoon plain nonfat yogurt
            1/2 tablespoon light mayonnaise
          1 tablespoon prepared horseradish

DIRECTIONS   Combine marinade ingredients in a shallow glass casserole. Place chicken fillets in marinade, turning once to coat. Cover and refrigerate 2 to 4 hours. Remove chicken from marinade.

Combine yogurt, mayonnaise, and horseradish in a small bowl. Spread one side of each toasted bread slice with the mayonnaise mixture. Place shredded lettuce on half of the slices.

Grill marinated fillets over medium-hot coals approximately 4 minutes on each side, or until chicken is done. Add to sandwich and serve.

SERVES: 5   SERVING SIZE: 1 sandwich   5.5 nutripoints

• French Bread Pizza •

    4 slices French bread
    2 ounces part-skim mozzarella cheese
  ²⁄₃ cup tomato sauce
  ¼ cup chopped onion
  ¼ cup chopped green pepper
  ¼ cup canned artichoke hearts, chopped
    2 teaspoons grated Parmesan cheese

DIRECTIONS Preheat oven to 350°F. Slice French bread into pieces 1 inch thick. Spread with tomato sauce that has been mixed with chopped, steamed vegetables. Top with mozzarella and Parmesan cheeses. Bake until cheese melts.

SERVES: 2   SERVING SIZE: 2 slices   6.0 nutripoints

• Open-Face Pita Sandwich •

  ¼ cup julienned carrots
  ¼ cup julienned zucchini
  ¼ cup sliced mushrooms
  ¼ cup julienned onion
  ¼ cup julienned bell pepper
      Salt
      Freshly ground black pepper
      Mrs. Dash
    4 teaspoons mustard
    2 pita breads
    4 slices tomato
    2 ounces shredded mozzarella cheese

DIRECTIONS Preheat oven to 375°F. Sauté vegetables in water or steam until tender. Drain and season to taste. Spread a thin layer of mustard on top of whole, unsplit pita. Top with vegetables, tomato slices, and cheese. Bake until cheese melts.

SERVES: 2   SERVING SIZE: 1 whole pita

                                                5.0 nutripoints

SALADS

————————— • Tossed Salad • —————————

   1 cup romaine lettuce leaves, torn
   ½ cup fresh spinach leaves, torn
   3 cherry tomatoes
   ⅛ cup purple cabbage, shredded
   2 cucumber slices
   1 mushroom, sliced

DIRECTIONS   Wash vegetables. Combine ingredients and toss.

   SERVES: 1   SERVING SIZE: 2 cups   51.5 nutripoints

————————— • Spinach Salad • —————————

   1½ cups spinach leaves, chopped
   2 fresh mushrooms, sliced
   1 radish, sliced
   ¼ tomato, chopped

DIRECTIONS   Wash vegetables. Combine ingredients and toss.

   SERVES: 1   SERVING SIZE: 2 cups   65.0 nutripoints

• Black Bean Dip •

1 cup canned black bean soup
1 clove garlic, pressed
2 tablespoons Worcestershire sauce
1 tablespoon salsa (picante sauce)
½ tablespoon black pepper
2 teaspoons celery seed

DIRECTIONS   Place all ingredients in food processor or blender and process until smooth. Add bean mixture to skillet and heat to reduce liquid volume. Remove from heat when mixture thickens. Refrigerate dip to allow mixture to continue to thicken. Serve with corn tortillas.

SERVES: 8   SERVING SIZE: 2 tablespoons

8.0 nutripoints

• Salad Greens with Balsamic Vinegar •

4 cups any combination of salad greens (red leaf lettuce, spinach, Boston lettuce, endive)
1 cup fresh basil leaves
Balsamic vinegar to taste
Equal to taste (optional)
Freshly ground black pepper to taste

DIRECTIONS   Wash and thoroughly dry the combination of leaves. Add just enough balsamic vinegar to satisfy your taste. You might like to try mixing Equal with the vinegar before adding it to the greens. Top with freshly ground pepper.

SERVES: 4   SERVING SIZE: 1 cup   42.0 nutripoints

———————————— • Slim Guacamole Dip • ————————————

    1 ripe avocado, chopped and mashed
    2 tablespoons fresh lime juice
  2–3 tablespoons salsa (picante sauce)
    1 ripe tomato, finely chopped
    2 tablespoons plain low-fat yogurt
  1/4 small yellow onion, finely chopped
  1/2 bell pepper, seeded and finely chopped
      Freshly ground black pepper to taste
  1/4 teaspoon ground cumin

DIRECTIONS   Mix all ingredients and serve with tortilla
chips.
  SERVES: 8   SERVING SIZE: 1/4 cup   7.5 nutripoints

———————————————— • Coleslaw • ————————————————

    3 cups green cabbage, shredded
    3 cups purple cabbage, shredded
    1 large onion, sliced
    2 carrots, shredded
    1 green pepper, seeded and sliced

DRESSING: 3/4 cup vinegar
            Sweet 'n' Low to taste*
        1/4 teaspoon salt
          1 teaspoon celery seed
        3/4 teaspoon dry mustard
        1/4 cup olive oil

DIRECTIONS   Mix first 5 dressing ingredients together and
bring to a boil. Add olive oil. Combine salad ingredients and
toss with hot dressing. Chill.
  SERVES: 8   SERVING SIZE: 1 cup   10.0 nutripoints

*If Equal used, do not add until salad is cool.

─────────────── • Tuna Salad • ───────────────

1 6½-ounce can water-packed tuna
1 stalk celery, diced
2 tablespoons fresh parsley, minced
⅛ cup onion, diced
¼ cup apple, diced
⅛ cup sweet pickle relish
½ cup grapes, cut in half
⅛ cup carrots, diced
¼ cup plain nonfat yogurt
⅛ cup light mayonnaise
1 tablespoon sesame seeds
¼ teaspoon dried dill
   Freshly ground pepper to taste

DIRECTIONS Mix all ingredients together. Chill and serve.

SERVES: 4   SERVING SIZE: ½ cup   5.0 nutripoints

─────────────── • Chicken Salad • ───────────────

3 cups cooked, diced chicken breast (grilled chicken recommended)
1½ cups celery, diced
½ cup scallions, diced
¼ cup fresh parsley, minced
1 cup water chestnuts, diced
1 apple, diced
2 tablespoons whole-grain mustard
½ cup low-fat buttermilk
2½ tablespoons light mayonnaise
2½ tablespoons plain nonfat yogurt
1½ tablespoons lemon juice
   Pinch of salt
   Freshly ground black pepper to taste

DIRECTIONS Mix first 6 ingredients and set aside. Mix remaining ingredients in a separate bowl and then add to chicken mixture.

SERVES: 15   SERVING SIZE: ½ cup   6.5 nutripoints

——————— • Potato Salad • ———————

6 1/2 cups unpeeled new potatoes, boiled, cooled, and diced
  2 hard-boiled egg whites, diced
  1 bunch scallions, chopped
1/8 cup sweet pickle relish
  1 tablespoon whole-grain mustard
2 1/2 tablespoons light mayonnaise
1 1/2 tablespoons orange juice concentrate
1/2 teaspoon rice wine vinegar
  1 tablespoon low-fat buttermilk
1/4 cup fresh parsley, minced
    Celery seed to taste
    Cayenne pepper to taste
    Freshly ground black pepper to taste
    Pinch of salt

DIRECTIONS Mix well, chill, and serve.
SERVES: 13 SERVING SIZE: 1/2 cup 9.0 nutripoints

——————— • Cold Mixed-Vegetable Salad • ———————

16 ounces frozen mixed vegetables (defrosted)
  1 6-ounce can kidney beans (drained)
  1 cup sliced water chestnuts (drained)
1/3 cup Bernstein's Low Calorie Italian salad dressing*
1/4 cup apple juice concentrate
  1 tablespoon rice wine vinegar
    Juice of 1/2 lemon
1–2 cloves garlic, pressed
    Freshly ground black pepper to taste

DIRECTIONS Combine vegetables and beans in a bowl.
Mix remaining ingredients separately. Pour mixture over
vegetables. Mix well and let marinate for at least 30 minutes.
Serve as a salad, or use on top of fresh greens.
SERVES: 6 SERVING SIZE: 1/2 cup 17.0 nutripoints

*Or substitute another low-calorie Italian dressing.

VEGETABLE DISHES

────── • South-of-the-Border Vegetarian Chili • ──────

```
    2  15-ounce cans black beans, rinsed and drained
    1  tablespoon cumin seed
1 1/2  teaspoons dried oregano
1 1/2  teaspoons dried basil
    1  tablespoon olive oil
    1  yellow onion, chopped
    1  green pepper, chopped
    1  yellow pepper, chopped
1 1/2  cups carrots, sliced
    2  cloves garlic, minced
    2  teaspoons paprika
  1/2  teaspoon cayenne pepper
    2  tablespoons chili powder
  1/4  teaspoon Morton Lite Salt
1 1/2  cups canned crushed tomatoes (salt-free), juice reserved
    2  fresh jalapeño peppers, minced (remove seeds)
  1/4  cup plain nonfat yogurt
    2  fresh tomatoes, chopped
```

DIRECTIONS In small nonstick skillet over medium heat, toast cumin seed, oregano, and basil, shaking pan occasionally until fragrant (5–10 minutes). Remove from heat.

In skillet over medium-high heat, heat oil until very hot. Add onion, peppers, carrots, garlic, toasted herbs, paprika, cayenne, chili powder, and Lite Salt. Sauté 5–10 minutes. Add canned tomatoes, some tomato juice, and jalapeño pepper. Bring to a boil. Add beans; continue to simmer. Add fresh tomatoes; heat thoroughly.

Top with yogurt to serve.

SERVES: 8   SERVING SIZE: 3/4 cup   13.0 nutripoints

————————— • Vegetable Medley • —————————

> ¼ cup julienned bell pepper
> ¼ cup julienned carrots
> ¼ cup julienned broccoli
> Salt
> Freshly ground pepper

DIRECTIONS Combine ingredients and steam or microwave until tender. Season to taste with McCormick's Salt Free Parsley Patch or Mrs. Dash.

SERVES: 1   SERVING SIZE: ¾ cup   48.5 nutripoints

————————— • Vegetable Stir-Fry • —————————

> 1 egg white
> 1 tablespoon sherry
> 1 tablespoon cornstarch
> 1 tablespoon peanut oil
> ¼ cup low-sodium soy sauce
> 1 cup sliced carrots
> ½ cup chopped scallions
> 1 clove garlic
> 1 small green pepper, thinly sliced
> 1 small red pepper, thinly sliced
> 1 cup zucchini, sliced
> 1 cup bok choy, shredded
> 1 cup fresh mushrooms, thinly sliced
> 1 cup broccoli, chopped
> 1 cup sliced water chestnuts
> ⅓ cup almonds, slivered

DIRECTIONS Combine egg white, sherry, and cornstarch; stir well.

Heat oil in a large skillet. Add soy sauce and carrots, stirring well. Stir-fry 2 minutes. Add scallions, garlic, and peppers; stir-fry an additional 2 to 3 minutes. Add zucchini, bok choy, mushrooms, broccoli, water chestnuts, and almonds; cook 2 to 3 minutes. Serve over hot rice.

SERVES: 6   SERVING SIZE: ¾ cup   13.5 nutripoints

——————— • Marinated Asparagus • ———————

32 fresh asparagus spears
1½ tablespoons Bernstein's Low Calorie Italian dressing
1½ tablespoons low-calorie vinaigrette dressing*
1 pimiento, cut into four long strips

DIRECTIONS Wash and trim asparagus spears. Steam until tender (or microwave). Drain. Place in flat container. Add salad dressings and marinate in refrigerator until cold. To serve: wrap 8 spears of asparagus in one long piece of pimiento. Tie pimiento into a bow if possible.

SERVES: 4   SERVING SIZE: 8 spears   38.5 nutripoints

——————— • Seasoned Turnip Greens • ———————

¼ cup water
2 cups chopped turnip greens
¼ teaspoon ground black pepper
Tobasco to taste (optional)
1 ounce turkey ham (optional)
2 tablespoons Butter Buds, not reconstituted

DIRECTIONS Bring water to a boil. Add turnip greens, pepper, and Tobasco and turkey ham, if using. Cover and simmer until tender, adding water as needed. When tender, add Butter Buds and serve.

SERVES: 4   SERVING SIZE: ½ cup   67.0 nutripoints

*May omit Bernstein's and use 3 tablespoons of another low-calorie vinaigrette dressing.

————————— • Home-Style Potatoes • —————————

  5 cups unpeeled new potatoes, cooked and diced
1 1/2 tablespoons olive oil
1 1/2 tablespoons water
  3/4 teaspoon paprika
  1/2 teaspoon garlic powder
  1/2 teaspoon ground black pepper
      Dash of cayenne pepper
      Pinch of salt
      Sprinkle of Parmesan cheese

DIRECTIONS Preheat oven to 425°F. Mix potatoes with oil, water, paprika, garlic powder, pepper, and salt. (Hands work best for mixing.) Spray a cookie sheet with a nonstick spray. Spread potato mixture on cookie sheet. Bake for at least 1 hour, or until done. Sprinkle lightly with Parmesan cheese.

SERVES: 9 SERVING SIZE: 1/2 cup 5.5 nutripoints

SEAFOOD DISHES

————————— • Scallop Kabobs • —————————

  6 ounces scallops*
  1/2 green pepper
  1/2 yellow pepper
  4 mushrooms
  4 cherry tomatoes
  1/4 onion
  4 skewers

DIRECTIONS Wash scallops. Cut vegetables into large pieces to be skewered. Skewer scallops and vegetables. Grill over open flame until done, about 5 minutes. (Indoor method: place under oven broiler until brown.)

  Serve with Scallop Sauce (see page 277).

SERVES: 2 SERVING SIZE: 2 skewers 16.0 nutripoints

* You may substitute chunks of chicken, swordfish, fresh tuna, beef, or venison for scallops.

—— • Red Snapper Veracruz (with wild rice) • ——

1 1½-pound red snapper, dressed
3½ tablespoons fresh lime juice
   Vegetable cooking spray
1 teaspoon olive oil
1 medium onion, thinly sliced
3 cloves garlic, minced
2½ cups peeled, chopped tomatoes (about 2 large tomatoes)
2 small fresh green chili peppers, seeded and halved, *or*
   1–2 tablespoons canned green chili peppers
2 cups cooked wild rice
   Fresh cilantro sprigs (optional)

DIRECTIONS Preheat oven to 400°F. Brush inside and outside of fish with lime juice. Place in a shallow roasting pan coated with vegetable oil spray, and set aside.

Coat a skillet with cooking spray; add oil, and place over medium heat until hot. Add onion and garlic; sauté 3 minutes. Add tomatoes and peppers; cook 5 minutes, stirring frequently.

Spoon sauce over fish; cover with foil and bake for 25 minutes. Place fish on bed of wild rice and garnish with fresh cilantro sprigs, if desired.

SERVES: 4   SERVING SIZE: 3 ounces fish, ⅓ cup sauce, and ½ cup rice   13.5 nutripoints

———————— • Lettuce-Wrapped Salmon • ————————

16 to 20 lettuce leaves
4 4- to 5-ounce salmon steaks
Juice of 1 lemon
Salt and pepper to taste

DIRECTIONS   Place 4 or 5 lettuce leaves in steamer; cover and steam over boiling water 1 minute, or until barely wilted. Drain on paper towels. Repeat with remainder of leaves.

Spread out 4 or 5 of the steamed lettuce leaves, slightly overlapping. Place one salmon steak on leaves, season with lemon juice, salt, and pepper to taste. Wrap lettuce around fish to enclose completely. Repeat with remaining steaks.

Place fish packets in steamer. Cover and steam until done (7–10 minutes). Remove cooked fish. Roll into heated serving dish. Ladle Herb Sauce (see recipe below) over fish.

SERVES: 4   SERVING SIZE: 1 4- to 5-ounce salmon steak

10.5 nutripoints

——————————— • Herb Sauce • ———————————

1 cup parsley leaves
1 clove garlic
1 teaspoon dried (or fresh) tarragon leaves
1 teaspoon sugar
8 ounces plain low-fat yogurt
Salt and pepper to taste
1 tablespoon lemon juice
Other spices as desired (dill, capers, etc.)

DIRECTIONS   Place parsley, garlic, tarragon, sugar, and ¼ cup of the yogurt in food processor; whirl to blend. Stir herb mixture into remaining ¾ cup yogurt. Add lemon juice, salt, and pepper. Spice as desired.

SERVES: 6   SERVING SIZE: ¼ cup   10.5 nutripoints

• Jambalaya* •

2 cups chopped onion
1 cup chopped celery
1 cup chopped green pepper
1 1/2 teaspoons minced garlic
1 1/2 teaspoons olive oil
2 1/2 cups low-sodium chicken stock
Cayenne pepper to taste
2 teaspoons Kitchen Bouquet
1 1/2 cups brown rice
1/2 cup wild rice
1 cup chopped scallions
1/2 cup chopped tomato

DIRECTIONS Sauté onion, celery, pepper, and garlic in olive oil to desired tenderness. Add chicken broth and cayenne, and bring to a boil. Add Kitchen Bouquet and rices. Return to boil. Cover and simmer for 10 minutes. Remove cover and stir. Continue cooking, uncovered, until rice is tender (approximately 20 minutes). Add more water if needed. Add scallions and chopped tomato. Serve. Freeze remainder of recipe in 1-cup servings.

SERVES: 12   SERVING SIZE: 1 cup   7.5 nutripoints

* May add chicken or lean beef if desired.

• Grilled Salmon with Yellow Bell Pepper Sauce •

            2 large yellow bell peppers
            3 tablespoons extra-virgin olive oil
            3 cloves garlic, minced
            2 shallots
          1/8 teaspoon white peppercorns
            1 tablespoon fresh thyme, chopped
          3–4 ounces dry white wine
         1 1/2 tablespoons lemon juice
            4 4- to 5-ounce salmon steaks*
               Red bell pepper strips
               Salt to taste
            4 fresh oregano sprigs

DIRECTIONS Roast yellow bell peppers in a 400°F. oven
or on grill until skins crack. Remove and let cool. Peel flesh
and remove seeds and membranes. Reserve bell pepper flesh.

Heat olive oil in a saucepan and sauté garlic and shallots
for approximately 1 minute. Add white peppercorns, thyme,
salt, and wine. Lower heat to simmer; add lemon juice and
cook until liquid is reduced by half.

Strain liquid into food processor. Add reserved bell pepper. Blend well.

Grill salmon steaks over hot coals until done, about 5
minutes per side.

Spoon bell pepper sauce onto each of 4 serving plates; top
with salmon steaks. Garnish with red bell pepper strips and
oregano.

SERVES: 4   SERVING SIZE: 1 4- to 5-ounce steak.

7.0 nutripoints

*Swordfish, halibut, or any firm-fleshed fish can be substituted.

• Crunchy Fish •

Lemon juice
3 fish fillets, about ½-inch thick (3½ ounces each)
½ cup Nutri-Grain nuggets, Bran Buds, or Grape-Nuts
cereal
1 tablespoon sesame seeds
1 tablespoon dried lemon peel
¼ cup flour
4 egg whites, beaten
Fresh parsley
Lemon slices

DIRECTIONS Preheat oven to 400°F. Rinse fish and pat
dry. (You may wish to marinate fish in lemon juice 30 minutes
before cooking.) Mix cereal, sesame seeds, and lemon peel in
a shallow pan. Put flour and egg whites in separate shallow
pans.

Thinly coat fish with flour, dip into egg whites, and then
into cereal-seed mixture. Arrange fish on ungreased baking
sheet; bake until done (5 minutes per ½ inch for fresh fish,
and 10 minutes per ½ inch if frozen; fish turns opaque).
Garnish with parsley and lemon.

SERVES: 3 SERVING SIZE: 1 3½-ounce fillet

6.5 nutripoints

MEAT AND POULTRY DISHES

• Aerobics Burger •

3 ounces lean ground round steak
1 whole wheat bun
¼ cup alfalfa sprouts
½ tomato
1 teaspoon mustard

DIRECTIONS Form beef into a patty. Grill beef over hot
coals or under oven broiler to desired doneness. Remove

excess grease by blotting with a paper towel. Assemble sandwich with remaining ingredients and serve.

SERVES: 1   SERVING SIZE: 1 3-ounce burger

5.0 nutripoints

• Beef Asada •
---

8 ounces lean beef flank steak
Salsa (picante sauce)
1 cup tomato, diced
4 whole wheat tortillas

STEAMED VEGETABLES:
1 cup onion, diced
1 cup green bell pepper, diced
1 cup yellow bell pepper, diced

SLIM GUACAMOLE DIP:
1/2 avocado, mashed
1 tablespoon lime juice
1–1 1/2 tablespoons salsa (picante sauce)
1/2 tomato, diced
1 tablespoon plain nonfat yogurt
2 1/2 tablespoons diced onion
1/4 bell pepper, diced
1/4 teaspoon freshly ground black pepper
1/8 teaspoon cumin seed

DIRECTIONS Marinate flank steak in salsa overnight.
Grill until done, 5–7 minutes per side. Slice across grain into
thin strips.

Steam (or microwave) vegetables until tender. Stir together
the guacamole ingredients.

To serve, place the diced tomato and beef strips on the
tortilla. Top with steamed vegetables and guacamole. Roll up
tortillas and serve.

SERVES: 4   SERVING SIZE: 1 filled tortilla

7.0 nutripoints

--------------------• Chicken Enchiladas •--------------------

1 onion, chopped
2 cups frozen corn
2 cups mushrooms, sliced
1 can (10¾-ounce) low-sodium cream of chicken (or low-sodium cream of mushroom) soup
1 cup plain yogurt
1 cup mozzarella cheese (divided use)
1 small can chopped green chili peppers
½ teaspoon cumin
½ teaspoon garlic powder
1 teaspoon chili powder
Black pepper to taste
1 cup cooked, diced chicken (try Tyson's frozen diced chicken)
10 corn tortillas

DIRECTIONS Preheat the oven to 350°F. Sauté onion, corn, and mushrooms (microwave works well). Add soup, yogurt, ½ cup cheese, chili peppers, and spices. Heat, but do not boil. Add chicken. Stir and heat 10 minutes. In a 9 × 13-inch pan, layer half of the mixture on 5 tortillas and then repeat. Top with remaining cheese. (You can make individual tortillas, if you prefer.) Bake for 20 minutes.

SERVES: 5   SERVING SIZE: 2 tortillas   5.0 nutripoints

———————— • Chicken Stir-Fry • ————————

      1   egg white
      1   tablespoon sherry
      1   tablespoon cornstarch
     12   ounces boneless chicken breast, skinned
      1   tablespoon peanut oil
    1/4   cup soy sauce (low-sodium)
      1   cup carrots, sliced
    1/2   cup sliced scallions
      1   clove garlic, minced
      1   small green pepper, thinly sliced
      1   small red pepper, thinly sliced
      1   cup zucchini, sliced
      1   cup bok choy, shredded
      1   cup fresh mushrooms, thinly sliced
      1   cup broccoli, chopped
      1   cup water chestnuts
    1/3   cup almonds, slivered

DIRECTIONS   Combine egg white, sherry, and cornstarch;
stir well. Cut chicken into bite-size pieces and add to sherry
mixture, tossing gently to coat. Let stand 1 hour.

   Heat oil in a large skillet. Remove chicken from marinade;
sauté chicken in oil until lightly browned. Add soy sauce and
carrots, stirring well. Cook 2 minutes. Add scallions, garlic,
and peppers; stir-fry an additional 2 to 3 minutes. Add zucchini, bok choy, mushrooms, broccoli, water chestnuts, and
almonds; cook 2 to 3 minutes. Serve over hot rice.

   SERVES: 6   SERVING SIZE: 1 cup   8.5 nutripoints

——————— • Lemon Chicken • ———————

1 tablespoon grated lemon rind
½ cup lemon juice
⅛ cup water
⅛ cup corn oil
2 teaspoons soy sauce
1 clove garlic, minced
½ teaspoon Morton's Lite Salt
½ teaspoon ground black pepper
6 4-ounce chicken breasts, skin removed
½ cup flour
1 teaspoon paprika

DIRECTIONS Mix together lemon rind and juice, water, oil, soy sauce, garlic, Lite Salt, and pepper. Pour over chicken. Cover and refrigerate at least 3 hours, or overnight.

Preheat oven to 400° F. Drain chicken, reserving marinade. Combine flour with paprika and coat chicken. Shake off excess. Place in single layer with tops down in shallow pan and bake for 30 minutes.

Turn chicken. Pour marinade over chicken; bake 30 minutes longer, or until tender, basting occasionally.

SERVES: 6   SERVING SIZE: 1 4-ounce chicken breast
3.5 nutripoints

——————— • Low-Fat Fried Chicken • ———————

⅓ cup flour
½ teaspoon salt
½ teaspoon paprika
¼ teaspoon cayenne pepper
¼ teaspoon onion powder or garlic powder
⅛ teaspoon black pepper
4 4-ounce pieces skinless, boneless chicken (3 ounces cooked)
1 tablespoon olive oil
¾ cup water

DIRECTIONS Combine flour and spices in plastic bag or in bowl. Coat chicken in seasoned flour. Heat tablespoon oil in large nonstick skillet. Quickly add chicken. Brown over medium heat 5 to 10 minutes per side, until golden brown on all sides. Preheat oven to 350° F. Remove chicken from skillet and place on a cookie sheet which has been sprayed with nonstick vegetable spray. Bake until done (approximately 30 minutes).

SERVES: 4   SERVING SIZE: 3 ounces cooked chicken
3.0 nutripoints

PASTA AND GRAIN DISHES

——• Angel Hair Pasta with Sunshine Sauce •——

          1 tablespoon olive oil
          1 clove garlic, minced
          2 14 ½-ounce cans plum tomatoes, diced
          2 cups fresh Roma tomatoes, diced
        ½ onion, chopped
          1 yellow pepper, seeded and chopped
            Pinch of salt
            Freshly ground pepper
            Italian seasoning to taste
          1 package (or cube) low-sodium chicken broth
          1 tablespoon sugar
          4 tablespoons fresh parsley, chopped
          1 tablespoon freshly grated Parmesan cheese
          2 peeled, sliced, and slivered yellow onions
    12–16 ounces angel hair pasta

DIRECTIONS   Over low flame heat ½ tablespoon olive oil in saucepan. Add garlic and cook until soft. Add tomatoes, chopped onion, yellow pepper, salt, pepper, Italian seasoning, chicken broth, and sugar. Stir and cook uncovered over medium heat 15 minutes. Add parsley and cheese. Remove from heat. Keep warm.

Line cookie sheet with foil. Spread slivered onions on sheet and toss lightly with remaining ½ tablespoon olive oil. Place under broiler and cook until onions are wilted and slightly brown.

Cook pasta; drain and rinse. Top pasta with sauce. Sprinkle with onions. Serve.

SERVES: 6   SERVING SIZE: 1½ cups   10.0 nutripoints

——————————— • Spinach Lasagna • ———————————

30 ounces frozen spinach
 2 egg whites
 8 large lasagna noodles
 6 cups Nutripoint Tomato Sauce (see page 276) or use
   bottled sauce
1½ cups 1-percent-fat cottage cheese, partially drained
 3 cups skim mozzarella cheese, sliced
¼ cup grated Parmesan cheese (Formagg brand)

DIRECTIONS This recipe requires one very large lasagna
pan. Defrost frozen spinach and drain very well. Mix with egg
white. Set aside. Cook lasagna noodles, drain, and rinse.
Preheat oven to 350° F. Layer ingredients as follows:

> 1½ cups sauce
> 4 lasagna noodles
> 1½ cups sauce
> ¾ cup cottage cheese
> 1½ cups mozzarella cheese
> 1½ cups spinach
> 4 lasagna noodles
> 1½ cups sauce
> ¾ cup cottage cheese
> 1½ cups mozzarella cheese
> 1½ cups spinach
> ¼ cup Parmesan cheese
> 1½ cups sauce

Cover pan with foil. Bake about 1 hour. Remove from
oven. Remove foil and let stand for 10 minutes. Serve. (This
dish freezes well.)
SERVES: 12   SERVING SIZE: 1 cup   9.0 nutripoints

———————• Herbed Lentils and Wild Rice •———————

2¼ cups chicken or vegetable broth
¾ cup lentils
1 onion, chopped
1 cup mushrooms, sliced
1 red bell pepper, chopped
½ cup wild rice
½ cup dry white wine
½ teaspoon dried basil, crushed
½ teaspoon dried oregano, crushed
½ teaspoon dried thyme, crushed
¼ teaspoon salt
⅛ teaspoon garlic powder
¼ teaspoon freshly ground black pepper
1 cup shredded mozzarella cheese (divided use)
½ cup pimiento, chopped

DIRECTIONS Preheat oven to 350° F. Combine all the ingredients except ½ cup mozzarella cheese and pimiento. Pour mixture into an ungreased 1½-quart casserole with a tight-fitting lid. Cover and bake, stirring twice, 1½ to 2 hours, or until lentils and rice are done.

Uncover casserole; top with the remaining ½ cup mozzarella cheese and pimiento. Bake 5 minutes, or until cheese melts.

SERVES: 4 SERVING SIZE: 1 cup   6.5 nutripoints

———————————— • Fresh Pasta Salad • ————————————

        1 cup fresh pasta
    ½–1 tablespoon extra-virgin olive oil
      ¼ cup fresh basil, shredded
        Squeeze of fresh lemon juice
      12 cherry tomatoes, halved
      ⅛ teaspoon salt (optional)
        Freshly ground black pepper

DIRECTIONS   Cook pasta. Drain. Toss immediately with
extra-virgin olive oil, basil, lemon juice, tomatoes, salt, and
pepper.
   SERVES: 8   SERVING SIZE: ¼ cup   4.5 nutripoints

FRUIT DISHES

———————————— • Fresh Fruit Slices • ————————————

      ¼ cantaloupe
      ¼ honeydew melon
      ½ cup sliced fresh strawberries

DIRECTIONS   Slice melon pieces and arrange with strawberries.
   SERVES: 2   SERVING SIZE: 1 cup   36.0 nutripoints

———————————— • Fruit Salad Plate • ————————————

        2 bananas, sliced
        2 kiwi fruit, sliced
      1½ cups fresh pineapple chunks
      2½ cups sliced fresh strawberries
        2 cups chopped Bibb lettuce

DIRECTIONS   Line 4 plates with the lettuce. Mix together
the fruit; arrange on lettuce.
   SERVES: 5   SERVING SIZE: 1 cup   14.5 nutripoints

——————————— • Rainbow Compote • ———————————

¼ cup fresh blueberries
¼ cup fresh raspberries
¼ cup sliced mango
¼ cup sliced fresh strawberries
4 sprigs fresh mint

DIRECTIONS   Layer fruit in small glass bowls and garnish with mint. Serve.

SERVES: 2   SERVING SIZE: ½ cup   18.0 nutripoints

——————————— • Fresh Fruit Platter • ———————————

12 red grapes
¼ cantaloupe, cut into large chunks
1 cup fresh pineapple chunks
½ kiwi fruit, sliced
½ skinned orange, cut into chunks
1 cup fresh strawberries
⅛ papaya, sliced
⅛ mango, sliced
Leafy lettuce

DIRECTIONS   Arrange fruit on platter lined with lettuce. Serve.

SERVES: 1   SERVING SIZE: 2½ cups   17.0 nutripoints

• Key Lime Mousse •

> 2 envelopes unflavored gelatin
> 1/4 cup cold water
> 1 cup boiling water
> 1 cup fresh lime juice
> 1 tablespoon grated lime rind
> 1/2 cup sugar
> 3 cups nonfat yogurt cheese*

DIRECTIONS   Dissolve gelatin in cold water. Add boiling water and stir until dissolved. Add lime juice, rind, and sugar. Stir well. Mix in yogurt cheese until smooth (food processor works well). Pour into a deep 9-inch pie pan, or pour into small individual-serving-size containers. Chill until firm.

SERVES: 10   SERVING SIZE: 1/2 cup   5.5 nutripoints

• Fruit-Yogurt Pie •

> 1 envelope unflavored gelatin
> 1/3 cup cold water
> 2 8-ounce containers low-fat fruit yogurt
> 2 egg whites
> 1/3 cup sugar
> 1 1/2 cups fresh berries
> 1 9-inch graham cracker pie crust

DIRECTIONS   In a small saucepan over low heat, soften gelatin in water. Cook and stir until gelatin dissolves. Remove from heat. Stir in yogurt. Chill until partially set (the consistency of unbeaten egg whites).

In a large bowl, beat the egg whites until soft peaks form. Add sugar, 1 tablespoon at a time, beating until stiff peaks form. Stir fruit into yogurt mixture and fold mixture into beaten egg whites. Turn into graham cracker pie crust. Chill 3 to 4 hours, or until firm.

SERVES: 12   SERVING SIZE: 1 small piece (1/12 of pie)
                               0.5 nutripoints

*Make yogurt cheese by draining plain nonfat yogurt in cheesecloth or coffee filter for 8 to 10 hours. 2 cups yogurt yield 1 cup yogurt cheese.

———————— • Poached Pears • ————————

RASPBERRY
PUREE: 1 cup frozen raspberries
         1–2 teaspoons cornstarch
           2 tablespoons cold water

           1 quart cranberry juice
           1 cinnamon stick
           6 black peppercorns
           1 clove
           2 pears, peeled with stems left on
           8 ounces plain low-fat yogurt, mixed
             with vanilla and honey to taste

DIRECTIONS   Heat raspberries in skillet. Strain to yield
only liquid raspberry juice. Dissolve cornstarch in cold water
and slowly add to raspberry juice. Stir well. Cook over medium heat until mixture thickens slightly.

Bring cranberry juice to a boil and add cinnamon stick,
peppercorns, and clove. Simmer peeled pears in liquid for 5
minutes, covered, then chill.

Cut poached pears in half and then into 1/8-inch-thick
slices, leaving them attached to the top of the pear. Spread
2 ounces yogurt on 4 plates. Fan pear slices on plate over the
yogurt. Squeeze raspberry puree from a bottle into several
horizontal lines on the yogurt surrounding the pear. Create
pattern by running a knife vertically through the lines of
raspberry puree from the bottom of the yogurt to the top.

SERVES: 4   SERVING SIZE: 1/2 pear   4.0 nutripoints

────────── • Bananas Flambé • ──────────

        4 small bananas
        1 tablespoon orange juice
        2 tablespoons reduced-calorie margarine
        2 tablespoons brown sugar
      1/4 teaspoon ground cinnamon
      1/4 cup 151-proof (flames best) rum
        1 quart low-fat frozen vanilla yogurt

DIRECTIONS Slice bananas in half lengthwise, then in
half again. Toss with orange juice and set aside. Combine
margarine with brown sugar in a large nonstick skillet. Cook
over medium heat, stirring constantly until sugar melts. Add
reserved bananas; cook 4 minutes. Sprinkle with cinnamon
and remove from heat. Pour rum over banana mixture. Ignite;
let flames die down. Serve immediately over frozen yogurt.

SERVES: 8 SERVING SIZE: 2 banana slices and 1/2 cup
yogurt   2.5 nutripoints

────────── • Blackberry Freeze • ──────────

        1 package frozen blackberries (no added sugar),
           semi-defrosted
    1 1/2 tablespoons orange juice concentrate
        1 orange, sliced

DIRECTIONS Place first two ingredients into blender or
food processor. Process until the mixture reaches the consistency of a sorbet. Garnish with fresh orange slices.

SERVES: 4 SERVING SIZE: 3/4 cup   8.5 nutripoints

———————————— • Banana Gladje • ————————————

  2 frozen bananas, cut into large pieces, semi-defrosted
3–4 tablespoons part-skim ricotta cheese (or 1 ounce
    Neufchâtel cheese)
⅛–¼ cup skim milk
    Fresh mint

DIRECTIONS   Place bananas into blender or food proces-
sor. Add remaining ingredients and process until smooth.
Garnish with fresh mint.
  SERVES: 3   SERVING SIZE: ⅓ cup   6.0 nutripoints

———————————— • Applesauce • ————————————

    4 large apples
    1 teaspoon cinnamon
  ½ teaspoon nutmeg
    Pinch of cloves
    Pinch of allspice
  ¼ cup water
  2–4 packages Sweet 'n' Low to taste
    2 teaspoons honey

DIRECTIONS   Core and peel apples. Add spices and water
to a small saucepan; cover and simmer until apples are tender—approximately 25 minutes. Stir in Sweet 'n' Low and
honey. Serve warm.
  SERVES: 4   SERVING SIZE: ½ cup   3.0 nutripoints

BREAKFAST DISHES

———————— • Bran Muffins • ————————

1½ cups Whole Wheat Total (or other bran cereal)
½ cup orange juice, boiling
4 egg whites (or ¼ cup egg substitute)
½ cup ½-percent-fat buttermilk
4 ounces orange juice concentrate
3 tablespoons safflower oil
1 large ripe banana, mashed
½ cup currants
2 tablespoons honey, brown sugar, or molasses
½ teaspoon vanilla extract
1 cup whole wheat flour
½ cup white flour
1½ teaspoons baking soda
2 teaspoons baking powder
¾ teaspoon cinnamon
¾ teaspoon nutmeg
Zest of 1 orange, chopped finely

DIRECTIONS   Preheat oven to 400° F. Combine cereal in
a large bowl with boiling orange juice. Let cool. Add the egg
whites, buttermilk, orange juice concentrate, oil, banana, currants, honey, and vanilla. Mix well. In a small bowl, combine
flours, baking soda, baking powder, and spices. Add to cereal
mixture and mix very well.* Spray a muffin tin with nonstick
spray. Spoon into muffin cups. Bake for 20 minutes, or until
done.

SERVES: 12   SERVING SIZE: 1 muffin   10.0 nutripoints

* Batter can be stored in refrigerator up to 2 weeks.

————————— • Oat Bran Muffins • —————————

1 ¼ cups oat bran cereal
1 cup whole wheat flour
¼ cup dried apricots, coarsely chopped
1 tablespoon baking powder
½ cup skim milk
½ cup orange juice
¼ cup molasses (or honey)
2 tablespoons vegetable oil
3 egg whites

DIRECTIONS Preheat oven to 425°F. Spray bottom and sides of 12 medium-size muffin cups with nonstick spray (or line with paper baking cups). Combine dry ingredients. Add milk, juice, egg whites, molasses, and oil. Mix just until dry mixture is moistened. Fill prepared muffin cups ¾ full. Bake for 15 minutes.

SERVES: 12   SERVING SIZE: 1 muffin   3.5 nutripoints

————————————— • French Toast • —————————————

1 egg yolk
2 egg whites
¹⁄₁₆ teaspoon salt
½ teaspoon vanilla extract
2 teaspoons brown sugar
Cinnamon to taste
3 slices cinnamon bread

DIRECTIONS Combine first six ingredients and beat well. Pour mixture into baking dish and add bread. Turn bread to coat with mixture. Spray nonstick skillet with nonstick spray. Add bread and cook over medium heat until golden brown on both sides.

SERVES: 2   SERVING SIZE: 1½ pieces toast

0.5 nutripoints

Serving suggestions
1. Serve with frozen fruit which has been heated in the microwave and sweetened to taste.
2. Top with vanilla-flavored low-fat yogurt.

• Garden Scrambled Eggs •

$\frac{1}{8}$ green pepper, diced
$\frac{1}{8}$ onion, diced
2 fresh mushrooms, diced
2 egg whites
1 egg yolk
$\frac{1}{8}$ cup low-fat cottage cheese

DIRECTIONS   Place first 3 ingredients in a microwave-safe container, cover, and microwave on medium setting until vegetables are tender, or spray a nonstick skillet with a nonstick spray and lightly sauté vegetables. Whip egg whites with yolk and cottage cheese. Scramble eggs in skillet with cooked vegetables until done.

SERVES: 1   SERVING SIZE: $\frac{3}{4}$ cup   5.5 nutripoints

• Fruited Cinnamon Cereal •

$\frac{3}{4}$ cup cooked old-fashioned oatmeal
$\frac{1}{4}$ apple, shredded
1 tablespoon raisins or chopped dried apricots
Cinnamon to taste

DIRECTIONS   Mix all ingredients together and serve.

SERVES: 1   SERVING SIZE: 1 cup   5.0 nutripoints

• Whole Grain Pancakes •

2 cups whole wheat flour
$\frac{1}{2}$ teaspoon baking soda
$\frac{1}{2}$ teaspoon Morton Lite Salt
2 egg whites
1 egg yolk
1 tablespoon oil
$1\frac{3}{4}$ cups orange juice

DIRECTIONS   Sift flour, baking soda, and Lite Salt together in a bowl.

Blend eggs, oil, and orange juice in a bowl. Add dry ingredients. Mix just until blended.

Heat nonstick skillet and spray with nonstick vegetable spray. Drop batter onto skillet to make small pancakes. Cook over medium heat until bubbles burst and bottoms are golden brown, about 2 minutes. Flip pancakes and brown other side.

SERVES: 6   SERVING SIZE: 4 pancakes   5.5 nutripoints

——————— • Hot Blueberry Topping • ———————

1 16-ounce package frozen, unsweetened blueberries (or 2 pints fresh blueberries)
1 tablespoon honey
  Sweet 'n' Low to taste
4 teaspoons cornstarch
4 teaspoons cold water
2 teaspoons orange juice

DIRECTIONS   Heat fruit in large pan (or in microwave). Add honey and Sweet 'n' Low. Dissolve cornstarch in cold water and slowly add to hot fruit mixture. Stir well. Mixture will look cloudy at this point. Add orange juice. Bring to a boil, which will clear mixture. Serve hot.

SERVES: 3–4   SERVING SIZE: ½ cup   2.5 nutripoints

——————— • Hot Peach Topping • ———————

1 16-ounce package frozen, unsweetened peaches (or 4 cups sliced fresh peaches)
1 tablespoon honey
  Sweet 'n' Low to taste
4 teaspoons cornstarch
4 teaspoons cold water
2 teaspoons orange juice
  Cinnamon to taste

DIRECTIONS   Heat fruit in large pan (or in microwave). Add honey and Sweet 'n' Low. Dissolve cornstarch in cold water and slowly add to hot fruit mixture. Stir well. Mixture will look cloudy at this point. Add orange juice and cinnamon. Bring to a boil, which will clear mixture. Serve hot.

SERVES: 3–4   SERVING SIZE: ½ cup   7.0 nutripoints

—————— • Hot Red Raspberry Topping • ——————

   1 16-ounce package frozen, unsweetened raspberries
     (or 2 pints fresh raspberries)
   1 tablespoon honey
    Sweet 'n' Low to taste
   4 teaspoons cornstarch
   4 teaspoons cold water
   2 teaspoons orange juice
    Cinnamon to taste

DIRECTIONS Follow directions for Hot Peach Topping.
Add cinnamon to taste.
   SERVES: 3–4 SERVING SIZE: ½ cup 9.0 nutripoints

—————————— • Honey Cream Cheese • ——————————

   8 ounces low-fat cream cheese (Neufchâtel)
   1 tablespoon honey
   1 package Equal
   1 tablespoon milk

DIRECTIONS Place ingredients in food processor. Mix
until smooth.
   SERVES: 8–16 SERVING SIZE: 1–2 tablespoons
         5.5 nutripoints

DRESSINGS AND SAUCES

———————— • Lite Spicy Mustard Dressing • ————————

  ½ cup of Dijon mustard
   2 cloves garlic, minced
    Juice of 2 lemons
   2 packages Equal
  ⅛ cup water (or plain nonfat yogurt, if desired)

DIRECTIONS Mix all ingredients. Refrigerate and serve.
   SERVES: 16 SERVING SIZE: 1 tablespoon
         0.5 nutripoints

———————— • Lite Zero Salad Dressing • ————————

1/2 cup tomato juice or V-8 (may add low-sodium canned
    tomatoes pureed in food processor to thicken)
 2 tablespoons fresh lemon juice
 1 tablespoon finely chopped onion (or dehydrated onion)
1/4 cup fresh finely chopped parsley
1/2 cup canned tomatoes (no added salt), chopped

DIRECTIONS   Combine ingredients in jar with tight lid and
shake well, or whiz in a blender.
   SERVES: 10   SERVING SIZE: 2 tablespoons

                                              1.0 nutripoints

———————— • Balsamic Vinegar Dressing • ————————

4 tablespoons low-fat buttermilk
1 tablespoon rice wine vinegar
1 tablespoon balsamic vinegar
1 teaspoon sugar
  Freshly ground black pepper and Morton Lite Salt to taste

DIRECTIONS   Mix ingredients well and serve.
   SERVINGS: 6   SERVING SIZE: 1 tablespoon

                                              0.0 nutripoints

———————— • Blue Cheese Dressing • ————————

   1/2 cup low-fat cottage cheese
   1/4 cup low-fat buttermilk
     1 tablespoon white vinegar
 1 1/2 tablespoons blue cheese salad dressing mix

DIRECTIONS   Blend all ingredients until smooth. Refrigerate for 1 hour to develop full flavor.
   SERVES: 8   SERVING SIZE: 2 tablespoons

                                              8.0 nutripoints

—————————— • Lite 16-Island Dressing • ——————————

1 cup plain nonfat yogurt
1 tablespoon Dijon mustard
2 tablespoons olive oil
½ teaspoon horseradish
1 tablespoon fresh lemon juice
1 teaspoon minced chives (or scallions)
2 tablespoons tomato paste or crushed tomatoes
1 tablespoon chopped fresh parsley
1 teaspoon dried basil*
Freshly ground black pepper to taste
Morton's Lite Salt to taste

DIRECTIONS   Combine all ingredients and mix until smooth.
    SERVES: 12   SERVING SIZE: 2 tablespoons

2.5 nutripoints

—————————— • Honey Yogurt Dressing • ——————————

1 cup plain nonfat yogurt
1⅔ tablespoons honey

DIRECTIONS   Mix well in a blender or food processor.
    SERVES: 16   SERVING SIZE: 1 tablespoon

2.0 nutripoints

—————————— • Lite Mayonnaise Mix • ——————————

¾ cup plain nonfat yogurt
¼ cup light mayonnaise

DIRECTIONS   Mix ingredients until smooth.
    SERVES: 16   SERVING SIZE: 1 tablespoon

1.5 nutripoints

*You might want to substitute spaghetti sauce for tomato paste, parsley, and basil.

——————————— • New Way Sour Cream • ———————————

     1 cup low-fat cottage cheese
     2 tablespoons fresh lemon juice
     1 tablespoon skim milk

DIRECTIONS   Mix all ingredients in a food processor and whiz until smooth.

SERVES: 8   SERVING SIZE: 2 tablespoons

6.5 nutripoints

——————————— • Lite Caper Dressing • ———————————

     ¼ cup light mayonnaise
     ⅔ cup plain low-fat yogurt
     3 tablespoons red wine vinegar
  2½–3 tablespoons capers, rinsed and minced
     2 tablespoons minced fresh chives
     2 tablespoons chopped fresh parsley
     2 tablespoons minced shallots
     1 clove garlic, minced
     1 tablespoon fresh chopped basil
     2 tablespoons Dijon mustard

DIRECTIONS   Combine all ingredients. Mix until smooth.

SERVES: 12   SERVING SIZE: 2 tablespoons

2.0 nutripoints

─────────── • Lite Vinaigrette Dressing • ───────────

    2 large cloves garlic, crushed
    2 tablespoons olive oil
    4 tablespoons mild vinegar (cider vinegar recommended)
1–2 tablespoons lemon juice
    2 tablespoons water
 1/2 teaspoon dry mustard
 1/4 teaspoon freshly ground black pepper
    1 teaspoon sugar or Equal to taste
 1/4 teaspoon salt

DIRECTIONS Combine ingredients and mix well.
  SERVES: 3   SERVING SIZE: 2 tablespoons

                                            1.5 nutripoints

Variations
  1. Substitute any fruit vinegar for cider vinegar.
  2. Add 4 diced artichoke hearts, a bit more dry mustard,
     and 1 tablespoon balsamic vinegar.

─────── • Lite Orange Vinaigrette Dressing • ───────

           1/2 cup orange juice concentrate
           1/4 cup olive oil
           1/4 cup apple cider vinegar
             2 teaspoons Dijon mustard
             2 egg whites, beaten
               Herbs as desired

DIRECTIONS Slowly add oil to orange juice while using a
hand beater. Add vinegar and mustard; beat again. Fold in
egg whites and herbs and serve.
  SERVES: 8   SERVING SIZE: 2 tablespoons

                                            2.5 nutripoints

─────────── • Lite Ranch Dressing • ───────────

    1 cup low-fat buttermilk
  ¾ cup plain low-fat yogurt
  ¼ cup light mayonnaise
    2 tablespoons chopped fresh parsley
2½ teaspoons minced fresh dill, or ¾ teaspoon dried
    2 teaspoons chopped fresh basil, or ¾ teaspoon
      dried
  ½ teaspoon Worcestershire sauce
1–2 cloves garlic, pressed
  ¾ teaspoon onion powder

DIRECTIONS Blend all ingredients. Chill at least 8 hours
before serving.

SERVES: 16   SERVING SIZE: 2 tablespoons

3.5 nutripoints

• Juniper Berry Marinade and Sauce
──────(For Venison, Quail, or Chicken) •──────

MARINADE:
- ½ cup olive oil
- 2–3 stalks celery, diced
- Salt and freshly ground pepper to taste
- 6 juniper berries, crushed
- Juice of 6 lemons
- 1 carrot, diced

SAUCE:
- 2 tablespoons cornstarch
- Cold water
- 1 cup warm low-sodium beef broth
- 1 teaspoon margarine
- 6 juniper berries, crushed
- Dash of salt
- Freshly ground pepper and other spices to taste

DIRECTIONS   Stir together marinade ingredients. Place meat of your choice in a large nonmetallic bowl and pour marinade over it. Set aside in refrigerator for 4 to 8 hours, turning the meat occasionally.

Mix cornstarch with small amount of cold water to form a paste; add slowly to beef broth. Place over medium heat and reduce until thick. Add margarine and crushed berries. Add salt, pepper, and spices to taste.

Marinate meat; grill meat; ladle ¼ cup sauce on top. Serve hot.

SERVES: 4   SERVING SIZE: ¼ cup   0.0 nutripoints

——• Hawaiian Marinade for Chicken or Fish •——

> ½ cup low-sodium soy sauce
> ½ cup pineapple juice
> ½ cup water
> 1 teaspoon minced garlic
> ½ tablespoon dry mustard
> ¼ cup sugar
> ⅛ cup vegetable oil (or olive oil)
> 1 kiwi fruit, peeled and mashed
> 1 cup fresh pineapple, cut into large chunks

DIRECTIONS Mix together all the ingredients. Place skin-less chicken breasts or fish in a shallow nonmettalic container and pour marinade over all. Set aside in the refrigerator for about 2 hours. Remove chicken or fish from marinade and grill. Meanwhile, simmer marinade in a saucepan until reduced and thickened. Ladle 1 ounce on top of chicken or fish, making sure that each plate gets a few chunks of fresh pineapple.

SERVES: 6   SERVING SIZE: Marinade for 6 4-ounce chicken
breasts or 6 4-ounce fish fillets
4.0 nutripoints

─────────── • Tomato Sauce • ───────────

    1 carrot
    2 stalks celery
    1 red or green bell pepper, halved and seeded
 1½ medium onions
    2 cloves garlic
    2 large tomatoes, skins removed
  ½ medium zucchini
       Small amount of olive oil
    6 cups crushed tomatoes

SPICES: 1 tablespoon Italian seasoning
          2 teaspoons basil
          2 teaspoons sugar
          1 tablespoon fennel seed, crushed
          1 bay leaf
         ⅛ cup chopped fresh parsley
          2 teaspoons oregano
          2 teaspoons salt
          2 teaspoons chili powder

DIRECTIONS   Using a food processor, chop the vegetables into small pieces. Heat olive oil in large saucepan and sauté vegetables until tender (about 10 to 12 minutes). Add the crushed tomatoes and the spices and let simmer about 2 hours.

SERVES: 12 cups   19.0 nutripoints

─────────── • Mango Sauce • ───────────

    1 shallot, minced
  ½ tablespoon margarine
    1 15-ounce can mangoes (no sugar), puréed
    2 tablespoons cornstarch
       Sherry to taste
    1 fresh mango, peeled and mashed

DIRECTIONS   Sauté shallot in margarine. Add pureed mango. Combine cornstarch with a small amount of cold water and add to pureed mixture. Bring to a boil. Add sherry to taste. Stir in fresh mango. Pour small amount of sauce over baked chicken breasts.

SERVES: 8   SERVING SIZE: ¼ cup   1.0 nutripoints

• Scallop Sauce •

⅛ cup diced onion
½ tablespoon minced garlic (or shallots)
½ tablespoon olive oil
1½ tablespoons sherry
½ cup ½-percent-fat milk
4 teaspoons low-sodium chicken bouillon
1 tablespoon fresh lemon juice
¼ teaspoon tarragon
½ teaspoon dill
½ teaspoon basil
Pinch of salt
Freshly ground pepper to taste
¼ cup fresh tomato, peeled and diced
3 fresh mushrooms, sliced
1–2 tablespoons cornstarch
½ cup cold water

DIRECTIONS   Sauté onion and garlic in olive oil. Add sherry, milk, bouillon, lemon juice, and spices. Steam tomato and mushrooms and add to mixture. Dissolve cornstarch in cold water and add to mixture to thicken. Serve over broiled or baked scallops.

SERVES: 6   SERVING SIZE: ¼ cup   1.0 nutripoints

———————— • Banana Mint Sauce • ————————

1 frozen banana
1 cup low-fat plain yogurt
Fresh mint leaves

DIRECTIONS Peel and break banana into pieces and freeze. Combine frozen banana, yogurt, and mint. Mix all ingredients in a food processor until smooth. Spoon over seasonal fruit.

SERVES: 16   SERVING SIZE: 2–4 tablespoons

6.5 nutripoints

FRUIT DRINKS

———————— • Strawberry Smoothie • ————————

½ cup low-fat milk
½ cup strawberries
2 packages Equal
3–4 ice cubes

DIRECTIONS Mix ingredients in blender until smooth.

SERVES: 1   SERVING SIZE: 1–1½ cups   13.5 nutripoints

———————— • Sunrise Cooler • ————————

3 cups freshly squeezed orange juice
1 cup frozen strawberries
2 cups sparkling mineral water
Ice cubes as desired

DIRECTIONS Pureé frozen strawberries in food processor. Mix with orange juice and freeze until just firm. Before serving add mineral water and pour over ice cubes.

SERVES: 8   SERVING SIZE: ½ cup   15.5 nutripoints

PART VII

NUTRIPOINT LISTS

THE LISTS THAT FOLLOW CONTAIN NUTRIPOINT RATINGS FOR MORE than 3,000 foods. The lists are in three parts:

Nutrigroup Ratings   page 285
Other Groups   page 370
Alphabetical Ratings   page 384

The Nutrigroup Ratings lists show the rating of every food within its Nutrigroup, highest to lowest. There are six basic Nutrigroups:

1. Vegetables
2. Fruits
3. Grains
4. Legumes/nuts/seeds
5. Milk/dairy
6. Meat/fish/poultry

There are five types of foods on the Nutrigroup Ratings lists:

1. Nutripoint recipes
2. Basic foods
3. Generic foods
4. Brand-name foods
5. Fast foods

There are also five Other Group lists:

1. Fats/oils
2. Sugar
3. Alcohol
4. Condiments
5. Miscellaneous

The following are notes and explanations concerning various aspects of the lists.

Nutripoint Recipes   These are easily identified because they always include the word *Nutripoint.* Two examples of such entries from the lists include "Red Snapper, Veracruz, Nutripoint" and "Dressing, Lite, Blue Cheese, Nutripoint." These are recipes we've created for dishes that are high in Nutripoints, and, of course, delicious. You'll find the recipes for them in the recipe section (page 225). (You'll also find these foods featured on the Nutripoint fourteen-day menus, beginning on page 209.)

Basic Foods   These are just what you would think: apples, whole wheat flour, milk, chicken breast, and so on. They're foods that are unprocessed.

Generic Foods   You'll notice that some of the foods on the list are neither brand names nor basic foods such as grapes. These foods are what we call *generic foods.* They have ratings based on USDA nutritional information. Some of these are foods that have had some processing, such as canned pumpkin or tomato sauce; others are what are known as *home recipes,* such as coleslaw. Home recipes are standard recipes that most people would use at home to prepare certain foods. Of course, your recipe for tuna noodle casserole might well differ from the USDA home recipe version, but to assume a certain standard is the only way to evaluate these foods.

Brand-Name Foods   These are foods that have been processed by a particular manufacturer who also provided the nutritional information used as the basis of analysis of these foods. These foods include everything from Birds Eye frozen whole leaf spinach to Gatorade.

Fast Foods   These are foods that are served by fast-food restaurants. We've included most of the major fast-food chains, from Arby's to McDonald's, and we've tried to include the most popular items on their menus, from salads, to burgers, to pizzas.

You'll notice that there are three columns for the food ratings. The *Nutripoints* column, obviously, is the rating of the food.

The *Food Name* column, of course, identifies the food.

The *Serving Size* column shows the amount of food that is rated. The measurements include cups, pieces, fluid ounces, ounces by weight, tablespoons, and teaspoons. Various explanations concerning serving sizes appear in the text.

Next to a food name you'll sometimes find an asterisk (*), a dagger (†), or a double dagger (‡). An asterisk means that the food is fortified, a dagger indicates that it contains too much cholesterol, and a double dagger warns the reader to exercise caution when eating a food because it may contain contaminants.

Fortification   You'll notice, particularly in the grain Nutrigroup, that many of the foods have an asterisk (*). This means that these foods derive at least 50 percent of their nutritional value from fortification. There are further discussions of this topic in the text (see pages 179–80), but I'll simply reiterate here that some controversy exists about the value of fortification. Often, nutrients have been removed through processing and then replaced artificially. While these foods do contain large amounts of certain nutrients, they're not "natural" in that they aren't as nature formulated them. In general, the fortified foods at the top of the list are far preferable to fortified foods lower on the list because the top foods (cereals usually) begin with a whole food and then fortify it. The foods lower down sometimes have sugar as a primary ingredient, with vitamins and minerals added to that.

My basic suggestion concerning fortified foods is that if you choose them, check the labels to be sure that the food is based on a real, basic food. One of the best tip-offs to a fortified food with little value is if the label contains any of the various terms for sugar (see page 103) listed among its first few ingredients.

Cholesterol Some foods, particularly those in the meat/poultry/fish Nutrigroup, have a dagger (†) indicating cholesterol. Again, this has been discussed more fully in the text (see pages 94–95, 170–171), but briefly, the notation means that these foods have a content of cholesterol per calorie of 1 milligram or more. This is a high concentration of cholesterol and, whatever the ranking of the food, I suggest that you avoid foods with the cholesterol mark.

Caution Some shellfish have a double dagger (‡), which indicates the possibility of contamination. While many of these foods are high in Nutripoints, care must be taken when eating them.

NUTRIGROUP RATINGS

VEGETABLE GROUP

Nutripoints	Serving Size	Food Name
79.0	1 cup	Turnip greens, chopped, cooked
75.0	2 cups	Spinach, raw, chopped
72.5	1 cup	Bok choy, raw, shredded
67.0	1 cup	Turnip greens, seasoned, Nutripoint
65.0	2 cups	Salad, spinach, Nutripoint
62.0	1 cup	Mustard greens, cooked
57.0	1 cup	Spinach, Whole Leaf, frozen, Birds Eye
56.5	1 cup	Beet greens, cooked
54.5	1 cup	Parsley, fresh
53.5	1 cup	Spinach, fresh, cooked
53.0	1 cup	Broccoli, raw
52.5	20 pieces	Watercress
51.5	2 cups	Salad, Tossed, Nutripoint
48.5	1 cup	Vegetable Medley, Nutripoint
48.0	1 cup	Mustard greens, frozen, cooked
47.5	2 cups	Lettuce, romaine
46.0	½ cup	Broccoli, frozen, Birds Eye
44.5	1 cup	Dandelion greens, raw
44.0	8 stalks	Asparagus, fresh
42.5	2 whole	Peppers, sweet red, raw
42.5	¾ cup	Spinach, frozen, cooked
42.5	1 cup	Collard greens, raw, chopped
42.0	1 cup	Swiss chard, cooked
42.0	1 cup	Collard greens, fresh, cooked

VEGETABLE GROUP

Nutripoints	Serving Size	Food Name
42.0	1 cup	Salad Greens, w/Balsamic Vinegar, Nutripoint
41.5	1 cup	Broccoli, Cauliflower, and Red Peppers, frozen, Birds Eye
40.5	1 cup	Cauliflower, raw
40.0	3/4 cup	Dandelion greens, cooked
40.0	1/2 cup	Collard greens, frozen, cooked
40.0	1/2 cup	Brussels sprouts, cooked
39.5	1 cup	Cress, garden, cooked
39.0	1 cup	Cabbage, common, raw, shredded
38.5	8 stalks	Asparagus, marinated, Nutripoint
38.5	1 cup	Broccoli, cooked
38.5	1 cup	Kale, chopped, cooked
37.5	2 whole	Green pepper, raw
37.5	1 cup	Cauliflower, cooked
36.0	1 cup	Broccoli, Carrots, and Cauliflower, frozen, Pictsweet
35.5	1 cup	Chicory greens, raw
35.5	3/4 cup	Spinach, Early Garden, canned, Del Monte
35.5	1 whole	Carrots, raw
34.0	2 cups	Lettuce, butterhead/Boston/Bibb, chopped
33.0	1 cup	Broccoli, Cauliflower, and Carrots, frozen, Green Giant
33.0	1 cup	Salad, tossed, no dressing
32.5	1 cup	Mushrooms, fresh
32.5	8 stalks	Asparagus, canned
31.5	1 cup	Cabbage, common, chopped, cooked
31.0	1/2 cup	Broccoli, Baby Carrots, Water Chestnuts, frozen, Birds Eye
31.0	1/2 cup	Okra, cooked
30.5	1 cup	Broccoli, Cauliflower, and Carrots, frozen, Birds Eye
30.5	10 leaves	Lettuce, loose-leaf
30.0	1 piece	Tomato, fresh
30.0	1/2 cup	Carrots, sliced, cooked
29.5	1 cup	Spinach, Leaf, no salt added, canned, Del Monte
29.5	1 cup	Cabbage, red, raw, shredded

VEGETABLE GROUP

Nutripoints	Serving Size	Food Name
29.0	1 cup	Radishes, raw
28.5	6 fluid ounces	Juice, Vegetable, no salt added, V-8
28.0	1/2 cup	Peas and carrots, frozen, cooked
27.0	1/2 cup	Brussels sprouts, frozen, cooked
27.0	8 stalks	Asparagus, frozen, cooked
26.5	1/2 cup	Squash, butternut, baked
26.0	6 fluid ounces	Juice, Vegetable, Spicy, V-8
26.0	1 cup	Okra, raw
26.0	6 fluid ounces	Juice, tomato, low-sodium
25.5	1/2 cup	Pumpkin, canned
25.0	1/2 cup	Brussels Sprouts, Baby, frozen, Seabrook Farms
25.0	1/2 cup	Peas and carrots, canned
24.5	1 cup	Squash, summer, cooked
24.5	1 cup	Cabbage, savoy, raw, shredded
24.5	1/2 cup	Broccoli, Sweet Peas, and Carrots, frozen, Green Giant
24.5	6 fluid ounces	Juice, Vegetable, V-8
24.5	2 cups	Kohlrabi, raw
24.5	6 fluid ounces	Juice, tomato
24.5	1 cup	Beans, green, cooked
24.0	10 stalks	Scallions
23.5	1 cup	Soup, Spinach, Clear, Nutripoint
23.0	1 cup	Cauliflower, frozen, Birds Eye
23.0	1/2 cup	Squash, Winter, Cooked, frozen, Birds Eye
23.0	1/2 cup	Tomatoes, canned
22.0	1/2 cup	Vegetables, mixed, canned
21.5	1 cup	Salad, tossed, w/tomato
21.0	1/2 cup	Mixed Vegetables, frozen, Veg-All
20.0	8 stalks	Celery, raw
20.0	1 piece	Cucumber, raw
20.0	1/2 cup	Spinach, Cut Leaf, in butter, frozen, Green Giant
20.0	1/4 cup	Tomato paste, canned
19.5	1 cup	Turnips, cooked
19.0	1/2 cup	Sauce, Tomato, Nutripoint
19.0	1 cup	Mushrooms, cooked
18.5	1 cup	Lettuce and tomato

VEGETABLE GROUP

Nutripoints	Serving Size	Food Name
18.5	1/2 cup	Mixed Vegetables, Natural Pack, canned, Libby's
18.0	1/2 cup	Kelp
18.0	1/2 cup	Turnips, raw
18.0	1/2 cup	Rutabagas, cooked
18.0	10 leaves	Lettuce, iceberg
18.0	1/2 cup	Vegetables, Custom Cuisine w/Dijon, frozen, Birds Eye
18.0	1/2 cup	Vegetables, mixed, frozen, cooked
18.0	1/2 cup	Vegetables, Mixed, frozen, Birds Eye
17.5	1/2 cup	Pumpkin, cooked
17.5	2 cups	Alfalfa sprouts, raw
17.5	1/2 cup	Sauce, tomato, canned
17.0	3/4 cup	Broccoli, Carrots, and Red Peppers, frozen, Birds Eye
17.0	1/2 cup	Bamboo shoots, raw
17.0	1 cup	Sauerkraut, canned
17.0	1/2 cup	Salad, Mixed Vegetable, Nutripoint
17.0	1/2 cup	Eggplant, cooked
17.0	1/2 cup	Broccoli, Corn, and Red Peppers, frozen, Birds Eye
16.5	1/2 serving	Wendy's Garden Salad (take-out)
16.5	1 cup	Bamboo shoots, canned
16.0	1/2 cup	Squash, winter, baked
16.0	2 whole	Leeks, raw
16.0	1 cup	Zucchini, raw
15.5	1 cup	Beans, Green, Cut, frozen, Birds Eye
15.5	1/2 cup	Sauce, Tomato, Thick and Zesty, Contadina
15.0	1 cup	Zucchini, cooked
15.0	6 fluid ounces	Juice, carrot
14.5	1 cup	Asparagus, 50-Percent Less Salt, canned, Green Giant
14.0	1 cup	Tomatoes, Peeled, Del Monte
14.0	1/2 cup	Asparagus, Cuts, canned, Green Giant
13.5	1/2 cup	Vegetable Stir-Fry, Nutripoint
13.5	1/2 cup	Beans, yellow snap, cooked
13.5	1 tablespoon	Wendy's Crushed Red Peppers

VEGETABLE GROUP

Nutripoints	Serving Size	Food Name
13.5	1 cup	Beans, green, cut, No Salt Added, canned, Del Monte
13.0	1 cup	Soup, Vegetable, No Salt, Health Valley
13.0	1 cup	Alfalfa Sprouts, Arrowhead Mills
13.0	1 cup	Mushrooms, canned, Green Giant
13.0	1/2 cup	Broccoli, Cauliflower, and Carrots w/Cheese Sauce, frozen, Birds Eye
13.0	1/2 cup	Broccoli, Cauliflower, and Carrots w/Cheese Sauce, Green Giant
13.0	1 cup	Beans, Green, Whole, canned, Del Monte
12.5	1/4 cup	Tomato Paste, Contadina
12.5	1 cup	Soup, Vegetable, Health Valley
12.5	1 whole	Artichoke, cooked
12.0	1/2 whole	Sweet potato/yam, baked
12.0	1/2 cup	Soup, Tomato, No Salt, Health Valley
12.0	3/4 cup	Juice, Tomato, Campbell's
12.0	1/2 cup	Brussels Sprouts w/Butter, frozen, Green Giant
12.0	1 cup	Soup, vegetable
11.5	1/2 cup	Parsnips, raw
11.5	1/2 cup	Squash, acorn, baked
11.5	1/2 cup	Soup, Tomato, Health Valley
11.0	1 cup	Soup, Chunky Five-Bean Vegetable, Health Valley
11.0	1/2 cup	Beets, cooked
10.5	1/2 cup	Sauce, Tomato, Del Monte
10.0	1/2 cup	Coleslaw, Nutripoint
9.5	1/2 cup	Sauce, Spaghetti, Pritikin
9.0	1/2 cup	Sauce, Tomato, Hunt's
9.0	1/2 cup	Potato Salad, Nutripoint
8.5	1/2 cup	Onion, raw (1 T = 1 tsp dried onion flakes)
8.5	1/4 cup	Shallots, raw
8.5	1/2 potato	Potato, baked
8.5	1 serving	Carl's Jr. Garden Salad (take-out)
8.5	1/2 cup	Parsnips, cooked
8.0	1/2 cup	Corn, frozen, cooked
8.0	1 cup	Beans, Green, 50-Percent Less Salt, canned, Green Giant

VEGETABLE GROUP

Nutripoints	Serving Size	Food Name
8.0	1/2 potato/yam	Sweet potato/yam, canned
8.0	1/2 cup	Celeriac, raw
7.5	1/2 cup	Mixed Vegetables, w/Butter, frozen, Green Giant
7.5	1/2 cup	Succotash, cooked
7.5	1 cup	Leeks, cooked
7.5	1/2 cup	Beets, canned, cooked
7.0	1/2 cup	Vegetables, Pasta Primavera Style, frozen, Birds Eye
7.0	1/2 cup	Succotash, frozen, cooked
7.0	1/2 cup	Tomatoes, Stewed, Hunt's
7.0	1 package	Corn, Little Ears, frozen, Birds Eye
6.5	1 cup	Soup, Tomato w/Vegetables, Progresso
6.5	1 cup	Soup, Vegetable, Pritikin
6.0	1/2 cup	Corn, Golden, Family Style, no salt, canned, Del Monte
6.0	1/2 cup	Broccoli, w/Butter Sauce, frozen, Green Giant
6.0	1/2 serving	Roy Rogers coleslaw
6.0	1/2 cup	Cauliflower, w/Cheese Sauce, frozen, Green Giant
6.0	1/2 cup	Corn, Sweet, frozen, Birds Eye
6.0	1/4 serving	Wendy's Chef Salad (take-out)
6.0	1/2 piece	Corn on cob, fresh, cooked
5.5	1/2 cup	Potatoes, Homestyle, Nutripoint
5.5	1/4 cup	Flour, potato
5.5	1 cup	Water chestnuts, canned
5.0	1 cup	Soup, Chunky Vegetable, Campbell's
5.0	1 cup	Soup, minestrone
5.0	1/2 cup	Corn, w/red and green peppers, canned
4.5	1 cup	Beans, Green, Kitchen Cut, canned, Green Giant
4.5	8 ounces	Soup, Vegetarian Vegetable, Campbell's
4.5	1/2 cup	Corn, creamed, canned
4.5	1 cup	Soup, vegetable beef
4.5	1/2 portion	Vegetables, Spring w/Cheese Sauce, frozen, Budget Gourmet

VEGETABLE GROUP

Nutripoints	Serving Size	Food Name
4.5	1/4 serving	Wendy's Hot Stuffed Potato
4.5	1/2 cup	Corn, canned
4.0	1/2 cup	Salad, spinach, w/egg/bacon/tomato
4.0	1/2 serving	Roy Rogers hot Topped Potato, plain
4.0	1/2 serving	Carl's Jr. Chef Salad (take-out)
4.0	1/2 potato	Sweet potatoes, candied
4.0	1/2 cup	Sauce, Spaghetti, Meatless, Aunt Millie's
4.0	1/2 cup	Sauce, Spaghetti, No Salt Added, Prego
4.0	1/4 portion	Eggplant rollettes, frozen, Celentano
3.5	1 cup	Beans, green, French Style Cut, canned, Green Giant
3.5	1/2 cup	Sauce, Spaghetti w/Peppers and Sausage, Aunt Millie's
3.5	1 cup	Soup, Minestrone, Campbell's
3.5	1/2 cup	Poi
3.5	1 cup	Soup, Chunky Minestrone, Campbell's
3.5	1/2 cup	Beets, pickled, canned
3.0	1/2 portion	Spinach au Gratin, frozen, Budget Gourmet
3.0	1/2 cup	Sauce, Spaghetti w/Mushrooms, Homestyle, Ragú
3.0	1/2 potato	Carl's Jr. Lite Potato
3.0	1/4 portion	Eggplant Parmigiana, frozen, Celentano
3.0	1/2 cup	Coleslaw
3.0	1/2 cup	Corn, 50-Percent Less Salt, canned, Green Giant
3.0	3 cups	Popcorn, Light, Orville Redenbacher's
3.0	1 cup	Soup, Vegetable, 1/3 Less Salt, Campbell's
3.0	2 whole	Pickles, Kosher Crunchy Dills, Half Salt, Vlasic
3.0	1/2 cup	Beans, Green, French Cut, in Butter, Green Giant
3.0	1/4 cup	Artichoke hearts, marinated
3.0	1/2 cup	Vegetables, Italian Style, frozen, Birds Eye
2.5	1/2 cup	Kentucky Fried Chicken, corn
2.5	1/2 cup	Soup, Tomato Minestrone, Couscous, NSF
2.5	1/2 cup	Corn, Whole Kernel, canned, Green Giant
2.5	1 cup	Carl's Jr. Lumber Jack Mixed Vegetable Soup
2.5	2 cups	Popcorn, Gourmet, Orville Redenbacher

VEGETABLE GROUP

Nutripoints	Serving Size	Food Name
2.5	1/2 cup	Soup, Vegetable Parmesan, Couscous, Nile Spice Foods
2.5	1/4 serving	Roy Rogers Hot Topped Potato, w/margarine
2.5	1 cup	Soup, tomato
2.5	1/2 cup	Vegetables, Japanese Style, frozen, Birds Eye
2.5	1 whole	Pickles, Sweet 'n Sour, Claussen
2.5	1/4 cup	Potatoes au gratin
2.0	1 cup	Soup, Vegetable, Campbell's
2.0	1/4 cup	Potatoes, scalloped
2.0	1/4 cup	Wendy's Deluxe Three-Bean Salad
2.0	1/2 cup	Corn, Whole Kernel, canned, Del Monte
2.0	1 cup	Soup Mix, Country Vegetable, Lipton
2.0	1/4 serving	Carl's Jr. Broccoli and Cheese Potato
2.0	1/4 cup	Potatoes, mashed, from flakes
2.0	1/2 portion	Cauliflower, w/Cheddar Cheese Sauce, frozen, Budget Gourmet
2.0	1/2 portion	Broccoli, w/Cheddar Cheese Sauce, frozen, Stouffer's
1.5	1/4 serving	Wendy's Hot Stuffed Potato w/Broccoli and Cheese
1.5	1/4 serving	Carl's Jr. Taco Salad (take-out)
1.5	1/2 cup	Corn, Niblets, in Butter, frozen, Green Giant
1.5	1/2 cup	Goulash
1.5	1/2 cup	Kentucky Fried Chicken, w/Coleslaw
1.5	1/4 piece	Taco Bell Tostada Red Sauce
1.5	1/2 portion	Cabbage roll, frozen dinner
1.5	1/2 cup	Taco salad
1.5	1/4 serving	Taco Bell Tostada Green Sauce
1.5	1/4 portion	Potato, Baked, w/Broccoli and Cheese, frozen, Weight Watchers
1.5	1/2 portion	Potatoes, Cheddared, w/Broccoli, frozen, Budget Gourmet
1.5	1/4 portion	Potato, Baked, Chicken Divan, frozen, Weight Watchers
1.5	1/4 cup	Broccoli, fried, w/breading
1.5	1 cup	Gazpacho
1.5	1 portion	Ratatouille, frozen dinner
1.0	1/2 cup	Soup, cream of asparagus

VEGETABLE GROUP

Nutripoints	Serving Size	Food Name
1.0	1/4 tostada	Tostada
1.0	1/4 cup	Potatoes, mashed, home recipe
1.0	1/4 cup	Okra, fried, w/breading
1.0	9 pieces	Potato Chips, Light, Ruffles
1.0	1 serving	McDonald's Side Salad
1.0	1/2 cup	Soup, Tomato, Low Sodium, with Tomato Pieces, Campbell's
1.0	1/4 cup	Wendy's California Coleslaw
1.0	1/2 cup	Carl's Jr. Cream of Broccoli Soup
1.0	1/4 serving	Carl's Jr. Sour Cream and Chive Potato
1.0	2 tablespoons	Catsup
1.0	4 pieces	French fries (18 pieces = 1/2 cup)
0.5	1/2 cup	Soup Mix, Green Pea, Cup-A-Soup, Lipton
0.5	1 cup	Soup, Tomato, Campbell's
0.5	2 cups	Popcorn, Natural Salt Free, Orville Redenbacher's
0.5	2 tablespoons	Catsup, Tomato, Del Monte
0.5	1/2 cup	Sauce, Spaghetti w/Mushrooms, Prego
0.5	1/4 serving	Taco Bell Taco Salad w/Salsa, w/o shell
0.5	2 whole	Pickles, Kosher Dill Spears, Vlasic
0.5	1/4 serving	Roy Rogers Hot Topped Potato w/Broccoli and Cheese
0.5	1/4 serving	Carl's Jr. Cheese Potato
0.5	1/2 cup	Vegetables, San Francisco Style, frozen, Birds Eye
0.5	2 tablespoons	Catsup, low-sodium/sugar
0.5	1 cup	Soup, Tomato, 1/3 Less Salt, Campbell's
0.5	1/4 serving	Carl's Jr. Fiesta Potato
0.5	1/2 cup	Sauce, Spaghetti, Prego
0.5	1/4 cup	Potatoes, hash browned
0.5	1/2 cup	Soup, potato
0.5	1/2 portion	Potatoes, Scalloped, frozen, Stouffer's
0.5	1/2 piece	Soufflé, Corn, frozen, Stouffer's
0.5	1/2 cup	Potatoes, Golden Crinkles, Ore-Ida
0.0	8 pieces	Potato Chips, Unsalted, Lay's
0.0	1/4 serving	Taco Bell Taco Salad, w/o shell
0.0	1/2 cup	Corn, Cream Style, Golden Sweet, canned, Del Monte

VEGETABLE GROUP

Nutripoints	Serving Size	Food Name
0.0	1/4 cup	Potatoes, Instant Mashed, Hungry Jack
0.0	1/2 cup	Sauce, Spaghetti, plain, Extra Thick and Zesty, Ragú
0.0	1/2 cup	Soup, Tomato, w/milk, 1/3 Less Salt, Campbell's
0.0	5 pieces	Potato chips
0.0	1/4 serving	Roy Rogers Hot Topped Potato w/Taco Beef and Cheese
0.0	1/4 cup	Potato sticks, shoestring
0.0	1/8 serving	Taco Bell Taco Salad w/Salsa, w/shell
0.0	8 pieces	Potato Chips, Lay's
0.0	1/2 cup	Sauce, Spaghetti, Flavored w/Meat, Ragú
0.0	1/4 serving	Wendy's Hot Stuffed Potato w/Sour Cream and Chives
0.0	1/4 serving	Roy Rogers Hot Topped Potato w/Sour Cream and Chives
0.0	1/2 cup	Sauce, Spaghetti, plain, Ragú
0.0	9 pieces	Potato Chips, Ruffles
−0.5	2 pieces	Onion rings, fried
−0.5	1/4 cup	Potatoes, Tater Tots, Ore-Ida
−0.5	1/4 serving	Wendy's Hot Stuffed Potato w/Bacon and Cheese
−0.5	1/2 cup	Corn, Cream Style, canned, Green Giant
−0.5	1/4 piece	Corn, fried, w/breading
−0.5	1/4 cup	Potatoes au Gratin, Betty Crocker
−0.5	3 tablespoons	Sauce, Traditional Pizza Quick, Ragú
−0.5	1/2 cup	Sauce, Spaghetti, Extra Thick and Zesty, Flavored w/Meat, Ragú
−0.5	1/2 cup	Soup, cream of celery
−0.5	1/4 serving	McDonald's Regular French Fries
−0.5	1/4 cup	Sauce, Spaghetti, Garden Tomato w/Mushrooms, Prego
−0.5	2 cups	Popcorn, Gourmet, Microwave, Orville Redenbacher
−0.5	1/4 cup	Potatoes, Instant Mashed, Betty Crocker
−0.5	1/4 cup	Sauce, Spaghetti, Extra Chunky Mushroom and Onion, Prego
−0.5	1 cup	Jack in the Box Side Salad

VEGETABLE GROUP

Nutripoints	Serving Size	Food Name
−0.5	1/4 cup	Cauliflower, fried, w/breading
−0.5	1/3 portion	Corn, Sweet, w/Butter Sauce, frozen, Budget Gourmet
−0.5	1/2 portion	Potatoes au Gratin, frozen, Stouffer's
−0.5	1/4 cup	Jack in the Box Mexican Chicken Salad
−0.5	1/4 serving	Carl's Jr. Bacon and Cheese Potato
−0.5	1/4 cup	Wendy's Old-Fashioned Corn Relish
−0.5	1/4 serving	Roy Rogers Hot Topped Potato w/Bacon and Cheese
−1.0	1/2 cup	Soup, Tomato w/Milk, Campbell's
−1.0	1/2 cup	Potato Chips, Light, Pringle's
−1.0	1 piece	Carl's Jr. Onion Rings
−1.0	1/4 cup	Sauce, Spaghetti, Meat Flavor, Prego
−1.0	1/2 serving	Potato Chips, Wise
−1.0	17 pieces	Corn Chips, Fritos
−1.0	1/4 cup	Potato salad, home recipe
−1.0	1 serving	Carl's Jr. Fried Zucchini
−1.0	1 cup	Soup, Creamy Natural Broccoli, Campbell's
−1.0	1/4 cup	Mushrooms, fried, w/breading
−1.0	1/4 cup	Squash, fried, w/breading
−1.0	8 pieces	Pickles, Bread 'n Butter, Cucumber Slices, Heinz
−1.0	1/4 cup	Soup, cream of mushroom
−1.0	1/2 cup	Soup, Creamy Natural Broccoli w/Milk, Campbell's
−1.0	1/4 cup	Soup, Cream of Mushroom, Campbell's
−1.0	1/4 cup	Roy Rogers Potato Salad
−1.0	1/4 cup	Jack in the Box Taco Salad
−1.5	2 pieces	Carl's Jr. Hash Browns Nuggets
−1.5	1/2 cup	Salad, chef, w/ham/cheese, w/o dressing
−1.5	1 cup	Soup, onion
−1.5	1/4 cup	Wendy's Red Bliss Potato Salad
−1.5	1/2 cup	Potato Chips, Sour Cream 'n Onion, Pringle's
−1.5	1 cup	Soup, Tomato-Rice, Old-Fashioned, Campbell's
−1.5	1/4 serving	Roy Rogers French Fries
−1.5	2 tablespoons	Ketchup, Heinz
−2.0	1/2 cup	Potato Chips, Pringle's

VEGETABLE GROUP

Nutripoints	Serving Size	Food Name
−2.0	1 serving	Jack in the Box Hash Browns
−2.0	1/2 serving	McDonald's Hash Brown Potatoes
−2.0	1/4 serving	Wendy's Hot Stuffed Potato w/Cheese
−2.0	1 cup	Soup, Cream of Mushroom, 1/3 Less Salt, Campbell's
−2.5	1/4 cup	Rhubarb, cooked, w/sugar
−2.5	1/4 cup	Jack in the Box Chef Salad
−2.5	1/4 piece	Pie, rhubarb, homemade
−2.5	2 tablespoons	Relish, Hot Dog, Vlasic
−2.5	1/2 cup	Soup, Creamy Natural Potato, w/milk, Campbell's
−2.5	1 cup	Soup Mix, Cream of Mushroom, Cup-A-Soup, Lipton
−2.5	1 cup	Soup Mix, Tomato, Cup-A-Soup, Lipton
−2.5	1/2 cup	Kentucky Fried Chicken, Mashed Potatoes
−2.5	1 whole	Pickles, Sweet Gherkins, Heinz
−3.0	1/2 cup	Soufflé, spinach
−3.0	1 cup	Soup, Cream of Celery, Campbell's
−3.5	2 tablespoons	Relish, Sweet, Heinz
−3.5	1 cup	Soup, French Onion, Campbell's
−3.5	2 whole	Pickles, dill
−4.0	2 whole	Pickles, Kosher, Claussen
−4.0	1/2 cup	Soup, Creamy Natural Potato, Campbell's
−4.5	1 cup	Soup, Cream of Mushroom, Campbell's
−5.0	1 whole	Pickles, sweet
−5.5	1 cup	Soup Mix, Onion, Lipton
−6.0	2 tablespoons	Pickle relish

FRUIT GROUP

Nutripoints	Serving Size	Food Name
29.0	1/4 melon	Melon, cantaloupe
23.5	1 cup	Fruit Slices, Fresh, Nutripoint
21.0	1 whole	Guava
20.5	1/2 papaya	Papaya
19.0	1 cup	Strawberries, fresh

FRUIT GROUP

Nutripoints	Serving Size	Food Name
19.0	3/4 cup	Currants, black
18.0	1/2 cup	Fruit, Rainbow Compote, Nutripoint
17.5	1/2 mango	Mango
17.0	1 whole	Kiwi fruit
17.0	1 cup	Strawberries, frozen, unsweetened
17.0	1/2 cup	Fruit Platter, Fresh, Nutripoint
16.0	6 whole	Litchi, fresh
15.5	1/2 cup	Fruit Drink, Sunrise Cooler, Nutripoint
15.5	1/2 cup	Mandarin oranges, canned, unsweetened
14.5	1/2 cup	Fruit Salad Plate, Nutripoint
14.0	1/4 melon	Melon, honeydew
14.0	1/2 cup	Plums, canned, unsweetened
13.5	1 whole	Orange, fresh
13.5	3 whole	Apricot, fresh
13.0	1 cup	Fruit Drink, Strawberry Smoothie, Nutripoint
13.0	1 whole	Tangerine
13.0	1/2 fruit	Grapefruit, fresh
13.0	1/2 cup	Blackberries, fresh
13.0	1/2 cup	Fruit salad, fresh
12.5	1 cup	Juice, cranberry, low-cal.
12.5	1 whole	Carambola (starfruit)
12.5	8 fluid ounces	Juice, Cranapple, Low-Cal., Ocean Spray
12.5	1/2 cup	Raspberries, fresh
11.5	6 fluid ounces	Juice, orange, fresh-squeezed
11.0	1 whole	Peach, fresh
11.0	6 fluid ounces	Juice, Orange, Tropicana
11.0	1/4 melon	Melon, casaba
11.0	6 whole	Apricots, dried
11.0	6 fluid ounces	Juice, Orange, Calcium Fortified, Minute Maid
11.0	6 fluid ounces	Juice, grapefruit, unsweetened
11.0	1/2 cup	Apricots, canned, unsweetened
11.0	6 fluid ounces	Juice, orange, frozen, reconstituted
10.5	6 fluid ounces	Juice, Orange, w/Calcium, Citrus Hill
10.5	1 cup	Watermelon
10.5	1/2 cup	Peaches, canned, unsweetened
10.5	1/2 portion	Apples, Glazed w/Raspberry Sauce, frozen, Budget Gourmet

FRUIT GROUP

Nutripoints	Serving Size	Food Name
10.5	8 fluid ounces	Juice, Cranberry, Low-Cal., Ocean Spray
10.0	6 fluid ounces	Juice, orange-grapefruit, unsweetened, canned
10.0	6 fluid ounces	Juice, Orange, frozen, Minute Maid
10.0	1 whole	Prickly pear
10.0	6 whole	Kumquat
10.0	1/2 cup	Fruit cocktail, canned, unsweetened
10.0	1 whole	Nectarine, fresh
10.0	1 cup	Cranberries, raw
10.0	5 whole	Loquat, fresh
9.5	6 fluid ounces	Juice, orange-pineapple
9.0	1/2 cup	Boysenberries, frozen
9.0	1/2 cup	Topping, Red Raspberry, Hot, Nutripoint
9.0	2 whole	Passion fruit, purple, fresh
8.5	3/4 cup	Blackberry Freeze, Nutripoint
8.5	1/2 cup	Strawberries, Halved, in Light Syrup, frozen, Birds Eye
8.0	6 pieces	Apricots, Dried, Sun-Maid
8.0	6 fluid ounces	Juice, Orange Sparkler, Sundance
8.0	6 fluid ounces	Juice, Grapefruit, Ocean Spray
8.0	1/2 cup	Pineapple, fresh
7.5	6 pieces	Apricots, Dried, Del Monte
7.5	1/2 cup	Cherries, sour, canned, unsweetened
7.5	1/2 cup	Blackberries, frozen, unsweetened
7.5	10 whole	Cherries, sour, raw
7.5	1 small	Banana
7.5	1 whole	Persimmon
7.0	6 fluid ounces	Juice, Cranberry Cocktail, Ocean Spray
7.0	1/2 cup	Topping, Peach, Hot, Nutripoint
7.0	6 fluid ounces	Juice, grapefruit, sweetened
7.0	1/2 cup	Blueberries, fresh
7.0	6 fluid ounces	Juice, Grapefruit Sparkler, Sundance
6.5	1/2 cup	Prunes, cooked, unsweetened
6.5	1/2 cup	Frozen Dessert, Peach, Vitari Soft Serve
6.5	1 whole	Peaches, canned in juice
6.5	1/2 cup	Strawberries, frozen, sweetened
6.5	1/2 cup	Peaches, Light Yellow Cling, w/Fruit Juice, canned, Libby's

FRUIT GROUP

Nutripoints	Serving Size	Food Name
6.0	3 pieces	Prunes, Whole, Sunsweet
6.0	1/3 cup	Banana Gladje, Nutripoint
6.0	2 whole	Plum, fresh
6.0	1 whole	Quince
6.0	1/2 plantain	Plantain, fresh
6.0	3/4 cup	Soup, Blueberry, Chilled, Nutripoint
6.0	6 fluid ounces	Juice, Grapefruit, Pink, Ocean Spray
6.0	4 pieces	Prunes, dried
6.0	6 fluid ounces	Juice, pineapple, unsweetened, canned
5.5	1/2 cup	Cherries, sweet, canned in water
5.5	1/2 cup	Plantain, cooked
5.5	6 fluid ounces	Juice, Grape, Unsweetened, frozen, Welch's
5.5	6 fluid ounces	Juice, grape, unsweetened
5.5	10 whole	Cherries, sweet, fresh
5.0	6 fluid ounces	Juice, Pineapple, Dole
5.0	1/4 cup	Strawberries, frozen, w/Heavy Syrup, Birds Eye
5.0	4 fluid ounces	Juice, prune, canned
5.0	2 pieces	Figs, dried
5.0	1/2 cup	Mandarin oranges, canned
5.0	1/2 cup	Fruit Cocktail, Hot, Nutripoint
5.0	1 ounce	Prunes, Pitted, Bite-Size, Sunsweet
5.0	4 pieces	Peaches, Dried, Sun-Maid
5.0	2 pieces	Peaches, dried, sulfured, uncooked
4.5	4 fluid ounces	Apricot nectar, canned
4.5	1/2 cup	Blueberries, frozen, unsweetened
4.5	1/4 cup	Currants, zante
4.5	1/2 cup	Frozen Dessert, Orange, Vitari Soft Serve
4.5	1/4 cup	Prunes, canned in heavy syrup
4.5	1 whole	Pear, fresh
4.5	8 fluid ounces	Fruit Drink, Low-Cal., Hawaiian Punch
4.5	6 fluid ounces	Juice, Apple, frozen, Seneca
4.5	6 fluid ounces	Juice, Kiwi Fruit, Sweetened, Kiwi Island
4.5	1/4 cup	Raspberries, frozen, sweetened
4.5	2 pieces	Figs, Mission, Sun-Maid
4.5	1/4 cup	Guacamole
4.5	20 grapes	Grapes, raw
4.5	1 medium	Apple, fresh

FRUIT GROUP

Nutripoints	Serving Size	Food Name
4.0	½ cup	Pineapple, Sliced, in Juice, canned, Del Monte
4.0	½ cup	Pineapple Chunks, in Juice, canned, Del Monte
4.0	2 pieces	Figs, Calimyrna, Sun-Maid
4.0	¼ avocado	Avocado, Florida
4.0	1 whole	Figs, fresh
4.0	½ serving	Pear, Poached, Nutripoint
4.0	½ cup	Pineapple, Sliced, in Juice, canned, Dole
4.0	4 fluid ounces	Juice, Prune, Sunsweet
4.0	¼ cup	Raisins
4.0	¼ cup	Prunes, cooked, w/sugar
4.0	6 fluid ounces	Peach nectar, canned
4.0	½ cup	Peaches, Yellow Cling, in Light Syrup, canned, Del Monte
4.0	6 fluid ounces	Papaya nectar, canned
4.0	5 pieces	Dates
3.5	1 whole	Pomegranate
3.5	6 fluid ounces	Fruit Drink, Citrus Punch, Sunny Delite
3.5	2 ounces	Mixed Fruits, Dried, Sun-Maid
3.5	½ cup	Applesauce, no sugar
3.5	6 fluid ounces	Juice, cranberry, sweetened
3.5	1 ounce	Fruit Bits, Dried, Sun-Maid
3.5	6 fluid ounces	Juice, Red Grape, Welch's
3.5	6 fluid ounces	Juice, Purple Grape, Welch's
3.5	½ cup	Pears, canned, no sugar
3.5	¼ cup	Currants, Zante, Sun-Maid
3.5	½ cup	Frozen Dessert, Wildberry, Vitari Soft Serve
3.0	6 fluid ounces	Fruit Drink, Guava, Ocean Spray
3.0	½ cup	Frozen Dessert, Strawberry, Vitari Soft Serve
3.0	½ cup	Applesauce, Nutripoint
3.0	½ cup	Applesauce, Natural Style, Mott's
3.0	2 tablespoons	Raisins, California Golden, Sun-Maid
3.0	2 pieces	Pears, dried
3.0	2 tablespoons	Raisins, Thompson Seedless, Natural, Sun-Maid
2.5	6 fluid ounces	Juice, Apple Sparkler, Sundance
2.5	½ cup	Apricots, canned in heavy syrup

FRUIT GROUP

Nutripoints	Serving Size	Food Name
2.5	6 fluid ounces	Fruit Drink, Crangrape, Ocean Spray
2.5	6 fluid ounces	Juice, apple
2.5	1/2 cup	Fruit Cocktail, in Light Syrup, Del Monte
2.5	2 ounces	Apples, Chunks, Dried, Sun-Maid
2.5	1/2 cup	Topping, Blueberry, Hot, Nutripoint
2.5	1/2 cup	Fruit Cocktail, in Light Syrup, Libby's
2.5	6 fluid ounces	Pear nectar, canned
2.5	6 fluid ounces	Juice, Apple, Mott's
2.5	1/4 avocado	Avocado, California
2.0	1/2 cup	Applesauce, Unsweetened, Musselman
2.0	6 fluid ounces	Juice, Grape, Sweetened, frozen, Welch's
2.0	1/2 cup	Cherries, sweet, frozen, sweetened
2.0	6 fluid ounces	Juice, White Grape, Welch's
2.0	6 fluid ounces	Juice, Raspberry Sparkler, Sundance
2.0	1/2 cup	Pineapple, Sliced, in Light Syrup, canned, Dole
2.0	1 ounce	Fruit leather
2.0	6 fluid ounces	Juice, Cranberry Sparkler, Sundance
2.0	6 fluid ounces	Juice, Kiwi-Lime Sparkler, Sundance
1.5	1/2 cup	Pears, Bartlett, in Light Syrup, canned, Del Monte
1.5	6 fluid ounces	Juice, Apple, from concentrate, Tree Top
1.5	6 fluid ounces	Juice, Cranapple, Ocean Spray
1.5	6 fluid ounces	Fruit Drink, Fruit Juicy Red, Hawaiian Punch
1.5	6 fluid ounces	Fruit Drink, Grape, Hi-C
1.5	1 bar	Frozen dessert, fruit bar
1.0	6 fluid ounces	Juice, Apple, from concentrate, frozen, Tree Top
1.0	1/2 cup	Pineapple, canned in heavy syrup
1.0	1 tablespoon	Taco Bell Guacamole
1.0	1/2 cup	Frozen Dessert, Chunky Strawberry, Frozfruit
1.0	1 cup	Gelatin, Cherry, Sugar-Free, Jell-O
1.0	1/2 cup	Fruit cocktail, canned, heavy syrup
1.0	6 fluid ounces	Juice, Apple, Lucky Leaf
1.0	1/2 cup	Cherries, sour, canned in heavy syrup
0.5	1 bar	Frozen Dessert, Fudgesicle
0.5	2 tablespoons	Jelly, Grape, Imitation, Smucker's
0.5	1/2 piece	McDonald's Garden Salad

FRUIT GROUP

Nutripoints	Serving Size	Food Name
0.0	½ cup	Cherries, sweet, canned, heavy syrup
0.0	6 fluid ounces	Juice, Cranberry Cocktail, frozen, Welch's
0.0	½ cup	Peaches, canned in heavy syrup
0.0	4 whole	Olives, Ripe, Lindsay
0.0	6 fluid ounces	Fruit Drink, Grape, frozen, Welchade
0.0	1 tablespoon	Jelly, fruit butters, all flavors
0.0	½ cup	Plums, canned in heavy syrup
−0.5	½ portion	Apples, Escalloped, frozen, Stouffer's
−0.5	1 bar	Frozen Dessert, Pineapple, Frozfruit
−0.5	¼ serving	McDonald's Chef Salad
−0.5	½ cup	Applesauce, w/sugar
−0.5	2 tablespoons	Jam, low-cal.
−1.0	1 piece	Luncheon meat, olive loaf
−1.0	1 ounce	Raisins, carob-covered
−1.0	½ piece	Pie, raspberry
−1.0	½ piece	Pie, banana cream
−1.0	¼ piece	Pie, mincemeat
−1.0	½ cup	Pears, canned in heavy syrup
−1.0	¼ piece	Burger King Apple Pie
−1.0	¼ cup	Apple crisp
−1.5	½ cup	Pie Filling, Apple, Lite, Thank You
−1.5	6 fluid ounces	Fruit drink, w/sugar
−1.5	½ piece	Pie, blackberry
−1.5	½ piece	Pie, strawberry
−1.5	½ cup	Frozen Dessert, Banana, Creamy, Frozfruit
−1.5	1 ounce	Raisins, chocolate-covered
−1.5	6 fluid ounces	Fruit Drink, Cranicot, Ocean Spray
−1.5	6 fluid ounces	Fruit Drink, Hawaiian Punch
−1.5	¼ serving	Banana split
−2.0	½ piece	Pie, Apple, frozen, Weight Watchers
−2.0	1 piece	Fruit leather, with sugar
−2.0	¼ piece	Pie, apple
−2.0	½ piece	Pie, peach
−2.0	½ piece	Pie, blueberry
−2.0	½ piece	Pie, berry
−2.0	¼ piece	McDonald's Apple Pie
−2.0	¼ piece	Pie, fruit
−2.0	1 tablespoon	Coconut

FRUIT GROUP

Nutripoints	Serving Size	Food Name
−2.0	1/4 piece	Pie, Cherry, Hostess
−2.0	1/4 piece	Pie, Blueberry, Hostess
−2.0	8 whole	Olives, black
−2.0	1 piece	Coconut, chocolate-covered
−2.0	1/4 piece	Pie, Cherry, in Natural Juice, Mrs. Smith's
−2.0	1/2 cup	Salad, Waldorf
−2.5	1/4 piece	Pie, Apple, in Natural Juice, Mrs. Smith's
−2.5	1/2 cup	Sherbet, orange
−2.5	1/4 piece	Jack in the Box Hot Apple Turnover
−2.5	1/4 piece	Pie, Peach, Mrs. Smith's
−2.5	1/2 portion	Mousse, Raspberry, frozen, Weight Watchers
−3.0	2 tablespoons	Sauce, cranberry, canned, sweetened
−3.0	1/2 piece	Pie, pumpkin, homemade
−3.0	1 bar	Frozen Dessert, Banana, Pudding Pops, Jell-O
−3.0	1 tablespoon	Jam, preserves, all flavors
−3.0	8 whole	Olives, Medium, Mammoth Queen, S&W
−3.0	1/2 cup	Pie Filling, Apple, Thank You
−3.0	1 cup	Fruit drink, limeade
−3.5	1/4 piece	Pie, cherry, w/cream cheese and sour cream
−3.5	1/2 piece	Pie, coconut cream
−3.5	1 tablespoon	Coconut, Shredded Premium, Baker's
−3.5	1 ounce	Coconut, raw
−3.5	2 pieces	Cherries, chocolate-covered
−4.0	1 tablespoon	Topping, Strawberry, Smucker's
−4.0	1 tablespoon	Coconut, dried, sweetened, shredded
−4.0	8 whole	Olives, green
−4.0	1/2 bar	Candy Bar, Coconut, Almond Joy
−4.0	1/2 cup	Pie Filling, Cherry, Thank You
−4.0	1/4 piece	Pie, lemon meringue
−4.0	1/2 cup	Gelatin, Strawberry-Banana, Royal
−4.5	6 fluid ounces	Fruit drink, lemonade
−4.5	1/4 cup	Sauce, Cranberry, Whole Berry, Ocean Spray
−5.0	6 fluid ounces	Lemonade, Minute Maid
−5.0	1/2 piece	Pie, cherry
−5.0	1/2 cup	Gelatin, Cherry, Jell-O
−5.0	1 tablespoon	Preserves, all varieties, Kraft
−5.5	6 fluid ounces	Fruit Drink, Punch, Capri Sun
−5.5	6 fluid ounces	Fruit Drink, Orange, Capri Sun

FRUIT GROUP

Nutripoints	Serving Size	Food Name
−5.5	2 tablespoons	Jelly, cranberry
−5.5	2 tablespoons	Jelly, Blackberry Spread, Smucker's
−5.5	1 tablespoon	Jelly, Grape, Welch's
−5.5	1 tablespoon	Jam, Grape, Welch's
−5.5	1 tablespoon	Preserves, Strawberry, Welch's
−6.0	1 tablespoon	Jam, Strawberry, Smucker's
−6.0	1 tablespoon	Preserves, Raspberry, Smucker's
−6.0	1 tablespoon	Marmalade, Orange, Smucker's
−6.0	1 tablespoon	Jelly, Concord Grape, Smucker's

GRAIN GROUP

Nutripoints	Serving Size	Food Name
64.5	1 cup	* Cereal, Whole Wheat Total, General Mills
57.5	1 cup	* Cereal, Total Corn Flakes, General Mills
56.0	1 cup	* Cereal, Product 19, Kellogg's
51.0	1/2 cup	* Cereal, Instant Total Oatmeal, w/skim milk, General Mills
51.0	2/3 cup	* Cereal, Just Right, Kellogg's
43.5	1/2 cup	* Cereal, All Bran Extra Fiber, Kellogg's
40.5	1/2 cup	* Cereal, Total Raisin Bran, General Mills
36.5	3/4 cup	* Cereal, Just Right w/Fruit and Nuts, Kellogg's
31.5	1/2 cup	* Cereal, Fiber One, General Mills
31.0	1/2 cup	* Cereal, 100% Bran, Nabisco
28.5	2/3 cup	* Cereal, Fruitful Bran, Kellogg's
27.5	1 ounce	Wheat Bran, Toasted, Kretschmer
27.0	1/3 cup	* Cereal, All Bran, Kellogg's
26.5	1/2 cup	Wheat bran
25.5	1/3 cup	* Cereal, Bran Buds, Kellogg's
23.5	1/2 cup	* Cereal, 100% Bran with Oat Bran, Nabisco
21.0	2/3 cup	* Cereal, Bran Flakes, Kellogg's
21.0	2/3 cup	* Cereal, 40+ Bran Flakes, Kellogg's
18.0	1 cup	* Cereal, Corn Flakes, Kellogg's
18.0	7/8 cup	* Cereal, Grape-Nuts Flakes, Post

*Fortified

GRAIN GROUP

Nutripoints	Serving Size	Food Name
18.0	3/4 cup	* Cereal, Honey Buc-Wheat Crisp, General Mills
17.5	2/3 cup	* Cereal, Natural Bran Flakes, Post
17.0	1 piece	* Candy Bar, Slim-Fast
17.0	1/2 cup	* Cereal, Natural Raisin Bran, Post
17.0	1/2 cup	* Cereal, Oat Squares, Quaker
16.0	1/2 cup	* Cereal, Crunchy Bran, Quaker
16.0	1/2 cup	* Cereal, Cinnamon-Apple Crisp, w/Fruit and Fibre, Post
15.5	2/3 cup	* Cereal, Nutri-Grain, Wheat, Kellogg's
15.5	1/2 cup	* Cereal, Fruit and Fibre w/Raisins/Peaches/Almonds, Post
15.5	1/2 cup	* Cereal, Fruit and Fibre w/Dates/Raisins/Walnuts, Post
15.5	3/4 cup	* Cereal, Raisin Bran, Kellogg's
15.5	3/4 cup	* Cereal, Bran Chex, Ralston
15.0	2/3 cup	* Cereal, Nutri-Grain, Biscuits, Kellogg's
15.0	1/2 cup	* Cereal, Fruit and Fibre w/Pineapple/Banana/Coconut, Post
14.0	2/3 cup	* Cereal, Common Sense Oat Bran w/Raisins, Kellogg's
14.0	1 cup	* Cereal, Special K, Kellogg's
14.0	1/2 cup	* Cereal, Cracklin' Oat Bran, Kellogg's
14.0	1/2 cup	* Cereal, Shredded Wheat Squares w/Raisins, Kellogg's
13.5	1/4 cup	* Cereal, Grape-Nuts, Post
13.5	2/3 cup	* Cereal, Common Sense Oat Bran, Kellogg's
13.5	2 bars	* Candy bar, Ideal Grain Apple, Thompson Foods
13.0	2/3 cup	* Cereal, Wheat Chex, Ralston
13.0	1 1/4 cups	* Cereal, Cheerios, General Mills
13.0	1/2 cup	* Cereal, Raspberry Fruit Wheats, Nabisco
13.0	1 cup	* Cereal, Fruit Loops, Kellogg's
13.0	1/2 cup	* Cereal, Blueberry Fruit Wheats, Nabisco
13.0	2/3 cup	* Cereal, Oat Flakes, Post
13.0	1/2 cup	* Cereal, Nut and Honey Crunch Biscuits, Kellogg's

*Fortified

GRAIN GROUP

Nutripoints	Serving Size	Food Name
12.5	1/2 cup	*Cereal, Müeslix, Bran Muesli, Kellogg's
12.5	1/2 cup	*Cereal, Frosted Mini-Wheats, Kellogg's
12.0	1 cup	*Cereal, Heartwise, Kellogg's
12.0	1/2 cup	*Cereal, Oat Bran, w/low-fat milk, Nabisco
12.0	1/4 cup	Wheat Germ, Kretschmer
12.0	1 cup	*Cereal, Wheaties, General Mills
11.5	1 cup	*Cereal, Honey Graham Oh's, Quaker
11.5	1/2 cup	*Cereal, Frosted Wheat Squares, Nabisco
11.5	1 cup	*Cereal, Rice Krispies, Kellogg's
11.5	2/3 cup	*Cereal, Nutri-Grain w/Wheat and Raisins, Kellogg's
11.5	1 cup	*Cereal, Team Flakes, Nabisco
11.0	2/3 cup	*Cereal, Life, Cinnamon, Quaker
10.5	1 whole	Muffin, Nutripoint
10.5	1 cup	*Cereal, Nutrific Oatmeal, Kellogg's
10.5	1/4 cup	Wheat germ
10.5	1 cup	Soup, Wild Rice, Nutripoint
10.5	1/2 cup	*Cereal, Clusters, General Mills
10.5	1 cup	*Cereal, Lucky Charms, General Mills
10.5	1 cup	*Cereal, Sun Flakes, Ralston
10.0	1/2 cup	*Cereal, Müeslix, 5-Grain Muesli, Kellogg's
10.0	1/3 cup	*Cereal, Oatbake, Kellogg's
10.0	1 1/2 cups	*Cereal, Kix, General Mills
10.0	1/2 cup	*Cereal, Raisin Nut Bran, General Mills
10.0	3/4 cup	*Cereal, Honey Nut Cheerios, General Mills
10.0	1/3 cup	*Cereal, Horizon Trail Mix, Post
10.0	1 cup	*Cereal, Corn Chex, Ralston
10.0	1 cup	*Cereal, Crispix, Kellogg's
10.0	1/2 cup	*Cereal, S.W. Graham Shredded Biscuits, Kellogg's
10.0	1 1/2 cups	Pasta, Angel Hair, w/Sunshine Sauce, Nutripoint
9.5	3/4 cup	*Cereal, Crispy Wheat 'n Raisins, General Mills
9.5	3/4 cup	*Cereal, Bran News, Ralston
9.5	1/2 cup	*Cereal, Oatmeal Raisin Crisp, General Mills
9.5	3/4 cup	*Cereal, Kenmei Rice Bran, Kellogg's

*Fortified

GRAIN GROUP

Nutripoints	Serving Size	Food Name
9.5	2/3 cup	* Cereal, Life, Quaker
9.5	2/3 cup	* Cereal, Nutri-Grain w/Almonds and Raisins, Kellogg's
9.5	1 cup	* Cereal, Apple Jacks, Kellogg's
9.5	1/2 cup	Cereal, Oats, Instant, w/Bran, w/low-fat milk, 3 Minute Brand
9.0	8 pieces	Cracker, Snackbread, High-Fiber, Ryvita
9.0	1 cup	Lasagna, Spinach, Nutripoint
9.0	1/2 cup	* Cereal, Muesli w/Raisins/Dates/Almonds, Ralston
9.0	1 1/8 cups	* Cereal, Rice Chex, Ralston
9.0	1 1/4 cups	* Cereal, Toasties Corn Flakes, Post
9.0	2 ounces	Bran, Rice
9.0	1 cup	* Cereal, Apple Cinnamon Oh's, Quaker
9.0	3/4 cup	* Cereal, Crunch Berries, Quaker
9.0	3/4 cup	* Cereal, Golden Grahams, General Mills
9.0	1/2 cup	* Cereal, S.W. Graham w/Cinnamon, Kellogg's
9.0	1/3 cup	Bran, Oat, Arrowhead Mills
9.0	3/4 cup	* Cereal, Cap'n Crunch, Peanut Butter, Quaker
8.5	1 cup	* Cereal, Alpha-Bits, Post
8.5	3/4 cup	* Cereal, Cap'n Crunch, Quaker
8.5	2/3 cup	* Cereal, Apple Raisin Crisp, Kellogg's
8.5	1 1/3 cups	* Cereal, Honey-Comb, Ralston
8.5	1/4 cup	Cereal, Hot, High-Fiber, Ralston
8.0	1 cup	* Cereal, Fruity Yummy Mummy, General Mills
8.0	1 cup	* Cereal, Smurf Magic Berries, Post
8.0	1 ounce	Wheat Germ, Honey Crunch, Kretschmer
8.0	7/8 cup	* Cereal, Super Golden Crisp, Post
8.0	1/2 cup	* Cereal, Muesli w/Raisins/Peaches/Pecans, Ralston
8.0	1 cup	* Cereal, Trix, General Mills
8.0	3/4 cup	* Cereal, Apple Cinnamon Cheerios, General Mills
8.0	1 cup	* Cereal, Corn Pops, Kellogg's
7.5	1 cup	* Cereal, Dinersaurs, Ralston

*Fortified

GRAIN GROUP

Nutripoints	Serving Size	Food Name
7.5	3 pieces	Cracker, Crispbread Fiber Plus, Wasa
7.5	3/4 cup	*Cereal, Cinnamon Toast Crunch, General Mills
7.5	1 cup	*Cereal, Cookie-Crisp, Ralston
7.5	1 cup	*Cereal, Malt-O Meal, w/water, cooked
7.5	1 cup	Jambalaya, Nutripoint
7.5	1/2 cup	*Cereal, C.W. Post, w/Raisins, Post
7.5	7/8 cup	*Cereal, Fruity Pebbles, Post
7.5	7/8 cup	*Cereal, Cocoa Pebbles, Post
7.5	2/3 cup	*Cereal, Honeybunches of Oats w/Almonds, Post
7.0	3/4 cup	*Cereal, Cocoa Krispies, Kellogg's
7.0	1/4 cup	*Cereal, C.W. Post, Post
7.0	3/4 cup	*Cereal, Almond Delight, Ralston
7.0	3 pieces	Pancakes, Lite, Buttermilk, Aunt Jemima
7.0	3/4 cup	*Cereal, Frosted Flakes, Kellogg's
7.0	1/2 cup	Cereal, Oat Bran, Quaker
6.5	1/2 cup	Cereal, Oat Bran, Instant, w/skim milk, 3 Minute Brand
6.5	2/3 cup	*Cereal, Honey Graham Chex, Ralston
6.5	1 cup	*Cereal, Cocoa Puffs, General Mills
6.5	3 slices	Bread, Hi-Fiber, Wonder
6.5	4 ounces	Pilaf, Vegetarian Amaranth, Health Valley
6.0	1 whole	Muffin, English, whole wheat
6.0	1/4 cup	Cereal, Hot, High-Fiber, w/milk, Ralston
6.0	1 ounce	Cereal, Oat Bran, Instant, w/water, 3 Minute Brand
6.0	1 piece	Pizza, French Bread, Nutripoint
6.0	1/4 cup	Flour, whole wheat
6.0	3 slices	Bread, Less, Mrs. Baird's
6.0	2 slices	Bread, Whole Wheat, Stone-Ground, The Sourdough
6.0	2 slices	Bread, whole wheat
6.0	1 ounce	Cereal, Shredded Wheat 'n Bran, Nabisco
5.5	1 cup	Cereal, Puffed Wheat, Quaker
5.5	4 pieces	Pancake, Whole Grain, Nutripoint
5.5	3 slices	Bread, Light Bran & Oat, Oatmeal Goodness

*Fortified

GRAIN GROUP

Nutripoints	Serving Size	Food Name
5.5	1 cup	Cereal, Oat Bran, Instant, w/whole milk, 3 Minute Brand
5.5	3 slices	Bread, Oat Bran n' Honey, Light, Roman Meal
5.5	1 cup	Cereal, Instant Oatmeal w/Peaches and Cream, Quaker
5.5	1 ounce	Quinoa, Dry, Arrowhead Mills
5.5	1/2 cup	Cereal, oatmeal, dry
5.5	1/2 cup	Rice, wild, cooked w/o salt
5.5	1/4 cup	Flour, Whole Wheat, Gold Medal
5.5	3 slices	Bread, diet, 40 cal./slice
5.0	2 slices	Bread, Wheat, Fresh Horizons
5.0	2 slices	Bread, mixed grain
5.0	2 tablespoons	McDonald's Croutons
5.0	1/2 serving	Sandwich, Open-Face Pita, Nutripoint
5.0	1 ounce	Amaranth, Dry, Arrowhead Mills
5.0	1 piece	Cereal, Shredded Wheat, large biscuit, Nabisco
5.0	6 pieces	Cracker, Rykrisp, Ralston
5.0	1 cup	Cereal, Oatmeal, Fruited Cinnamon, Nutripoint
5.0	1 bar	* Candy Bar, Tiger's Milk Nutrition
5.0	1 whole	Muffin, Raisin Oat Bran, Health Valley
5.0	2 slices	Bread, sprouted wheat
5.0	2 slices	Bread, 5 Bran, Home Pride
5.0	2/3 cup	Cereal, Spoon-Size Shredded Wheat, Nabisco
4.5	2/3 cup	Rice, Whole Grain Brown, Uncle Ben's
4.5	1/2 cup	* Cereal, Malt-O Meal, Quick, w/whole milk
4.5	2 slices	Bread, Whole Wheat, Thin, Pepperidge Farm
4.5	1/2 cup	Pasta Salad, Fresh, Nutripoint
4.5	1 cup	* Cereal, Cream of Wheat, Quick, Nabisco
4.5	1 whole	Tortilla, whole wheat
4.5	2 cups	Cereal, puffed wheat
4.5	2 slices	Bread, Wheat, Lite 35, Earth Grains
4.5	2 slices	Bread, Whole Wheat, Stone-Ground, Country Hearth

*Fortified

GRAIN GROUP

Nutripoints	Serving Size	Food Name
4.5	1/2 cup	*Cereal, Instant Cream of Wheat, w/low-fat milk, Nabisco
4.5	1 whole	Roll, whole wheat
4.5	1 whole	Muffin, English, w/raisins
4.5	2 ounces	Wheat, Whole Grain, Dry, Arrowhead Mills
4.5	1/2 cup	Cereal, whole wheat, cooked
4.5	1/2 cup	Rice, Wild, Sherry, frozen, Green Giant
4.5	2 slices	Bread, cracked wheat
4.5	1 bar	*Breakfast Bar, Honey Nut, Carnation
4.5	1/2 cup	Ravioli
4.5	1 whole	Muffin, English, Roman Meal
4.5	2 slices	Bread, Roman Meal
4.5	2 slices	Bread, Triticale
4.5	3/4 cup	Cereal, Oats, Old-Fashioned, Quaker
4.5	2 slices	Bread, pumpernickel
4.0	1/2 cup	Pasta Accents, Cheddar Cheese, Green Giant
4.0	1/2 cup	Rice, brown, cooked w/o salt
4.0	2 slices	Bread, whole rye
4.0	1 whole	Muffin, English
4.0	2 slices	Bread, wheat germ
4.0	1/2 portion	Lasagna, low-cal. frozen meal
4.0	1 bar	*Breakfast Bar, Chocolate, Carnation
2.0	1/2 cup	Spaghetti, w/sauce
4.0	1/4 cup	Flour, rye, whole grain
4.0	3 pieces	Cracker, Crispbread Golden Rye, Wasa
4.0	1/2 cup	Rotini Cheddar, Garden Gourmet, Green Giant
4.0	2 pieces	Cereal, Whole Wheat, Weetabix
4.0	2 whole	Tortilla, corn
4.0	1 ounce	Cereal, Oats, Steel-Cut, Arrowhead Mills
4.0	1/2 cup	Spaghetti, high-protein
4.0	1 whole	Bread, pita, whole wheat
4.0	1 ounce	Cereal, Seven Grain, Stone-Buhr
4.0	1 bar	Granola Bar, Chewy Fruit and Nut, Jack La Lanne

*Fortified

GRAIN GROUP

Nutripoints	Serving Size	Food Name
4.0	1/4 cup	Flour, Ezekiel, Arrowhead Mills
4.0	1 whole	Muffin, English, Pepperidge Farm
4.0	1/2 cup	Noodles, whole wheat
4.0	10 pieces	Cookies, Animal, Oat Bran, Health Valley
4.0	2 slices	Bread, 100% Whole Wheat, Wonder
4.0	1/2 cup	Macaroni and Spaghetti, Enriched, Prince
4.0	1 waffle	Waffles
4.0	2 slices	Bread, raisin
4.0	2 slices	Bread, Wheat Berry, Honey, Earth Grains
4.0	1 whole	Bagel, whole wheat
4.0	1/4 cup	Flour, Triticale, Whole, Arrowhead Mills
4.0	1/2 cup	Rice, Spanish
3.5	1/2 cup	Rice, Brown, Natural Long Grain, Mahatma
3.5	2 slices	Bread, Bran'nola, Oroweat
3.5	2 slices	Bread, Protogen Protein, Thomas'
3.5	2 slices	Bread, Wheat, Stone-Ground, Earth Grains
3.5	2 slices	Bread, 100% Whole Wheat, Home Pride
3.5	1/2 cup	Pasta Accents, w/Garlic Seasoning, Green Giant
3.5	1/4 cup	Flour, Whole Wheat, Pillsbury
3.5	1 whole	Bagel, pumpernickel
3.5	1 dinner	Spaghetti Dinner w/Meatballs, frozen, Morton
3.5	1 ounce	Macaroni, dry (2 ounces = 1 cup cooked)
3.5	1/2 cup	Macaroni, cooked, no salt (1 cup = 2 ounces dry)
3.5	1/2 cup	Pilaf, Breakfast, Seven Whole Grains and Sesame Seeds, Kashi
3.5	2 slices	Bread, bran
3.5	2 slices	Bread, Sandwich, Salt-Free, Earth Grains
3.5	1 piece	Biscuit Mix, Multigrain, Arrowhead Mills
3.5	1/4 cup	* Cereal, Alpen
3.5	1/4 cup	Flour, whole buckwheat
3.5	1 whole	Muffin, English, cracked wheat
3.5	2 slices	Bread, Original Bran'nola, Arnold

*Fortified

GRAIN GROUP

Nutripoints	Serving Size	Food Name
3.5	2 slices	Bread, Honey Wheat Berry, Arnold
3.5	1 whole	Muffin, Oat Bran, Nutripoint
3.5	1/4 cup	Corn Meal, Yellow Enriched, Aunt Jemima
3.5	1/2 cup	Linguine, Spinach, High-Protein, Buitoni
3.5	1/2 cup	Rice, Brown, Instant, Minute
3.5	1 whole	Roll, rye
3.5	6 pieces	Breadsticks
3.5	1 1/2 waffles	Waffles, Common Sense Oat Bran, Eggo
3.5	2 slices	Bread, Honey Nut and Oat Bran, Roman Meal
3.5	1 1/4 ounces	Cereal, Instant Oatmeal w/Apples and Cinnamon, Quaker
3.5	3 pieces	Cracker, Crispbread Hearty Rye, Wasa
3.5	2 slices	Bread, Oatmeal and Bran, Oatmeal Goodness
3.5	1/2 cup	Macaroni, cooked, all shapes, Mueller's
3.5	1 whole	Muffin, bran, w/raisins and nuts
3.5	2 slices	Bread, Oatmeal and Sunflower Seeds, Oatmeal Goodness
3.5	2 slices	Bread, low-sodium
3.5	1/4 cup	Corn meal, dry
3.5	1 whole	Muffin, Extra Crisp, Arnold
3.5	2 pancakes	Pancake Mix, Complete Buttermilk, Aunt Jemima
3.5	1/2 piece	Pizza Hut Supreme Hand-Tossed Pizza
3.5	1 whole	Bread, pita
3.5	1/2 cup	Noodles, spinach
3.0	1/2 cup	Macaroni, Superoni, Prince
3.0	2 slices	Bread, Wheat Berry, Home Pride
3.0	1/2 cup	Spaghetti, cooked (1 cup = 2 ounces dry)
3.0	4 pieces	Cracker, Crispbread Dark Rye, Ryvita
3.0	1/2 cup	Rice, Brown Pilaf, w/Vegetables and Herbs, Pritikin
3.0	2 slices	Bread, Wheat and Oatmeal, Oatmeal Goodness
3.0	2 slices	Bread, Seven Grain, Home Pride
3.0	2 cups	Cereal, Puffed, Seven Whole Grains and Sesame Seeds, Kashi
3.0	2 whole	Biscuit, Extra Rich Buttermilk, Hungry Jack

GRAIN GROUP

Nutripoints	Serving Size	Food Name
3.0	6 pieces	Cracker, Seasoned, Rykrisp
3.0	2 slices	Bread, Oat Bran, Honey, Earth Grains
3.0	1/4 cup	Flour, All-Purpose Enriched, Pillsbury
3.0	2 ounces	Linguine, Buitoni, (2 ounces dry = 3/4 cup cooked)
3.0	1/2 piece	Pizza Hut Pepperoni Pan Pizza
3.0	1 whole	Roll, cracked wheat
3.0	2 slices	Bread, Honey Wheat Berry, Pepperidge Farm
3.0	1/2 cup	Rice, white, regular, w/salt
3.0	1/2 cup	Cereal, Oats, Quick, w/low-fat milk, Quaker
3.0	1 ounce	Rotini, Rainbow, Creamette, Borden
3.0	2 slices	Bread, Grape-Nuts, Oroweat
3.0	1/2 bun	Bun, submarine/hoagie
3.0	2 slices	Bread, Sprouted Wheat, Pepperidge Farm
3.0	1/2 cup	Pilaf, Couscous, Casbah
3.0	1/4 cup	Flour, White, All-Purpose Plain, Martha
3.0	2/3 cup	Rice, white, instant, cooked
3.0	1/4 cup	Flour, All-Purpose, Gold Medal
3.0	2 slices	Bread, Rye, Family, Pepperidge Farm
3.0	8 pieces	Cracker, whole wheat
3.0	3 cookies	Cookies, Fruit Chunks, Health Valley
3.0	1/2 cup	Spaghetti, San Giorgio
3.0	1/2 cup	Rice, white, regular, cooked, w/o salt
3.0	2 slices	Bread, White, Butter-Top, Home Pride
3.0	1 whole	Muffin, bran
3.0	1/4 cup	Flour, white
3.0	1 slice	Bread, Health Nut, Oroweat
3.0	1 whole	Muffin, English, Health Nut, Oroweat
3.0	2 slices	Bread, White, Brick Oven, Arnold
3.0	1/2 portion	Cavatelli, frozen, Celentano
3.0	1/2 cup	Spaghetti, Ronzoni
3.0	2 slices	Bread, French
3.0	1 cup	Grits, cooked
3.0	2 slices	Bread, Rye, Light, Earth Grains
3.0	2 slices	Bread, Old-Fashioned Buttermilk, Country Hearth
3.0	1 ounce dry	Noodles, egg, cholesterol-free, no yolks

GRAIN GROUP

Nutripoints	Serving Size	Food Name
3.0	¼ cup	Bulgar, dry
3.0	1 piece	Pizza Hut Cheese Thin 'n Crispy Pizza
3.0	2 slices	Bread, Oatmeal, Pepperidge Farm
3.0	½ cup	Macaroni Ribbons, Spinach, Creamette, Borden
2.5	½ piece	Pizza Hut Cheese Pan Pizza
2.5	2 ounces	Linguine, San Giorgio (2 ounces dry = ¾ cup cooked)
2.5	½ portion	Spaghetti, w/Meat Sauce, frozen, Weight Watchers
2.5	2 slices	Bread, Italian
2.5	3 pieces	Cracker, Norwegian Crispbread, Thick Style, Kavli
2.5	½ cup	Lasagna
2.5	½ portion	Pasta Primavera, frozen, Weight Watchers
2.5	6 pieces	Cracker, Crispbread Dark, Finn
2.5	1 cup	Cereal, Puffed Rice, Quaker
2.5	½ cup	Macaroni, Elbow, Creamette, Borden
2.5	½ cup	Spaghetti, Creamette, Borden
2.5	2 slices	Bread, Rye, Jewish, Real Unseeded, Levy's
2.5	¼ cup	Cracker Meal, Keebler
2.5	2 slices	Bread, sourdough
2.5	½ portion	Lasagne Primavera, frozen, Celentano
2.5	2 whole	Roll, Sourdough, French Extra, Earth Grains
2.5	½ roll	Roll, French, Brown 'n Serve, Pepperidge Farm
2.5	½ portion	Spaghetti, low-cal., frozen dinner
2.5	2 pieces	Cracker, Crispbread Breakfast, Wasa
2.5	¼ cup	Flour, soybean
2.5	1 ounce	Spaghetti Substitute, Spinach, Deboles
2.5	1 ounce	Noodles, Egg, Veggie, Hodgson Mill
2.5	1 whole	Muffin, English, Regular, Thomas'
2.5	2 slices	Bread, Whole Wheat, Brick Oven, Arnold
2.5	1 ounce	Noodles, Spaghetti, Whole Wheat, Hodgson Mill
2.5	2 slices	Bread, Oatnut, Oroweat
2.5	2 slices	Bread, Bran'nola Rice Bran, Oroweat

GRAIN GROUP

Nutripoints	Serving Size	Food Name
2.5	2 pancakes	Pancake Mix, Original Complete, Aunt Jemima
2.5	2 slices	Bread, Honey Wheat Berry, Oroweat
2.5	1/2 cup	Rice, Minute Rice
2.5	1/4 cup	Flour, Rye, Medium, Pillsbury
2.5	1 whole	Roll, sourdough
2.5	1 whole	Roll, French or Vienna
2.5	1 piece	Roll, diet
2.5	1 cup	Farina, cooked
2.5	8 pieces	Cracker, Crispbread Light Natural, Krispen
2.5	1/2 cup	Rice, Brown, Quick, Vegetable Herb, Arrowhead Mills
2.5	1/2 cup	Rice, Converted, Uncle Ben's
2.5	1 piece	Cracker, matzo
2.5	3/4 cup	Cereal, cream of rice, cooked
2.5	2 slices	Bread, white
2.5	2 ounces	Linguine, Thin, Ronzoni (2 ounces dry = 3/4 cup cooked)
2.5	2 slices	Bread, White, Wonder
2.5	6 pieces	Breadsticks, plain, Keebler
2.5	1 muffin	Muffin mix, Oat Bran, Wheat-Free, Arrowhead Mills
2.5	1/2 cup	Fettucini, Garden Gourmet, frozen, Green Giant
2.5	1/4 cup	Cereal, Familia, w/Fruit and Nuts
2.0	1/2 cup	Rice, Long Grain Enriched, Mahatma
2.0	1/2 cup	Rice, Extra Long Grain Enriched, Carolina
2.0	2 rolls	Kentucky Fried Chicken w/Roll
2.0	1/2 cup	Rice, pilaf
2.0	1/2 piece	Pizza Hut Hand-Tossed Cheese Pizza
2.0	1 ounce	Noodles, Egg, Whole Wheat, Hodgson Mill
2.0	1 ounce	Noodles, Spinach, Whole Wheat, Hodgson Mill
2.0	1 whole	Muffin, English, Honey Wheat, Thomas'
2.0	1/2 cup	Noodles, Egg, Mueller's
2.0	2 slices	Bread, Bran'nola Multi-Bran, Oroweat
2.0	1 ounce	Ramen, Natural Whole Wheat, Westbrae

GRAIN GROUP

Nutripoints	Serving Size	Food Name
2.0	2 cups	Cereal, puffed rice
2.0	1/2 piece	Pizza Hut Super Supreme Pan Pizza
2.0	1 whole	Roll, Frankfurter, Wonder
2.0	1 whole	Bun, white hamburger
2.0	2 whole	Bagel, plain, Lender's
2.0	1 whole	Bagel, Raisin 'n Honey, Lender's
2.0	1 whole	Roll, hard
2.0	1/2 cup	Spaghetti, w/meat sauce
2.0	1 whole	Bagel
2.0	1/2 piece	Pizza Hut Supreme Pan Pizza
2.0	1 muffin	Muffin Mix, Bran, Original Wheat, Arrowhead Mills
2.0	1/2 cup	Bread crumbs
2.0	1/2 portion	Lasagna, Zucchini, Lean Cuisine, Stouffer's
2.0	6 pieces	Cracker, Melba Toast, White, Old London
2.0	1/2 piece	Pizza Hut Supreme Thin 'n Crispy Pizza
2.0	1 whole	Roll, white
2.0	1/2 cup	Ramen, Natural Mushroom, Westbrae
2.0	6 pieces	Breadsticks, Onion, Keebler
2.0	4 pieces	Cracker, Crispbread Lite Rye, Wasa
2.0	2 whole	Biscuit, Butter, Pillsbury
2.0	1 whole	Tortilla, flour
2.0	2 slices	Bread, Pumpernickel, Arnold
2.0	1/2 piece	Pizza Hut Super Supreme Hand-Tossed Pizza
2.0	1/2 piece	Pizza Hut Super Supreme Thin 'n Crispy Pizza
2.0	1/2 piece	Pizza, Cheese, French Bread, Lean Cuisine, Stouffer's
2.0	2 slices	Bread, oatmeal
2.0	1 piece	Cornbread, Southern, Nutripoint
2.0	1 ounce	Ramen, Natural Spinach, Westbrae
2.0	1/2 cup	Croutons
2.0	1/2 portion	Ravioli, Mini, frozen, Celentano
2.0	2 cups	Popcorn, air-popped
2.0	1/4 piece	Pizza Hut Supreme Personal Pan Pizza
2.0	1 cup	Cereal, oatmeal, cooked, prepared w/water

GRAIN GROUP

Nutripoints	Serving Size	Food Name
2.0	2 waffles	Waffles, Blueberry, Aunt Jemima
2.0	2 slices	Bread, potato
2.0	1 portion	Linguini, Seafood, frozen, Weight Watchers
2.0	1 bar	Breakfast bar
2.0	1/4 piece	Pizza Hut Pepperoni Personal Pan Pizza
2.0	1/4 cup	Cereal, Orangeola w/Bran and Whole Fruit, Health Valley
1.5	2 whole	Biscuit, Country Style, Pillsbury
1.5	1/2 cup	Rice, Rice-A-Roni, Spanish
1.5	2 slices	Bread, gluten
1.5	1 piece	Domino's Large 16-Inch Cheese Pizza
1.5	1 cup	Wendy's Pasta Deli Salad
1.5	1/2 cup	Bread Crumbs, plain, Progresso
1.5	1 roll	Roll, sweet, w/fruit
1.5	1 whole	Bun, Hot Dog, Arnold
1.5	1 1/4 ounces	Cereal, Instant Oatmeal w/Maple and Brown Sugar, Quaker
1.5	1/2 portion	Rice, Fried, w/Chicken, frozen, Chun King
1.5	2 pieces	Cracker, Honey Graham, Health Valley
1.5	1/2 portion	Lasagne, frozen, Celentano
1.5	1/4 cup	Granola, Maple Nut, Arrowhead Mills
1.5	1/2 cup	Spaghetti, w/meatballs
1.5	1 1/2 waffles	Waffles, Nutri-Grain, frozen, Eggo
1.5	4 pieces	Cracker, rice cake
1.5	1/2 portion	Fettucini, w/Meat Sauce, Slim, frozen, Budget Gourmet
1.5	1/2 piece	Pizza Hut Pepperoni Hand-Tossed Pizza
1.5	1 whole	Roll, Frankfurter, Side-Sliced, Pepperidge Farm
1.5	1/2 piece	Pizza Hut Pepperoni Thin 'n Crispy Pizza
1.5	1 piece	Pizza, Cheese, frozen, Weight Watchers
1.5	1/2 cup	Egg noodles, cooked (1.125 cups = 2 ounces dry)
1.5	1/2 portion	Lasagna, w/Bread, frozen, Morton
1.5	6 pieces	Biscuit, Uneeda
1.5	1/2 cup	Pretzels, Keebler
1.5	2 rolls	Roll, Dinner, Wheat Loaf, Pipin' Hot

GRAIN GROUP

Nutripoints	Serving Size	Food Name
1.5	½ piece	Domino's Large 16-Inch Sausage and Mushroom Pizza
1.5	6 pieces	Breadsticks, Sesame, Keebler
1.5	¼ cup	Granola, no sugar
1.5	½ piece	Pizza, Combo, Deluxe, frozen, Weight Watchers
1.5	⅓ portion	Lasagna, Three-Cheese, frozen, Budget Gourmet
1.5	½ portion	Pasta Shells and Beef, frozen, Budget Gourmet
1.5	2 rolls	Roll, Dinner, White Loaf, Pipin' Hot
1.0	11 pieces	Cracker, Wheat Vegetable, Stone-Ground, Hain
1.0	½ piece	Domino's Large 16-Inch Veggie Pizza
1.0	6 pieces	Breadsticks, Garlic, Keebler
1.0	½ piece	Domino's Large 16-Inch Ham Pizza
1.0	½ cup	Stuffing Mix, Herb Seasoned, Pepperidge Farm
1.0	10 pieces	Cracker, Low-Sodium, Saltine
1.0	4 pieces	Cracker, Oat Bran Krisp, Ralston
1.0	2 waffles	Waffles, Original, Aunt Jemima
1.0	4 pieces	Cracker, Melba Toast
1.0	1 whole	McDonald's English Muffin w/Butter
1.0	½ portion	Pasta Casino, frozen, Stouffer's
1.0	1 piece	Pizza, w/cheese
1.0	1 ounce	Pretzels, Twists, Rold Gold
1.0	½ portion	Lasagna, w/Meat Sauce, frozen, Weight Watchers
1.0	10 pieces	Cracker, Melba Toast, plain, Keebler
1.0	10 pieces	Cracker, Melba Toast, Onion, Keebler
1.0	10 pieces	Cracker, Melba Toast, Garlic, Keebler
1.0	4 pieces	Cracker, Amaranth Graham, Health Valley
1.0	½ piece	Pizza, French Bread Pepperoni, Stouffer's
1.0	½ piece	Pizza, Sausage, frozen, Weight Watchers
1.0	½ portion	Lasagna, Italian Cheese, frozen, Weight Watchers
1.0	50 pieces	Crackers, oyster, small

GRAIN GROUP

Nutripoints	Serving Size	Food Name
1.0	1/2 cup	Croutons, Cheddar and Romano Cheese, Pepperidge Farm
1.0	1 biscuit	Biscuit, baking powder/Buttermilk Flour from mix
1.0	2 pieces	Cracker, Sea Toast, Keebler
1.0	1 pancake	Pancake, cornmeal
1.0	1/2 cup	Fettucini, cooked (1 cup = 2 ounces dry)
1.0	1/2 portion	Rice, Fried, w/Pork, frozen, Chun King
1.0	8 pieces	Cracker, Saltine
1.0	1 cake	Cake, Elfin Loaves, Blueberry, frozen, Keebler
1.0	1 piece	Cornbread
1.0	1/2 piece	Pizza, Pepperoni, frozen, Weight Watchers
1.0	1 1/2 waffles	Waffles, Homestyle, frozen, Eggo
1.0	1/4 cup	Granola, Heartland
1.0	1 piece	Pizza, Cheese, Deluxe, frozen, Totino's
1.0	1 pancake	Pancake, buckwheat
1.0	2 biscuits	Biscuit, Buttermilk, Big Country, Pillsbury
1.0	5 pieces	Nachos, cheese/hot peppers
1.0	1 biscuit	Biscuit
1.0	1/4 cup	Noodles and Cheese Dinner, Deboles
1.0	6 pieces	Cracker, 7 Grain Vegetable, Stone-Ground Wheat, Health Valley
1.0	15 pieces	Tortilla Chips, Light Nacho Cheese, Doritos
1.0	1 whole	Carl's Jr. English Muffin w/Margarine
1.0	1/4 cup	Cereal, 100% Natural, Quaker
1.0	1/4 cup	Noodles, chow mein
1.0	1/2 piece	Domino's Large 16-Inch Pepperoni Pizza
1.0	50 pieces	Crackers, Oyster, Small, Keebler
1.0	1/4 cup	Pasta and Sauce, Marinara, Hain
1.0	1/2 portion	Pasta Oriental, frozen, Stouffer's
1.0	1 tart	Pop-Tarts, Frosted, Strawberry, Kellogg's
1.0	1 whole	Muffin, oatmeal
0.5	20 pieces	Crackers, Cheese Nips, Nabisco
0.5	1/2 portion	Lasagna, w/Meat Sauce, frozen, Stouffer's
0.5	1/4 cup	Cereal, Country Morning
0.5	1/2 cup	Pasta Salad, Italian, Cool Side, Lipton
0.5	1 pancake	Pancake, whole wheat

GRAIN GROUP

Nutripoints	Serving Size	Food Name
0.5	1 pancake	Pancake, plain
0.5	10 pieces	Cracker, Premium Saltine
0.5	1/2 piece	Pizza, French Bread Deluxe, frozen, Weight Watchers
0.5	1/2 piece	Pizza, Cheese, Frozen, Tree Tavern
0.5	1 pancake	Pancake, w/fruit
0.5	1 muffin	Muffin, cornbread
0.5	10 pieces	Pretzels, 3-ring
0.5	1/2 portion	Spaghetti w/Beef and Mushroom Sauce, frozen, Stouffer's
0.5	1 bar	Granola Bar, Chewy Chocolate Chip, Quaker
0.5	10 pieces	Cracker, rice, small
0.5	1/2 piece	Domino's Large 16-Inch Deluxe Pizza
0.5	1 tart	Pop-Tarts, Blueberry, Kellogg's
0.5	10 pieces	Cracker, Melba Toast, Sesame, Keebler
0.5	2 whole	Danish, Swiss Cheese, Borden
0.5	1/2 portion	Lasagna, Vegetable, Single Serving, frozen, Stouffer's
0.5	1/2 piece	Pizza, French Bread, Cheese, frozen, Stouffer's
0.5	1/2 piece	Pizza, French Bread, Vegetable Deluxe, frozen, Stouffer's
0.5	1/2 piece	Pizza, Cheese, French Bread, frozen, Weight Watchers
0.5	50 pieces	Pretzels, sticks
0.5	1 cake	Cake, Elfin Loaves, Apple Cinnamon, frozen, Keebler
0.5	1 cake	Cake, Elfin Loaves, Banana, frozen, Keebler
0.5	10 pieces	Cracker, soda
0.5	1/2 portion	Linguini, w/Shrimp, frozen, Budget Gourmet
0.5	12 pieces	Crackers, Oat Thins, Nabisco
0.5	1 bar	Candy Bar, Rice Krispies, Kellogg's
0.5	1/4 cup	Cereal, Natural, Heartland
0.5	1/4 portion	Lasagna, w/Italian Sausage, frozen, Budget Gourmet

GRAIN GROUP

Nutripoints	Serving Size	Food Name
0.5	1 piece	Pizza, 9-slice, frozen, Celentano
0.5	1/2 portion	Rigatoni, Baked, w/Meat Sauce and Cheese, frozen, Stouffer's
0.5	15 pieces	Tortilla chips
0.5	2 biscuits	Biscuit, Flaky, Hungry Jack
0.5	1 1/2 slices	French Toast, Nutripoint
0.5	1 piece	Pizza, Cheese, Chef Boyardee
0.5	1 tart	Pop-Tarts, Frosted Cherry w/Smucker's Fruit, Kellogg's
0.5	4 pieces	Cracker, Graham, Honey Maid
0.5	1 piece	Pizza, Thick Crust, frozen, Celentano
0.5	1/2 cup	Rice, Chicken Rice-A-Roni
0.5	7 pieces	Cracker, Oat Bran Graham, Health Valley
0.5	1 muffin	Muffin
0.5	1/2 cup	Bread, stuffing
0.5	1/2 piece	Domino's Large 16-Inch Double Cheese Pepperoni Pizza
0.5	26 pieces	Crackers, Oyster, Large, Keebler
0.5	1 piece	Pizza, Party Cheese, frozen, Totino's
0.5	1/2 portion	Lasagna, w/Meat Sauce, Slim, frozen, Budget Gourmet
0.5	1/2 portion	Lasagna, Single Serving, frozen, Stouffer's
0.0	1/2 cup	Rice, Rice-A-Roni
0.0	1/2 portion	Pasta Alfredo, w/Broccoli, frozen, Budget Gourmet
0.0	1/4 cup	Cereal, Natural, w/Raisins, Heartland
0.0	1 roll	Roll, sweet, w/fruit, frosted
0.0	1/2 portion	Pizza, Pepperoni, French Bread, frozen, Weight Watchers
0.0	1/4 cup	Macaroni and cheese
0.0	2 pieces	Cracker, graham, plain
0.0	2 tablespoons	McDonald's Chow Mein Noodles
0.0	1/2 cup	Macaroni and Cheese Dinner, Deluxe, Kraft
0.0	1/4 cup	Cereal, 100% Natural, Raisin and Date, Quaker
0.0	1 bun	Bun, cinnamon
0.0	2 cookies	Cookies, Commodore, Keebler

GRAIN GROUP

Nutripoints	Serving Size	Food Name
0.0	1 roll	Roll, sweet, w/fruit and nuts, frosted
0.0	1/2 cup	Ravioli, frozen, Celentano
0.0	1/2 portion	Spaghetti, w/Meat Sauce, frozen, Stouffer's
0.0	1/2 portion	Pasta and Cheese, frozen, Celentano
0.0	2 waffles	Waffles, Buttermilk, Jumbo, Downyflake
0.0	1 cup	Popcorn, caramel
0.0	1/4 serving	Taco Bell Nachos Bellgrande
0.0	1/2 portion	Pizza, French Bread, Pepperoni and Mushroom, frozen, Stouffer's
0.0	1 piece	Pizza, Cheese, frozen, Celeste
0.0	1 piece	Pizza, Cheese, Round, Family Style, Ellio's
0.0	6 pieces	Cracker, Harvest Wheat, Keebler
0.0	1/4 cup	Granola
0.0	1/2 cup	Macaroni salad
0.0	1/2 cup	Shells and Cheese Dinner, Velveeta
0.0	1 ounce	Pizza, Combos
0.0	1/2 portion	Macaroni and Cheese, frozen, Budget Gourmet
0.0	1 serving	Carl's Jr. Hot Cakes w/Margarine
0.0	1/2 portion	Rice, w/Oriental Vegetables, frozen, Budget Gourmet
0.0	1/2 piece	Pizza, Pepperoni, frozen, Ellio's
0.0	2 cups	Popcorn, cooked w/oil
0.0	1/2 cup	Noodles, Egg, Ronzoni
0.0	1 piece	Bread, garlic
0.0	1 muffin	Muffin, blueberry
0.0	1 piece	Gingerbread
0.0	1 ounce	Wendy's Taco Chips
−0.5	1/2 piece	Cake, upside down, pineapple
−0.5	1 piece	Cake, white
−0.5	1/2 danish	Carl's Jr. Danish (all varieties)
−0.5	16 pieces	Cracker, Wheat Thins, Nabisco
−0.5	1 piece	Bread, banana
−0.5	1/4 cup	Graham Crumbs, Keebler
−0.5	1 piece	Cake, Carrot, frozen, Weight Watchers
−0.5	6 pieces	Cracker, Triscuit, Nabisco

GRAIN GROUP

Nutripoints	Serving Size	Food Name
−0.5	1/4 serving	Roy Rogers Pancake Platter w/Syrup and Butter
−0.5	1 piece	Pizza, Pepperoni, Chef Boyardee
−0.5	1 bar	Granola bar
−0.5	15 pieces	Tortilla Chips, Nacho Cheese, Doritos
−0.5	1/2 cup	Stuffing Mix, American New England, Stove Top
−0.5	3 pieces	Cracker, Cheese and Peanut Butter, Keebler
−0.5	1/2 serving	McDonald's Biscuit w/Biscuit Spread
−0.5	1/2 serving	Taco Bell Nachos
−0.5	1/4 serving	Roy Rogers Pancake Platter w/Syrup/Butter/Ham
−0.5	1/2 portion	Linguini, Clam Sauce, frozen, Stouffer's
−0.5	18 pieces	Tortilla Chips, Doritos
−0.5	1/2 portion	Linguini, w/Scallops and Clams, Slim, frozen, Budget Gourmet
−0.5	1 piece	Cracker, Petite Butter Crescents, Pepperidge Farm
−0.5	1/2 serving	McDonald's Hotcakes w/Butter and Syrup
−0.5	15 pieces	Corn chips
−0.5	1/2 serving	Jack in the Box Pancake Platter
−0.5	1 muffin	Muffin, w/fruit and/or nuts
−0.5	1/4 piece	Taco Bell Mexican Pizza
−0.5	1 whole	Tamales, in Chili Sauce, Old El Paso
−1.0	1/2 danish	Wendy's Apple Danish
−1.0	4 pieces	Cracker, Toast and Peanut Butter, Keebler
−1.0	1/4 serving	Roy Rogers Pancake Platter w/Syrup/Butter/Bacon
−1.0	8 pieces	Cracker, Ritz
−1.0	1/2 piece	Pizza, w/sausage
−1.0	1 cup	Spaghetti, w/Meatballs in Tomato Sauce, Chef Boyardee
−1.0	1/2 portion	Pasta Mexicali, frozen, Stouffer's
−1.0	1/2 portion	Fettucini, Chicken, frozen, Weight Watchers
−1.0	1/2 serving	Taco Bell Meximelt
−1.0	1 cookie	Cookies, sugar

GRAIN GROUP

Nutripoints	Serving Size	Food Name
−1.0	1 muffin	Muffin Mix, Corn, Betty Crocker
−1.0	1 muffin	Muffin Mix, Bran Date, "Jiffy"
−1.0	1 roll	Roll, sweet, cinnamon bun, frosted
−1.0	1 muffin	Carl's Jr. Bran Muffin
−1.0	1/2 danish	McDonald's Raspberry Danish
−1.0	1 piece	Fruitcake
−1.0	1 piece	Snack Cake, Lights, Hostess
−1.0	4 pieces	Cracker, Hearty Wheat, Pepperidge Farm
−1.0	1 muffin	Muffin Mix, Corn, "Jiffy"
−1.0	1/2 piece	Shortcake, sponge type w/fruit
−1.0	1 muffin	Muffin Mix, Corn, Old-Fashioned, frozen, Pepperidge Farm
−1.0	1/4 piece	Burger King French Toast Sticks
−1.0	1 pancake	Pancake and Waffle Mix, Blue Corn
−1.0	2 pancake	Pancake and Waffle Mix, Extra Light, Hungry Jack
−1.0	1 bar	Granola Bar, Chewy Honey and Oats, Quaker
−1.0	1/4 cup	Pudding, rice
−1.0	45 pieces	Cracker, Original Tiny Goldfish, Pepperidge Farm
−1.0	1/4 cup	Pasta salad, home recipe
−1.0	1/2 biscuit	Roy Rogers Biscuit
−1.0	2 pieces	Hush puppies
−1.5	1/2 danish	McDonald's Cinnamon Raisin Danish
−1.5	2 pancakes	Pancake and Waffle Mix, Buttermilk, Hungry Jack
−1.5	10 pieces	Crackers, Animal, Barnum's
−1.5	1/2 danish	Roy Rogers Cheese Danish
−1.5	7 cookies	Cookies, Nilla Wafers
−1.5	1 ounce	Corn Puffs, Cheese, Cheez Doodles, Borden
−1.5	1 doughnut	Doughnut, whole wheat
−1.5	1/4 roll	Roy Rogers Crescent Roll
−1.5	1 piece	Bread, Date, Pillsbury
−1.5	1/2 cup	Stuffing
−1.5	1/2 piece	Egg roll
−1.5	4 cookies	Cookies, Lemon Creme, Keebler

GRAIN GROUP

Nutripoints	Serving Size	Food Name
−1.5	1/4 serving	Roy Rogers Pancake Platter w/Syrup/Butter/Sausage
−1.5	1 bar	Granola Bar, w/Roasted Almonds, Nature Valley
−1.5	1 muffin	Muffin Mix, Blueberry, Wild, Betty Crocker
−1.5	1/2 cup	Stuffing Mix, Cornbread, w/Butter, Stove Top
−1.5	1 roll	Roll, Sweet, Apple, frozen, Weight Watchers
−1.5	1 muffin	Muffin Mix, Blueberry, Wild, Duncan Hines
−1.5	2 cookies	Cookies, oatmeal
−1.5	10 pieces	Crackers, animal
−1.5	1 turnover	Turnover, fruit
−1.5	1 piece	Carl's Jr. French Toast Dips
−1.5	2 cookies	Cookies, O.F. Oatmeal, Keebler
−1.5	1/2 portion	Macaroni and Cheese, Casserole, frozen, Morton
−1.5	1/2 danish	McDonald's Apple Danish
−1.5	2 cookies	Cookies, Chocolate Fudge Sandwich, Keebler
−1.5	1/4 cup	Pasta and Sauce, Swiss, Creamy, Hain
−1.5	1/2 tamale	Tamale
−1.5	2 cookies	Cookies, Keebies, Keebler
−1.5	2 cookies	Cookies, O.F. Sugar, Keebler
−1.5	1/2 danish	Wendy's Cinnamon w/Raisin Danish
−1.5	2 cookies	Cookies, French Vanilla Creme, Keebler
−1.5	25 pieces	Cheese Puffs, Cheetos
−1.5	2 cookies	Cookies, Pitter Patter, Keebler
−1.5	1 piece	Cake, Angel Food, Duncan Hines
−1.5	1/4 portion	Pasta Carbonara, frozen, Stouffer's
−1.5	1/2 danish	Wendy's Cheese Danish
−1.5	1/4 piece	Roy Rogers Strawberry Shortcake
−1.5	5 cookies	Cookies, Vanilla Wafers, Keebler
−1.5	1/2 biscuit	Wendy's Buttermilk Biscuit
−1.5	1 ounce	Wendy's Cheddar Chips
−1.5	1/2 muffin	Carl's Jr. Blueberry Muffin
−1.5	1 bar	Granola Bar, Chewy Fruit, Quaker
−2.0	1/2 portion	Macaroni and Cheese, frozen, Stouffer's

GRAIN GROUP

Nutripoints	Serving Size	Food Name
−2.0	1/2 danish	Roy Rogers Apple Danish
−2.0	1/2 danish	Danish, Apple, Pillsbury
−2.0	1/2 serving	Taco Bell Cinnamon Crispas
−2.0	2 cookies	Cookies, O.F. Double Fudge, Keebler
−2.0	1 bar	Granola Bar, Oats 'n Honey, Nature Valley
−2.0	2 cookies	Cookies, Homeplate, Keebler
−2.0	2 cookies	Cookies, molasses
−2.0	1/2 portion	Fettucini Primavera, frozen, Stouffer's
−2.0	2 cookies	Cookies, applesauce
−2.0	1 piece	Cake, banana, w/frosting
−2.0	1 piece	Cake, Crumb, Hostess
−2.0	1 piece	Cake, crumb
−2.0	1/2 danish	McDonald's Iced Cheese Danish
−2.0	1 slice	Wendy's French Toast
−2.0	1/2 cup	Roy Rogers Macaroni
−2.0	1/2 piece	Cake, coffee
−2.0	2 cookies	Cookies, O.F. Chocolate Chip, Keebler
−2.0	1 piece	Bread, Carrot, Nut, Pillsbury
−2.0	1/2 piece	Pizza, w/pepperoni
−2.0	1 piece	Cake, Chocolate, frozen, Weight Watchers
−2.0	1 cookie	McDonald's McDonaldland Cookies
−2.0	4 cookies	Cookies, Buttercup, Keebler
−2.0	1/2 danish	Roy Rogers Cherry Danish
−2.0	1/2 piece	Chocolate eclair
−2.0	1 piece	Cake, German Chocolate, frozen, Weight Watchers
−2.0	1 piece	Cake, Banana, Sara Lee
−2.0	1/2 piece	Roy Rogers Brownie
−2.0	1/2 cup	Pudding, bread
−2.0	1/4 bar	Dairy Queen Fudge Nut Bar
−2.0	1/2 turnover	Turnover, Blueberry, frozen, Pepperidge Farm
−2.0	1 doughnut	Doughnut, cake w/o frosting
−2.0	1/2 cup	Egg Noodles, Creamette, Borden
−2.0	2 pieces	Fig Newton, Nabisco
−2.0	1 piece	Shortcake, Strawberry, frozen, Weight Watchers

GRAIN GROUP

Nutripoints	Serving Size	Food Name
−2.0	2 cookies	Cookies, macaroon
−2.0	1/2 piece	Cake, sponge, w/whipped cream and fruit
−2.0	1 piece	Snack Cake, Ding Dong, Hostess
−2.5	1 piece	Snack Cake, Drake's Devil Dogs
−2.5	1 doughnut	Doughnut, glazed
−2.5	1/2 pastry	Danish pastry
−2.5	1 piece	Pie Crust Mix, Betty Crocker
−2.5	1 roll	Roll, Sweet, Cinnamon, w/Icing, Pillsbury
−2.5	1 croissant	Croissant
−2.5	1 piece	Cake, Black Forest, frozen, Weight Watchers
−2.5	1/2 doughnut	Doughnut, chocolate, w/chocolate icing
−2.5	1/2 piece	Cake, carrot w/cream cheese frosting
−2.5	1 popover	Popover
−2.5	1 cookie	McDonald's Chocolaty Chip Cookies
−2.5	1 piece	Cake, angel food, plain
−2.5	2 cookies	Cookies, Oatmeal Cremes Sandwich, Keebler
−2.5	1 piece	Pie Crust, Pet Ritz
−2.5	1 doughnut	Doughnut, cake w/frosting
−2.5	1/2 roll	Roll, sweet
−2.5	3 pieces	Shortbread, Lorna Doone
−2.5	2 cookies	Cookies, sandwich, chocolate/vanilla
−2.5	1 piece	Cake, Pound, Blueberry Topping, frozen, Weight Watchers
−2.5	2 cookies	Cookies, Oreo, Nabisco
−2.5	1 slice	French toast
−3.0	1/2 doughnut	Doughnut, Old-Fashioned, Glazed, Earth Grains
−3.0	1 piece	Twinkies, Hostess
−3.0	1 cookie	Cookies, O.F. Granola, Large, Pepperidge Farm
−3.0	1 ounce	Candy, Cracker Jacks
−3.0	1 piece	Brownie, Walnut, Betty Crocker
−3.0	1 piece	Pie crust
−3.0	1/2 doughnut	Doughnut, jelly
−3.0	1/2 doughnut	Doughnut, chocolate creme filled
−3.0	1/2 doughnut	Doughnut, custard filled

GRAIN GROUP

Nutripoints	Serving Size	Food Name
−3.0	1 piece	Snack Cake, Drake's Ring Ding Jr.
−3.0	1/2 doughnut	Doughnut, Devil's Food, Earth Grains
−3.0	1/2 piece	Cake, German chocolate
−3.0	3 cookies	Cookies, Oatmeal Raisin, Pepperidge Farm
−3.0	6 cookies	Cookies, vanilla wafer
−3.0	1/2 piece	Cake, torte
−3.0	2 cookies	Cookies, Chips Deluxe, Keebler
−3.0	1/4 serving	Roy Rogers Breakfast Crescent Sandwich w/Sausage
−3.0	1/2 piece	Cake, Bundt Pound Supreme, Pillsbury
−3.0	1/2 cookie	Carl's Jr. Chocolate Chip Cookie
−3.0	1 piece	Cupcake, Chocolate, Hostess
−3.0	1 piece	Brownie, Chocolate, frozen, Weight Watchers
−3.0	1/2 piece	Cake, Devil's Food, Deluxe, Duncan Hines
−3.0	1/2 piece	Cake, chocolate w/o frosting (12-piece/cake)
−3.0	1/2 cookie	Wendy's Chocolate Chip Cookie
−3.0	1/2 piece	Cake, Boston Cream, Supreme, Pepperidge Farm
−3.0	1/4 danish	Burger King Great Danish
−3.0	1 piece	Sopaipilla
−3.0	1/2 piece	Cake, chocolate w/frosting (12 piece/cake)
−3.5	1/2 piece	Cake, Dutch Apple Streusel Swirl, Pillsbury
−3.5	1/4 serving	Roy Rogers Breakfast Crescent Sandwich
−3.5	1/2 piece	Snack Cake, Suzy Q's
−3.5	1/4 serving	Roy Rogers Breakfast Crescent Sandwich w/Bacon
−3.5	2 cookies	Cookie Dough, Chocolate Chip, Pillsbury
−3.5	1/4 serving	Roy Rogers Breakfast Crescent Sandwich w/Ham
−3.5	1/2 piece	Cake, angel food, w/glaze
−3.5	1 piece	Brownie, w/o frosting
−3.5	1 piece	Cake, Golden Layer, Pepperidge Farm
−3.5	1 piece	Chocolate Eclair, Good Humor
−3.5	1 piece	Cake, Chocolate Fudge Snack, Sara Lee
−3.5	2 cookies	Cookies, Chocolate Chip, Duncan Hines

GRAIN GROUP

Nutripoints	Serving Size	Food Name
−3.5	½ piece	Cake, sponge, w/icing
−3.5	1 cookie	Cookies, Chocolate Chip Oatmeal, Pillsbury
−3.5	½ piece	Cake, German Chocolate, Moist, Betty Crocker
−3.5	1 piece	Brownie, w/frosting
−3.5	3 cookies	Cookies, Milano Distinctive, Pepperidge Farm
−3.5	2 cookies	Cookies, Peanut Butter 'n Fudge, Duncan Hines
−3.5	1 piece	Cupcake, w/o frosting
−3.5	½ piece	Carl's Jr. Chocolate Cake
−4.0	½ piece	Cake, Chocolate Mint Plus, Pillsbury
−4.0	3 cookies	Cookies, Chocolate Chip, Pepperidge Farm
−4.0	1 piece	Cake, Pound, Original, Sara Lee
−4.0	3 cookies	Cookies, Chessmen, Pepperidge Farm
−4.0	2 cookies	Cookies
−4.0	2 cookies	Cookies, chocolate chip
−4.0	2 cookies	Cookies, Sandwich, Mystic Mint, Nabisco
−4.0	1 piece	Cupcake, w/frosting
−4.0	3 cookies	Cookies, Bordeaux, Pepperidge Farm
−4.0	½ piece	Mousse, Chocolate, Light, Sara Lee
−4.5	3 cookies	Cookies, Pirouettes, choc-laced, Pepperidge Farm
−4.5	1 piece	Cake, sponge
−5.0	1 piece	Cake, pound
−5.5	2 pieces	Snack Cake, Apple Delight, Little Debbie
−5.5	½ piece	Cheesecake, Classic Snack, Sara Lee
−6.5	2 pieces	Snack Cake, Oatmeal Creme Pie, Little Debbie
−7.0	2 pieces	Snack Cake, Peanut Butter Bar, Little Debbie
−8.5	2 pieces	Snack Cake, Star Crunch, Little Debbie

LEGUME/NUT/SEED GROUP

Nutripoints	Serving Size	Food Name
18.0	2 cups	Bean sprouts, mung, fresh
17.0	1 1/2 cup	Soup, French Market, Nutripoint
14.0	1 cup	Peas, Green, No Salt Added, canned, Del Monte
14.0	1 cup	Peas, frozen, cooked
14.0	1 1/2 cups	Soup, Minestrone, Health Valley
13.5	1 cup	Beans, navy, cooked
13.5	1 cup	Soup, Lentil, Nutripoint
13.0	3/4 cup	Chili, South-of-the-Border Vegetarian, Nutripoint
12.0	1 cup	Peas, Green, frozen, Birds Eye
11.0	1 cup	Pigeon peas, green, cooked
10.5	2 cups	Bean Sprouts, Mung, Arrowhead Mills
10.0	1/2 cup	Soup, Split Pea, Green, Health Valley
9.5	3/4 cup	Beans, lima, cooked
9.0	1 cup	Peas, black-eyed, canned
8.5	1/2 cup	Beans, kidney, cooked
8.5	4 ounces	Vegeburger, Loma Linda
8.5	3/4 cup	Beans, cooked
8.5	1 cup	Peas, black-eyed, cooked
8.0	1/4 cup	Dip, Black Bean, Nutripoint
8.0	1 cup	Lentils, cooked
8.0	1/2 cup	Soup, Lentil, Health Valley
8.0	1 cup	Cowpeas, cooked
8.0	1/2 cup	Peas, split
8.0	1/2 cup	Beans, garbanzo, cooked
7.5	1/2 cup	Beans, baked, w/tomato sauce
7.5	1 ounce	Soybeans, Dry, Arrowhead Mills
7.5	1 cup	Peas, canned
7.5	1 cup	Soup, Black Bean, Health Valley
7.5	8 fluid ounces	Milk, Soy, Soyamel, Worthington
7.0	2 ounces	Bologna, Slices, frozen, Loma Linda
7.0	3/4 cup	Soybeans, cooked
6.5	1/2 cup	Beans, pinto, cooked
6.5	2 ounces	Beef, Roast, Slices, frozen, Loma Linda
6.5	1 cup	Lentils and Rice, Herbed, Nutripoint
6.5	1/2 cup	Peas, Sweet, 50-Percent Less Salt, canned, Green Giant

LEGUME/NUT/SEED GROUP

Nutripoints	Serving Size	Food Name
6.5	1/2 cup	Peas, Sweet, canned, Green Giant
6.5	2 ounces	Turkey, Slices, frozen, Loma Linda
6.5	1 cup	Soup, Lentil Curry, Couscous, Nile Spice Foods
6.0	1/2 cup	Peas, Sweet, Early Garden, canned, Del Monte
5.5	2 ounces	Chicken, Slices, frozen, Loma Linda
5.5	1 ounce	Beans, Adzuki, Dry, Arrowhead Mills
5.5	2 ounces	Salami, Slices, frozen, Loma Linda
5.5	1 cup	Soup, lentil
5.5	1/2 portion	Enchiladas, Mexican, Legume
5.0	1/2 cup	Tofu
5.0	1 piece	Frankfurter, Linketts, Loma Linda
5.0	1 cup	Soup, black bean
5.0	1/2 cup	Chili, bean
5.0	1 ounce	Soybean nuts, roasted, salted
4.5	1/2 portion	Mexican Style Dinner, frozen, Morton
4.5	1 cup	Soup, lentil, w/ham
4.5	1/4 cup	Seeds, sunflower, unsalted
4.5	1 cup	Peas, Early June, canned, Le Sueur
4.0	1/2 cup	Beans, Kidney, Best Light, canned, Bush's
4.0	1 cup	Soup, Split Pea, Natural, Hain
4.0	1/2 portion	Enchiladas, beef/cheese
4.0	1/2 serving	Taco Bell Bean Burrito w/Green Sauce
4.0	1/2 serving	Taco Bell Bean Burrito w/Red Sauce
4.0	1 cup	Soup, pea
4.0	1 cup	Soup, Hot and Sour, Nutripoint
4.0	1/2 cup	Chili, Vegetarian, canned, Worthington
4.0	3 ounces	Soyburger patty
4.0	1/2 cup	Butter Beans, frozen, Pictsweet
4.0	1 cup	Soup, Minestrone, Progresso
3.5	1 piece	Hamburger Patty, Grillers, frozen, Morningstar Farms
3.5	2 pieces	Sausage Patty, Breakfast, frozen, Morningstar Farms
3.5	2 tablespoons	Dip, bean
3.5	3 pieces	Bacon, Breakfast Strip, frozen, Morningstar Farms

LEGUME/NUT/SEED GROUP

Nutripoints	Serving Size	Food Name
3.5	1 ounce	Soybeans, roasted, unsalted
3.5	1 cup	Soup, bean
3.5	3 pieces	Sausage, Breakfast Links, frozen, Morningstar Farms
3.5	1 cup	Beans, Refried, Old El Paso
3.5	1/2 cup	Beans, Boston baked
3.0	1/2 cup	Chili w/Lentils, Vegetarian, Health Valley
3.0	1/2 cup	Beans, w/pork
3.0	1/2 piece	Soyburger, w/bun
3.0	1 cup	Chili w/Beans, Spicy Vegetarian, Health Valley
3.0	1/2 cup	Beans, Chili, Loma Linda
2.5	1/2 cup	Beans, Vegetarian Style, Van Camp's
2.5	8 ounces	Soup, Green Pea, Campbell's
2.5	1/2 piece	Burrito, bean/cheese
2.5	1/2 cup	Soup, Split Pea, Green, Progresso
2.5	1 ounce	Seeds, pumpkin and squash, roasted, unsalted
2.5	1 ounce	Seeds, pumpkin and squash, roasted, salted
2.5	1 serving	Taco Bell Pintos and Cheese, w/Green Sauce
2.5	1 serving	Taco Bell Pintos and Cheese w/Red Sauce
2.0	1/2 cup	Soup, Chunky Old-Fashioned Bean 'n Ham, Campbell's
2.0	1/4 cup	Trail mix
2.0	1 cup	Milk, Soy, Natural, Edensoy
2.0	2 tablespoons	Seeds, Sunflower, Hulled, Arrowhead Mills
2.0	1/2 cup	Beans, refried
2.0	1/2 portion	Beans, w/Frankfurters Dinner, frozen, Morton
2.0	1/2 cup	Beans, Lima, Baby, w/Butter, frozen, Green Giant
2.0	1/2 piece	Sandwich, peanut butter, whole wheat
2.0	1/4 cup	Seeds, pumpkin and squash
2.0	1/2 serving	Taco Bell Burrito Supreme w/Red Sauce
2.0	1/2 serving	Taco Bell Burrito Supreme w/Green Sauce
2.0	2 ounces	Nut Meat, Nuteena, Loma Linda
2.0	1/2 cup	Beans, w/Pork, Van Camp's

LEGUME/NUT/SEED GROUP

Nutripoints	Serving Size	Food Name
2.0	1/2 portion	Chili, Vegetarian, w/Rice, frozen, Stouffer's Right Choice
1.5	1/2 cup	Beans, w/Pork in Tomato Sauce, Campbell's
1.5	1/2 cup	Beans, w/Pork, Showboat, Bush's
1.5	1 cup	Salad, three-bean
1.5	25 pieces	Peanuts, oil roasted, unsalted
1.5	2 tablespoons	Peanut Butter, Chunky, No Salt, Health Valley
1.5	2 tablespoons	Peanut Butter, Chunky, Health Valley
1.5	1/2 piece	Sandwich, peanut butter, white bread
1.5	1 ounce	Sesame butter, tahini
1.5	1 piece	Vegi-Patties, frozen, Lifestream
1.5	12 pieces	Cashews, dry roasted, unsalted
1.5	18 pieces	Almonds, raw
1.5	1 ounce	Cashews, Dry Roasted, Unsalted, Planters
1.5	1/2 serving	Taco Bell Beef Burrito w/Green Sauce
1.5	1 ounce	Peanuts, Dry Roasted, Unsalted, Planters
1.0	1/2 cup	Beans, Home Style, Campbell's
1.0	25 pieces	Peanuts, oil roasted, salted
1.0	1 ounce	Peanuts, Dry Roasted, Salted, Planters
1.0	1 tablespoon	Peanut butter, unsalted
1.0	1 ounce	Mixed nuts, dry roasted, unsalted
1.0	1 tablespoon	Peanut Butter, No Salt Added, Natural, Smucker's
1.0	1 ounce	Pine Nuts, Pignolia
1.0	1 tablespoon	Peanut butter, low-sodium
1.0	1 ounce	Butternuts
1.0	1 tablespoon	Peanut Butter, Natural, Smucker's
1.0	1 ounce	Peanuts, Spanish, Salted, Planters
1.0	1/2 serving	Taco Bell Beef Burrito w/Red Sauce
1.0	1/2 cup	Chili, bean/beef
1.0	1 cup	Milk, Soy, Natural Creamy Original, Vitasoy
1.0	1 ounce	Mixed nuts, oil roasted, salted
1.0	1 ounce	Pistachios, raw
1.0	1 ounce	Peanuts, Cocktail, Planters
1.0	25 pieces	Peanuts, Dry Roasted, Salted, Frito-Lay
1.0	1/4 piece	Burrito Dinner, frozen, Patio
0.5	1 tablespoon	Peanut butter

LEGUME/NUT/SEED GROUP

Nutripoints	Serving Size	Food Name
0.5	1 ounce	Cashews, dry roasted, salted
0.5	1 cup	Milk, Nondairy, Soy, West Soy
0.5	1 tablespoon	Almond butter, salted
0.5	1 ounce	Cashews, oil roasted, unsalted
0.5	1/2 piece	Sandwich, peanut butter/jelly, whole wheat bread
0.5	1/2 cup	Beans, Baked, Barbeque, B&M
0.5	1 ounce	Peanuts, honey roasted
0.5	1/2 piece	Taco, bean/cheese
0.5	1/2 portion	Burrito, Bean/Beef, Green, frozen, Patio
0.5	8 fluid ounces	Milk, Soy, Solait, Miller Farms
0.5	1/2 portion	Burrito, Bean/Beef, Red Chili, frozen, Patio
0.5	1/2 portion	Enchiladas, chicken w/sour cream sauce
0.5	1/2 piece	Sandwich, peanut butter/jelly, white bread
0.5	8 pieces	Macadamia nuts, oil roasted, salted
0.5	12 pieces	Walnuts, black
0.5	1 ounce	Filberts, oil roasted, salted
0.5	1 ounce	Almonds, Blanched, Blue Diamond
0.5	1 ounce	Cashews, oil roasted, salted
0.5	1 ounce	Cashew butter, salted
0.5	12 pieces	Almonds, oil roasted, salted
0.0	6 pieces	Brazil nuts, unsalted
0.0	1/2 portion	Burrito, Red Hot, frozen, Patio
0.0	1/2 piece	Burrito, beef/cheese
0.0	12 pieces	Walnuts, English or Persian
0.0	2 pieces	Cracker, peanut butter sandwich
0.0	1 tablespoon	Peanut Butter, Creamy, Skippy
0.0	1/4 portion	Mexican Dinner, frozen, Patio
0.0	1 cup	Milk, Soy, Soymoo, Health Valley
0.0	15 pieces	Pecans, unsalted, raw
0.0	1 tablespoon	Peanut Butter, Creamy, Jif
0.0	1 tablespoon	Peanut Butter, Super Chunk, Skippy
0.0	1 piece	Tofu Burger, frozen, Island Spring Oriental
0.0	1/2 portion	Burrito, Chicken, frozen, Weight Watchers
0.0	1/4 cup	Seeds, sesame
0.0	1/4 cup	Pistachios, dry roasted, salted
0.0	1/2 portion	Burrito, Bean/Beef, frozen, Patio
0.0	1/2 portion	Burrito, Beefsteak, frozen, Weight Watchers

LEGUME/NUT/SEED GROUP

Nutripoints	Serving Size	Food Name
0.0	1/3 portion	Mexican Style Combo Dinner, frozen, Patio
0.0	1 tablespoon	Peanut Butter, Crunchy, Peter Pan
0.0	1/2 piece	Enchiladas, bean/cheese
0.0	1 piece	Candy Bar, Peanut, Planters
−0.5	1/2 portion	Fiesta Dinner, frozen, Patio
−0.5	1/2 portion	Combination Dinner, frozen, Patio
−0.5	1 ounce	Candy, peanut butter morsels
−0.5	1 ounce	Walnuts, Baking, Blue Diamond
−0.5	1 ounce	Pecans, oil roasted, salted
−1.0	5 ounces	Burrito, Beef/Bean, Patio
−1.0	4 fluid ounces	Cream, Soy, Solait, Miller Farms
−1.0	1 ounce	Peanuts, yogurt-covered
−1.0	1/2 cup	Beans, Refried, w/Sausage, Old El Paso
−1.0	1/3 portion	Mexican Combination Dinner, frozen, Swanson
−1.0	1 ounce	Peanuts, chocolate-covered
−1.0	6 pieces	Almonds, chocolate-covered
−1.0	2 pieces	Cookies, peanut butter
−1.0	1/3 portion	Enchiladas, Cheese Ranchero, Van de Kamp's
−1.5	1 ounce	Filberts, dry roasted, salted
−1.5	1 serving	Jack in the Box Taco
−1.5	1 ounce	Nuts, Mixed, w/Peanuts, Planters
−1.5	2 pieces	Candy bar, Twix Peanut Butter
−1.5	6 pieces	Almonds, sugar-coated
−2.0	1/2 cup	Frozen Dessert, Low-Fat, Tofutti
−2.0	1/2 serving	Jack in the Box Super Taco
−2.0	1 ounce	Candy, Reese's Pieces
−2.5	1 ounce	Candy, caramel w/nuts, chocolate-covered
−3.0	1 ounce	Candy, peanut brittle
−3.0	1 ounce	Candy bar, milk chocolate w/peanuts
−3.5	1 piece	Candy, peanut butter cup
−3.5	1/2 piece	Pie, pecan
−3.5	1 ounce	Candy bar, milk chocolate w/almonds

MILK/DAIRY GROUP

Nutripoints	Serving Size	Food Name
23.5	3/4 cup	*Egg, Scrambled, Garden, Egg Beaters, Nutripoint
17.5	1/2 cup	*Egg Substitute, Egg Beaters, Fleischmann's
13.5	10 fluid ounces	*Milk Drink, Diet, Lite, Sego
13.0	1/2 cup	*Egg Substitute, Egg Beaters, Vegetable Omelette Mix, Fleischmanns
13.0	8 fluid ounces	*Milk Drink, Slim-Fast
12.0	1 cup	*Instant Breakfast, w/low-fat milk, no sugar, all flavors, Carnation
11.5	2 cups	Milk, Instant Nonfat Dry, Carnation
11.0	8 fluid ounces	*Milk Drink, Ultra Slim-Fast
10.5	1 piece	Cheese Substitute, Pasteurized Process, Formagg
10.5	8 ounces	Yogurt, Nonfat, Light, all flavors, Dannon
10.5	1/4 cup	Milk, nonfat dry
10.0	1/2 serving	*Egg Substitute, Egg Watchers, Tofutti
10.0	1/2 cup	*Egg Substitute, Scramblers
9.5	1 cup	Milk, skim
9.5	1/2 cup	Milk, canned, skim, evaporated
9.5	1 cup	Buttermilk, skim
9.0	5 ounces	Yogurt, Frozen TCBY
9.0	1 cup	Yogurt, Nonfat, plain, Dannon
9.0	3/4 cup	Milk, Evaporated, Skimmed, Carnation
8.0	1 cup	Milk, low-fat (1-percent)
8.0	1 cup	Yogurt, Nonfat Ultimate, all flavors, Weight Watchers
8.0	4 fluid ounces	*Sustacal
7.5	6 fluid ounces	*Milk Drink, Diet, Sego
7.5	1 cup	Milk, Low-Fat (2-percent), Hi-Calcium, Borden
7.0	8 ounces	Yogurt, low-fat, plain
6.5	1/4 cup	Cream, Sour, New Way, Nutripoint
6.5	1/4 cup	Sauce, Banana Mint, Nutripoint
6.0	1/2 cup	*Instant Breakfast, Chocolate, Carnation
6.0	4 ounces	*Egg Substitute, Egg Beaters, Cheez, Fleischmann's
6.0	6 whites	Egg white
6.0	4 fluid ounces	*Ensure Plus

*Fortified

MILK/DAIRY GROUP

Nutripoints	Serving Size	Food Name
6.0	1 cup	Milk, low-fat (2-percent), protein fortified
6.0	1/2 cup	*Instant Breakfast, Vanilla, Carnation
5.5	6 fluid ounces	*Ensure
5.5	1/2 cup	Mousse, Key Lime, Nutripoint
5.5	3/4 cup	Egg, Scrambled, Garden, Nutripoint
5.5	1/2 portion	Cannelloni, Florentine, frozen, Celentano
5.5	1/2 cup	Casserole, Five-Cheese, Nutripoint
5.5	1/2 cup	Cheese, cottage, dry
5.5	8 ounces	Yogurt, Low-Fat, plain, Dannon
5.5	1/4 cup	Cheese, Cream, Honey, Nutripoint
5.0	1 cup	Buttermilk, regular
4.5	1/2 cup	*Egg Substitute, Second Nature
4.5	6 fluid ounces	*Milk Drink, Nutrament
4.5	1/2 cup	Cheese, cottage, low-fat (1-percent)
4.5	1 ounce	Wendy's Imitation Parmesan Cheese
4.5	1 cup	Yogurt, Nonfat, Peach, Weight Watchers
4.0	1 ounce	Cocoa Mix, Hot, Sugar-Free, Swiss Miss
4.0	8 ounces	Yogurt, Nonfat, Light, all flavors, Yoplait
4.0	1/2 cup	Cocoa Mix, Chocolate Flavor Ovaltine
4.0	8 ounces	Yogurt, Nonfat, Lite, Plain, Colombo
3.5	1/2 cup	Mousse, Cheesecake, Sans Sucre De Paris
3.5	2 ounces	Cheese, low-cal.
3.5	16 fluid ounces	*Milk Drink, Alba
3.0	4 ounces	Cheese, cottage, low-fat (2-percent)
3.0	2 cups	Cocoa Mix, Hot, Sugar-Free, Carnation
3.0	1 cup	Pudding, low-cal.
2.5	8 ounces	Yogurt, Nonfat, Lite, Vanilla, Colombo
2.5	2 pieces	Cheese, Reduced Calorie, Laughing Cow
2.5	1 cup	Cocoa Mix, Sugar-Free, Quik, Nestle
2.5	1/3 cup	Banana Flambé, Nutripoint
2.5	8 ounces	Yogurt, whole milk, plain
2.5	1 cup	Milk, whole (3.3-percent)
2.5	1 cup	Milk, chocolate, low-fat (1-percent)
2.5	6 fluid ounces	Milk, chocolate, low-fat (2-percent)
2.0	1/2 portion	Manicotti, frozen, Celentano
2.0	6 ounces	Yogurt, fruit
2.0	1 cup	Milk, whole (3.7-percent)
2.0	1/2 portion	Shells, Stuffed, frozen, Celentano

*Fortified

MILK/DAIRY GROUP

Nutripoints	Serving Size	Food Name
2.0	6 ounces	Yogurt, Low-Fat, Fresh Flavors, all flavors, Dannon
2.0	1/2 cup	Pudding, Sustacal
2.0	1/4 cup	Dressing, Honey Yogurt, Nutripoint
2.0	6 ounces	Yogurt, Nonfat, Yoplait 150
2.0	1 cup	Pudding Mix, Vanilla, Sugar-Free, Instant, Jell-O
2.0	4 1/2 ounces	Yogurt, Extra Smooth Fruit, all flavors, Dannon
1.5	1 cup	Yogurt, Low-Fat, Swiss Style, plain, Lite-Line, Borden
1.5	1/4 piece	Shells, frozen, Broccoli Stuffed, Celentano
1.5	1 cup	Soup, cream
1.5	4 ounces	Yogurt, frozen
1.5	1 cup	Milk, goat
1.5	1/2 cup	Cheese, cottage
1.5	1 ounce	Wendy's Imitation Cheese, Salad Bar
1.5	1/2 cup	Cheese, Cottage, Low-Fat, Weight Watchers
2.0	1/2 cup	Yogurt, frozen, Low-Fat, Peaches and Cream, Blue Bell
1.5	1 cup	Ice Cream, Extra Light, Blue Bell
1.0	1/2 cup	Milk, canned, evaporated, unsweetened
1.0	1/2 cup	Milk, Evaporated, Carnation
1.0	1 ounce	Cheese, Cheddar Flavor, Sharp, Borden
1.0	1 tablespoon	Malted milk powder
1.0	1/4 cup	Cream, Sour, Blend, Weight Watchers
1.0	1/4 cup	Pudding, banana
1.0	1/2 portion	Shells, Stuffed, 3-Cheese, frozen, Le Menu
1.0	1 cup	Cocoa Mix, Hot, 70 Calorie, Carnation
1.0	1/2 portion	Ravioli, Baked, Cheese, frozen, Weight Watchers
1.0	4 ounces	Yogurt, Low-Fat, Fruit on Bottom, all flavors, Dannon
1.0	1/2 portion	Enchiladas, Cheese Dinner, frozen, Patio
0.5	1 cup	Yogurt Drink, Low-Fat, Dan'Up, all flavors, Dannon

MILK/DAIRY GROUP

Nutripoints	Serving Size	Food Name
0.5	4 ounces	Yogurt, Low-Fat, Nuts/Raisins/Fruit, Dannon
0.5	2 ounces	Cheese, ricotta, low-fat
0.5	2 tablespoons	Dressing, yogurt
0.5	1 ounce	Cheese, mozzarella, low-fat
0.5	1/3 portion	Manicotti, Cheese, w/Meat Sauce, frozen, Budget Gourmet
0.5	1/2 portion	Manicotti, 3-Cheese, Tomato Sauce, Le Menu
0.5	1 ounce	Cheese, Parmesan
0.5	1/2 portion	Ravioli, Cheese, Slim, frozen, Budget Gourmet
0.5	1/2 portion	Cannelloni, Cheese, Lean Cuisine, frozen, Stouffer's
0.5	1 piece	Pie, Fruit Yogurt, Nutripoint
0.5	1 ounce	Cheese, Swiss, Reduced Fat, Kraft
0.5	1 ounce	Cheese, Mozzarella, Skim, Land O Lakes
2.0	1/2 cup	Yogurt, frozen, Low-Fat, Raspberry, Blue Bell
0.5	8 ounces	Yogurt, Plain, Colombo
0.0	1/2 portion	Manicotti, Cheese, frozen, Weight Watchers
0.0	2 ounces	Cheese, American, Pasteurized Process, Lipton
0.0	1 ounce	Cheese, Mozzarella, Low-Fat, Borden
0.0	1/2 serving	Ice cream sundae, strawberry
0.0	1 cup	Chocolate, hot
0.0	4 ounces	Yogurt, Low-Fat, Nuts/Raisins/Vanilla, Dannon
0.0	1 ounce	Cheese, Parmesan, Imitation, Grated, Formagg
0.0	1/2 piece	Sandwich, grilled cheese, white bread
0.0	2 pieces	Cheese, Laughing Cow
0.0	1/2 portion	Tortellini, Cheese, w/Tomato Sauce, frozen, Stouffer's
0.0	4 ounces	Dairy Queen Frozen Dessert
0.0	4 fluid ounces	Yogurt, Frozen 97% Fat Free, Strawberry Passion, Colombo

MILK/DAIRY GROUP

Nutripoints	Serving Size	Food Name
—0.5	4 fluid ounces	Yogurt, Frozen, 96% Fat Free, Vanilla Dream, Colombo
—0.5	1/2 cup	Milk, Instant Natural Malted, Carnation
—0.5	4 ounces	Yogurt, Low-Fat, Strawberry, Borden
—0.5	1/2 cup	Yogurt, frozen, Almond Amaretto, Brice's
—0.5	4 ounces	Yogurt, Low-Fat, Cherry Vanilla, Borden
—0.5	4 ounces	Yogurt, Low-Fat, Peach, Borden
—0.5	1/2 cup	Milk, chocolate
—0.5	1/2 portion	Enchiladas, Cheese Ranchero, frozen, Weight Watchers
—0.5	4 ounces	Yogurt, Low-Fat, Strawberry, Yoplait
—0.5	4 ounces	Yogurt, Low-Fat, Boysenberry, Yoplait
—0.5	1 ounce	Cheese, Pasteurized Process, Reduced Sodium, Lite-Line
—0.5	4 fluid ounces	Ice Cream, Simple Pleasures, (w/Simplesse)
—0.5	1/2 portion	Pasta Shells, Cheese Stuffed, w/Meat Sauce, Stouffer's
—0.5	1 ounce	Cheese, Swiss
—0.5	1/2 cup	Pudding, tapioca
—0.5	3 fluid ounces	Yogurt, Frozen, 94% Fat Free, Caramel Pencan Chunk, Colombo
—0.5	1 ounce	Cheese, Gjetost
—1.0	1/2 cup	Milkshake, vanilla
—1.0	1 ounce	Cheese, American, Light n'Lively, Kraft
—1.0	1 ounce	Cheese, provolone
—1.0	1 ounce	Cheese, Swiss, Light n'Lively, Kraft
—1.0	1/2 cup	Ice milk, vanilla
—1.0	1/2 portion	Enchiladas Ranchero, Cheese, frozen, Weight Watchers
—1.0	4 ounces	Yogurt, Banana Custard Style, Yoplait
—1.0	1 piece	McDonald's Soft Serve Cone
—1.0	1 ounce	Cheese, Edam
—1.0	1/2 piece	Dairy Queen Cone, medium
—1.0	1 ounce	Cheese, Monterey Jack, Reduced Fat, Kraft
—1.0	1 ounce	Cheese, Camembert
—1.0	1 ounce	Cheese, Cheddar, Mild, Reduced Fat, Kraft
—1.0	3 fluid ounces	Yogurt, Frozen, 94% Fat Free, Bavarian Chocolate Crunch, Colombo

MILK/DAIRY GROUP

Nutripoints	Serving Size	Food Name
—1.0	1/2 cup	Soup, cheese
—1.0	1/2 serving	Ice cream sundae, hot fudge
—1.0	1/2 piece	Pie, Boston cream
—1.0	1/2 serving	Burger King Chocolate Shake
—1.0	1/2 cup	Milkshake, chocolate
—1.0	1 ounce	Cheese, Gruyère
—1.0	1/4 cup	Cream, Sour, Slender Choice
—1.0	1 ounce	Wendy's Potato Chili Cheese
—1.5	2 ounces	Cheese, Mozzarella, Low Fat, Alpine Lace
—1.5	1/4 cup	Dairy Queen Parfait
—1.5	1/4 cup	Dairy Queen Malt, medium
—1.5	1/2 serving	Egg McMuffin, McDonalds
—1.5	1 ounce	Cheese spread
—1.5	1 ounce	Cheese, mozzarella
—1.5	1 cup	Cocoa Mix, Hot, Regular, Swiss Miss
—1.5	1/2 cup	Pudding, vanilla
—1.5	1 ounce	Cheese Food Substitute, Low Cholesterol, Lite-Line
—1.5	1/4 serving	Egg McMuffin, w/Sausage, McDonalds
—1.5	1/4 cup	Cream, Sour, Light, Dairy Blend, Land O Lakes
—1.5	1 ounce	Cheese, Mozzarella, Skim, Kraft
—1.5	1 piece	Frozen Dessert, Chocolate Pudding Pops, Jell-O
—1.5	1/2 serving	McDonald's Strawberry Sundae
—1.5	1/4 cup	Dairy Queen Freeze (1 cup)
—1.5	3 fluid ounces	Yogurt, Frozen, 90% Fat Free, Peanut Butter Cup, Colombo
—1.5	3 fluid ounces	Yogurt, Frozen 92% Fat Free, Mocha Swiss Almond, Colombo
—1.5	1 ounce	Cheese, Gouda
—1.5	1/2 serving	McDonald's Hot Fudge Sundae
—1.5	1/2 serving	McDonald's Hot Caramel Sundae
—1.5	1 ounce	Cheese, brick
—1.5	1/2 cup	Carl's Jr. Shakes, regular size
—1.5	2 tablespoons	Cream, nondairy, imitation, liquid (vegetable oil)
—1.5	1/4 serving	Dairy Queen Heath Blizzard

MILK/DAIRY GROUP

Nutripoints	Serving Size	Food Name
−1.5	¼ serving	Dairy Queen Chipper Sandwich
−1.5	1 ounce	Cheese, Swiss, Borden
−1.5	1 ounce	Cheese, American, Pasteurized Process, Kraft
−1.5	1 ounce	Cheese, Parmesan, Grated, Kraft
−1.5	½ serving	Roy Rogers Strawberry Sundae
−1.5	1 ounce	Cheese, Muenster
−1.5	2 ounces	Cheese, Monterey Jack, Low Fat, Alpine Lace
−1.5	½ piece	Ice cream cone, vanilla
−1.5	1 ounce	Cheese, Monterey Jack
−1.5	1 piece	Mousse, Chocolate, frozen, Weight Watchers
−2.0	½ piece	Pie, Pumpkin Custard, Mrs. Smith's
−2.0	1 piece	Frozen Dessert, Vanilla, Lite Bar, Dove
−2.0	½ cup	Ice Cream, Dutch Chocolate, Borden
−2.0	4 ounces	Yogurt, Strawberry All Natural, Breyer's
−2.0	1 ounce	Cheese, Romano
−2.0	1 ounce	Cheese, blue
−2.0	¼ cup	Cream, Nondairy, Mocha Mix
−2.0	½ cup	Yogurt, Soft Frozen Peach, Yoplait
−2.0	2 ounces	Cheese, ricotta
−2.0	1 ounce	Cheese, Swiss, Natural, Kraft
−2.0	1 ounce	Cheese, Colby
−2.0	½ serving	Ice cream sundae, caramel
−2.0	½ piece	Cheesecake, Strawberry, frozen, Weight Watchers
−2.0	½ cup	Ice Milk, Chocolate, Borden
−2.0	1 ounce	Cheese, cheddar
−2.0	½ cup	Cocoa Mix, Chocolate, Quik, Nestle
−2.0	1 cup	Pudding Mix, Americana Tapioca, Jell-O
−2.0	½ piece	Cake, cheese, w/fruit topping
−2.0	½ cup	Ice cream, regular fat, vanilla
−2.0	½ cup	Eggnog
−2.0	½ serving	Carl's Jr. Sunrise Sandwich w/Bacon
−2.0	2 fluid ounces	Milk, sweetened condensed, canned
−2.0	½ serving	Roy Rogers Vanilla Shake
−2.0	4 ounces	Yogurt, Pineapple All Natural, Breyer's

MILK/DAIRY GROUP

Nutripoints	Serving Size	Food Name
−2.0	½ cup	Ice milk, Vanilla, Borden
−2.0	1 ounce	Cheese, Brie
−2.0	1 ounce	Cheese, pimiento
−2.0	¼ cup	Ice Cream, Vanilla, Rich
−2.0	½ serving	Roy Rogers Strawberry Shake
−2.0	½ serving	Roy Rogers Chocolate Shake
−2.0	½ cup	Ice Milk, Strawberry, Borden
−2.0	½ cup	Milk Drink Mix, Strawberry, Quik, Nestle
−2.0	½ serving	Roy Rogers Caramel Sundae
−2.0	¼ cup	Milk, Sweetened, Condensed, Carnation
−2.0	1 piece	Yogurt, frozen, Low-Fat, Chocolate, Tuscan Pop
−2.0	1 ounce	Cheese, Swiss, Low Fat, Alpine Lace
−2.0	¼ cup	Wendy's Chocolate Pudding
−2.0	½ piece	Cheesecake, frozen, Weight Watchers
−2.5	1 ounce	Cheese, feta
−2.5	¼ cup	Dairy Queen Shake, medium
−2.5	½ serving	Roy Rogers Hot Fudge Sundae
−2.5	½ cup	Ice Cream, Nondairy, Vanilla, Mocha Mix
−2.5	1 ounce	Cheese, Muenster, Land O Lakes
−2.5	1 ounce	Cheese, Swiss, Low-Sodium, Kraft
−2.5	½ serving	Dairy Queen Sundae, medium
−2.5	½ piece	Pie, Boston Cream Classic, Betty Crocker
−2.5	½ serving	Burger King Vanilla Shake
−2.5	½ piece	Ice Cream Bar, Nondairy, Chocolate-Covered, Mocha Mix
−2.5	½ piece	Pie, yogurt
−2.5	½ piece	Wendy's Breakfast Sandwich
−2.5	1 cup	Pudding Mix, Vanilla, Jell-O
−2.5	1 ounce	Cheese, Swiss, Sargento
−2.5	1 ounce	Cheese, American, Borden
−2.5	1 piece	Ice cream sandwich
−2.5	¼ serving	Carl's Jr. Sunrise Sandwich w/Sausage
−2.5	½ piece	Ice Cream Sandwich, Good Humor
−2.5	1 piece	Pie, Boston Cream, frozen, Weight Watchers
−2.5	¼ cup	Wendy's Butterscotch Pudding
−2.5	1 ounce	Cheese, Swiss, processed

MILK/DAIRY GROUP

Nutripoints	Serving Size	Food Name
−2.5	1 piece	Dairy Queen DQ Sandwich
−2.5	1 ounce	Cheese Spread, Pasteurized Process, Slices, Velveeta
−3.0	1/2 cup	Topping, Lite, Cool Whip
−3.0	1 ounce	Cheese, Cheddar, Low-Sodium, Tillamook
−3.0	1 ounce	Cheese, American, processed
−3.0	1/4 cup	Cream, half-and-half
−3.0	1/2 cup	Soufflé, cheese
−3.0	1/2 piece	Pie, vanilla cream
−3.0	1/2 piece	Ice Cream Bar, Chocolate Peanut Butter, Milk Chocolate, Häagen-Dazs
−3.0	1 ounce	Cheese, Neufchâtel, Philadelphia Brand
−3.0	1 ounce	Cheese Spread, Pasteurized Process, Velveeta
−3.0	1/2 serving	McDonald's Chocolate Milk Shake
−3.0	1/2 serving	McDonald's Vanilla Milk Shake
−3.0	1 ounce	Cheese, Cheddar, Tillamook
−3.0	2 tablespoons	Cream, nondairy, imitation, powder
−3.0	1/4 cup	Milk, Condensed, Sweetened, Eagle Brand
−3.0	1/2 serving	McDonald's Strawberry Milk Shake
−3.0	1 ounce	Cheese, Limburger
−3.0	1/2 piece	Jack in the Box Cheesecake
−3.0	1/2 piece	Cake, cheese, plain
−3.0	1 ounce	Cheese, Roquefort
−3.0	1 ounce	Cheese, Cheddar, Naturally Mild, Kraft
−3.0	1 ounce	Cheese, Natural Colby, Kraft
−3.0	1/2 piece	Sandwich, egg salad, whole wheat bread
−3.5	1/2 cup	Ice Cream, Sorbet and Cream, Key Lime, Häagen-Dazs
−3.5	1/2 cup	Ice Cream, Vanilla, Louis Sherry
−3.5	6 fluid ounces	Ice cream soda
−3.5	1 ounce	Cheese, Mozzarella, Casino, Kraft
−3.5	1/2 cup	Ice Cream, Vanilla, Soft Serve
−3.5	1/2 cup	Pudding, chocolate
−3.5	1/2 piece	Sandwich, egg salad, white bread
−3.5	1 ounce	Cheese, Gouda, Kraft
−3.5	1 ounce	Cheese, Cheddar, Sharp, Cracker Barrel
−3.5	1/4 cup	Ice Cream, Coffee, Häagen-Dazs

MILK/DAIRY GROUP

Nutripoints	Serving Size	Food Name
−3.5	1 ounce	Cheese, Monterey Jack, Kraft
−3.5	1/2 piece	Dairy Queen Dipped Cone, medium
−3.5	1/2 piece	Wendy's Frosty Dairy Dessert
−3.5	1 ounce	Cheese Spread, Cheez Whiz, Kraft
−3.5	2 tablespoons	Cream, Nondairy, Coffee Mate, Carnation
−3.5	1 piece	Ice Cream Bar, Eskimo Pie
−3.5	1/4 cup	Dairy Queen Mr. Misty Freeze
−3.5	1/4 cup	Ice Cream, Chocolate/Chocolate Chip, Häagen-Dazs
−3.5	1/4 serving	Jack in the Box Scrambled Egg Platter
−3.5	1/4 piece	Dairy Queen Buster Bar
−3.5	1/2 piece	Pie, custard
−3.5	1/4 cup	Dairy Queen Peanut Buster Parfait
−3.5	1/4 cup	Cream, sour
−3.5	1/2 cup	Ice Cream, Strawberry, Borden
−3.5	1 ounce	Candy bar, milk chocolate
−3.5	1/2 cup	Dairy Queen Mr. Misty Float
−3.5	4 ounces	Pudding, Chocolate Pudding Snacks, Jell-O
−3.5	1/2 piece	Dairy Queen Dilly Bar
−3.5	1/2 cup	Yogurt, Low-Fat, Strawberry, Light N'Lively
−3.5	1/2 serving	Burger King Breakfast Croissan'wich w/Ham
−4.0	1 ounce	Cheese, Monterey Jack, Casino Brand
−4.0	1/2 cup	Custard
−4.0	2 tablespoons	Cream, nondairy, imitation, liquid
−4.0	1/4 cup	Ice Cream, Vanilla, Häagen-Dazs
−4.0	1/2 cup	Ice Cream, French Vanilla, Meadow Gold
−4.0	1/4 cup	Sauce, custard
−4.0	1/2 cup	Dairy Queen Float
−4.0	1/2 cup	Sherbet, Orange, Borden
−4.0	1 ounce	Cheese, Swiss, Pasteurized Process, Kraft
−4.0	1/2 piece	Ice Cream Bar, Vanilla/Milk Chocolate/Almonds, Häagen-Dazs
−4.0	1/2 cup	Ice Cream, Vanilla, Party Time, Knudsen
−4.0	1/2 serving	McDonald's Egg McMuffin
−4.0	1/4 cup	Ice Cream, Vanilla Swiss Almond, Häagen-Dazs
−4.0	1/2 cup	Ice Cream, Buttered Pecan, Borden

MILK/DAIRY GROUP

Nutripoints	Serving Size	Food Name
−4.0	1/4 cup	Ice Cream, Chocolate, Schrafft's
−4.0	4 ounces	Pudding, Chocolate, Snack Pack, Hunt's
−4.0	4 ounces	Pudding, Vanilla, Snack Pack, Hunt's
−4.0	1/2 serving	Burger King Scrambled Egg Platter w/Bacon
−4.0	1/4 serving	Burger King Scrambled Egg Platter w/Sausage
−4.0	1/2 piece	Ice Cream Bar, Vanilla, Milk Chocolate, Häagen-Dazs
−4.0	1/2 serving	Burger King Breakfast Croissan'wich w/Bacon
−4.0	1 ounce	Cheese, Neufchâtel
−4.5	1/4 cup	Cheese fondue
−4.5	1/2 serving	Burger King Scrambled Egg Platter
−4.5	1/4 piece	Quiche, cheese/bacon
−4.5	4 pieces	Fried cheese sticks
−4.5	1/2 serving	McDonald's Biscuit w/Bacon/Egg/Cheese
−4.5	1/4 cup	Topping, Nondairy, Cool Whip, Birds Eye
−4.5	2 tablespoons	Cream, Nondairy, Cremora
−5.0	1/2 cup	Ice Cream, Butter Pecan, Meadow Gold
−5.0	2 tablespoons	Cheese, cream
−5.0	1/4 serving	Roy Rogers Egg and Biscuit Platter w/Ham
−5.5	1/2 serving	Burger King Breakfast Croissan'wich w/Sausage
−5.5	1/4 serving	Roy Rogers Egg and Biscuit Platter
−5.5	1/4 serving	Roy Rogers Egg and Biscuit Platter w/Sausage
−5.5	1/4 cup	Sauce, cheese
−5.5	1/4 serving	Roy Rogers Egg and Biscuit Platter w/Bacon
−5.5	1/4 cup	Topping, Whipped, La Creme
−5.5	2 tablespoons	Cream, sour, imitation
−6.0	2 tablespoons	Cream, coffee, light
−6.0	1/4 cup	Topping, Extra Creamy Cool Whip, Birds Eye
−6.0	1/2 piece	Quiche, cheese
−6.5	1/4 cup	Cream, whipped
−6.5	2 tablespoons	Cream, whipping, light

MILK/DAIRY GROUP

Nutripoints	Serving Size	Food Name
−7.0	½ serving	Wendy's Omelet #1 (Eggs, Ham, Cheese)
−7.0	2 tablespoons	Cream, heavy
−7.0	½ cup	Egg foo young
−8.0	½ serving	Egg, omelet, w/ham/cheese (1 serving = 3 eggs)
−9.0	¼ cup	Egg salad
−10.0	½ serving	Wendy's Omelet #3 (Eggs, Ham, Cheese, Onion)
−10.0	½ serving	Wendy's Omelet #2 (Eggs, Ham, Cheese/Mushroom)
−10.5	1 egg	Egg, deviled (1 piece = whole egg)
−11.0	2 eggs	Carl's Jr. Scrambled Eggs
−11.5	2 eggs	Egg, poached
−11.5	2 eggs	Egg, hard
−11.5	2 eggs	Egg, boiled
−11.5	1 serving	Wendy's Omelet #4 (Eggs, Mushroom/Green Peppers/Onion)
−12.5	1 egg	Egg, fried
−13.5	1 egg	Egg, scrambled
−15.0	2 yolks	Egg yolk
−19.5	1 serving	McDonald's Scrambled Eggs

MEAT/FISH/POULTRY GROUP

Nutripoints	Serving Size	Food Name
16.0	2 kabobs	Scallop Kabob, Nutripoint
13.5	6 ounces	‡ Clams, mixed species, raw
13.5	3 ounces	Red Snapper Veracruz, Nutripoint
13.0	12 oysters	‡ Oysters, eastern, raw
12.0	6 ounces	‡ Clams, raw
10.5	4 ounces	Salmon, Lettuce-Wrapped, w/Herb Sauce, Nutripoint
8.5	4 ounces	Venison, baked
8.5	1 cup	Chicken Stir-Fry, Nutripoint

†Cholesterol: excessively high
‡Caution: high risk for contamination

MEAT/FISH/POULTRY GROUP

Nutripoints	Serving Size	Food Name
8.0	1 cup	Clams, canned
8.0	4 oysters	‡ Oysters, Pacific, raw
8.0	1/2 cup	Tuna, Chunk Light, in Water, Low-Sodium, Chicken of the Sea
7.5	3/4 cup	Tuna, canned in water
7.5	6 ounces	Pike, baked
7.5	3 ounces	Salmon, steamed/poached
7.5	4 ounces	Halibut, baked
7.0	6 ounces	Red snapper, baked
7.0	1 piece	Beef, Carne Asada, Nutripoint
7.0	1/2 cup	Tuna, Chunk Light, in Water, Bumble Bee
7.0	6 ounces	Bass, freshwater, baked
7.0	3 ounces	† Beef liver, fried
7.0	4 ounces	Halibut, w/Yellow Bell Pepper Sauce, Nutripoint
7.0	3 ounces	Oysters, broiled, w/butter
6.5	6 ounces	Venison, w/Juniper Berry Sauce, Nutripoint
6.5	1/2 cup	Tuna, Solid White, in Water, Bumble Bee
6.5	3 ounces	Abalone
6.5	1/2 cup	Salmon, canned in water
6.5	3 ounces	Swordfish, baked
6.5	3 ounces	Tuna, fresh, broiled
6.5	3/4 cup	Chicken Salad, Nutripoint
6.5	3 ounces	Fish, Crunchy, Nutripoint
6.5	3/4 cup	Tuna, Chunk Light, in Water, Chicken of the Sea
6.0	1/2 portion	Chicken Primavera, frozen, Celentano
6.0	6 ounces	Clams, steamed/boiled
6.0	4 ounces	Quail, w/o skin
6.0	6 ounces	Sole, baked
6.0	1/2 cup	Tuna, Lite Chunk Light, in Water and Oil, Chicken of the Sea
5.5	4 pieces	Ham, Slices, Jubilee, Oscar Mayer
5.5	1/2 cup	Tuna, Solid White, in Water, Star-Kist
5.5	4 ounces	Pheasant, w/o skin
5.5	4 ounces	Sturgeon, steamed
5.5	3/4 cup	Soup, chicken gumbo

†Cholesterol: excessively high

MEAT/FISH/POULTRY GROUP

Nutripoints	Serving Size	Food Name
5.5	½ cup	Tuna, Solid White, in Water, Chicken of the Sea
5.5	3 ounces	Moose
5.5	1½ cups	Soup, Chicken, Home Style, Progresso
5.5	3 ounces	Salmon, baked/broiled
5.5	3 ounces	Chicken, Cajun, Nutripoint
5.0	1 burger	Hamburger, Aerobics, Nutripoint
5.0	½ cup	Tuna, Diet Albacore, Chunk White, in Water, Low-Sodium, Chicken of the Sea
5.0	3 ounces	Clams, smoked, canned in oil
5.0	4 ounces	Ham, lean, baked, canned, 4-percent fat
5.0	½ cup	Tuna Salad, Nutripoint
5.0	1 portion	Ham Dinner, frozen, Morton
5.0	1 serving	McDonald's Chicken Salad Oriental
5.0	3 ounces	Trout, baked
5.0	½ portion	Beef Teriyaki, frozen, Chun King
5.0	2 pieces	Enchiladas, Chicken, Nutripoint
4.5	3 ounces	Clams, breaded, fried
4.5	2 ounces	† Liverwurst
4.5	6 ounces	† Crab, hard-shell, steamed
4.5	¾ cup	Salmon, Pink, Chunk, Skinless and Boneless, in Water, Chicken of the Sea
4.5	3 pieces	Sardines, canned in oil
4.5	1 cup	Soup, clam chowder, New England milk base
4.5	4 ounces	Chicken, Grilled w/Mango Sauce, Nutripoint
4.5	3 ounces	Abalone, floured, fried
4.5	4 ounces	Smelt, rainbow, baked
4.5	4 ounces	Ocean perch, baked
4.5	1 cup	Soup, Chicken, w/Ribbon Pasta, Pritikin
4.5	3 pieces	Bacon, Canadian Style, Oscar Mayer
4.5	3 ounces	Turkey, light meat, baked, w/o skin
4.0	3 ounces	Chicken breast, baked, w/o skin
4.0	3 ounces	Beef round steak, lean, broiled
4.0	½ piece	Sandwich, chicken salad, whole wheat bread

†Cholesterol: excessively high

MEAT/FISH/POULTRY GROUP

Nutripoints	Serving Size	Food Name
4.0	1 cup	Soup, beef
4.0	½ cup	Salmon, Pink, Bumble Bee
4.0	3 ounces	Anchovy, canned
4.0	4 ounces	Shark, mixed species, raw
4.0	3 ounces	† Beef heart, braised
4.0	1 piece	Beef, Sliced, frozen, Morton
4.0	4 ounces	Snails
4.0	1 whole	Sandwich, Turkey, Nutripoint
4.0	1 cup	Soup, Chunky Beef, Campbell's
4.0	2 ounces	† Braunschweiger
4.0	3 ounces	Beef flank steak, lean, broiled
4.0	½ cup	Tuna, Tonno, Solid Light, in Oil, Chicken of the Sea
4.0	6 ounces	Scallops, baked/broiled
4.0	5 ounces	Orange roughy, raw
4.0	1 portion	Turkey, w/Dressing, frozen, Morton
4.0	4 ounces	Perch fillet, baked/broiled
4.0	3 ounces	Mackerel, baked
4.0	1 portion	Turkey Dinner, frozen, Morton
4.0	½ cup	Tuna, Albacore Solid White, in Oil, Chicken of the Sea
4.0	3 ounces	Beef top loin, lean, broiled
3.5	6 pieces	Sardines, canned, in tomato sauce
3.5	3 ounces	† Veal cutlet/steak, lean, braised
3.5	1 cup	Soup, seafood gumbo
3.5	3 ounces	Fish, smoked
3.5	3 ounces	Lamb roast, leg, baked
3.5	3 ounces	Flounder, baked
3.5	3 ounces	Halibut fillet, batter-fried
3.5	1 cup	Beef stew
3.5	½ cup	Salmon, Red, Chunk, Skinless and Boneless, Chicken of the Sea
3.5	½ portion	Beef, frozen dinner
3.5	½ piece	Sandwich, chicken salad, white bread
3.5	1 serving	Carl's Jr. Chicken Salad (take-out)
3.5	½ piece	Sandwich, tuna salad, whole wheat bread
3.5	4 ounces	Cod, baked
3.5	3 ounces	Beef tenderloin fillet, lean, broiled

†Cholesterol: excessively high

MEAT/FISH/POULTRY GROUP

Nutripoints	Serving Size	Food Name
3.5	4 ounces	Turkey, White, canned, Premium Chunk, Swanson
3.5	3 ounces	Beef chuck roast, lean, braised
3.5	3 ounces	Turkey, light/dark meat, baked, w/o skin
3.5	1/2 portion	Turkey, frozen dinner
3.5	3 pieces	Turkey Breast Slices, Louis Rich
3.5	1/2 cup	Tuna, Chunk Light, in Oil, Chicken of the Sea
3.5	4 ounces	Chicken, Marinated, Hawaiian, Nutripoint
3.5	1/2 piece	Burrito, chicken
3.5	3 pieces	Luncheon meat, honeyloaf
3.5	4 ounces	Chicken, Lemon, Nutripoint
3.5	1 cup	Tuna noodle casserole
3.5	1 portion	Chicken Oriental, frozen, Healthy Choice
3.5	1 portion	Chicken Parmigiana, frozen, Healthy Choice
3.0	1 portion	Chicken, Sweet and Sour, frozen, Healthy Choice
3.0	1 portion	Beef Sirloin Tips, frozen, Healthy Choice
3.0	1 cup	Oyster stew
3.0	4 ounces	Chicken, Fried, Low-Fat, Nutripoint
3.0	3 ounces	Squirrel
3.0	3 ounces	Rabbit, wild
3.0	3 ounces	Turkey, dark meat, baked, w/o skin
3.0	3 ounces	Hamburger patty, lean, broiled
3.0	1/2 cup	Salmon, Red Sockeye, Bumble Bee
3.0	1 cup	Chicken a la King w/Rice, Dining Lite
3.0	1 cup	Beef w/macaroni and tomato sauce
3.0	1/2 piece	Sandwich, tuna salad, white bread
3.0	3 ounces	Lamb shoulder, lean, baked
3.0	5 ounces	Catfish, baked
3.0	1/2 cup	Tuna salad
3.0	1/2 piece	Hamburger w/bun/lettuce/tomato (fast-food)
3.0	3 ounces	Pork chop, loin, lean, baked
3.0	3 ounces	Turkey roll, light meat
3.0	3 ounces	Rabbit, domestic, breaded, fried
3.0	5 ounces	Grouper, baked
3.0	1/2 portion	Beef, Pepper Oriental, frozen, Chun King
3.0	3 ounces	Salmon, smoked

MEAT/FISH/POULTRY GROUP

Nutripoints	Serving Size	Food Name
3.0	1 piece	Sausage patty
3.0	1/2 portion	Chicken Imperial, frozen, Chun King
2.5	3 pieces	Beef jerky
2.5	3 ounces	Chicken breast, fried, w/o bread, w/skin
2.5	4 ounces	Ocean Perch Fillet, frozen, Gorton's
2.5	1/2 cup	Tuna helper, prepared
2.5	3 ounces	Beef rib eye, lean, broiled
2.5	1/2 cup	Chicken fricassee
2.5	1/2 portion	Ham, frozen, dinner
2.5	1 piece	Green pepper, stuffed w/meat
2.5	3 ounces	Beef porterhouse steak, lean, broiled
2.5	6 ounces	Lobster, steamed/boiled
2.5	6 ounces	Sushi/raw fish
2.5	1/2 portion	Chicken, low-cal., frozen dinner
2.5	1 portion	Chicken Tenderloins in Barbecue Sauce, frozen, Stouffer's Right Course
2.5	1 cup	Soup, Turkey Vegetable, Campbell's
2.5	1 portion	Chicken and Pasta Divan, Healthy Choice
2.5	1/2 serving	Jack in the Box Club Pita
2.5	3 ounces	Carp, smoked
2.5	1/2 piece	Sandwich, turkey, whole wheat bread
2.5	4 ounces	Haddock, baked
2.5	3 ounces	Chicken leg, baked, w/o skin
2.5	1 piece	Taco, beef/cheese
2.5	3 ounces	Beef T-bone steak, lean, choice, broiled
2.5	3 1/2 ounces	Turkey, light meat and skin, baked
2.0	3 ounces	Rabbit, stewed
2.0	1/2 cup	Chicken salad
2.0	1 cup	Soup, Chicken Vegetable, Couscous, Nile Spice Foods
2.0	6 ounces	Mussels, cooked
2.0	1/2 piece	Sandwich, chicken, whole wheat bread
2.0	1/2 portion	Fish Dinner, frozen, Morton
2.0	3 ounces	Salmon, baked, w/butter
2.0	1/2 serving	Jack in the Box Chicken Fajita Pita
2.0	3 ounces	Beef round steak, medium fat, broiled
2.0	1 portion	Lasagna, Tuna/Spinach/Noodles/Vegetables, frozen, Stouffer's
2.0	1 cup	Soup, Chicken Vegetable, Campbell's

MEAT/FISH/POULTRY GROUP

Nutripoints	Serving Size	Food Name
2.0	3 ounces	Chicken thigh, fried, w/o breading
2.0	1 cup	Wendy's Taco Beef Salad
2.0	3 ounces	Chicken liver, stewed
2.0	4 ounces	Whiting, baked/broiled
2.0	1 portion	Chicken, w/Vegetables and Vermicelli, frozen, Stouffer's
2.0	3/4 cup	Chicken w/dumplings
2.0	1 serving	Shrimp étouffée (1 serving = 1 1/2 cups)
2.0	1/2 portion	Beef Salisbury steak, frozen dinner
2.0	1/2 piece	Fish, w/Chips, frozen, Morton
2.0	4 ounces	Luncheon meat, turkey ham
2.0	1 portion	Beef, Pot Roast, Homestyle, frozen, Stouffer's Right Course
2.0	1/2 piece	Sandwich, chicken, white bread
2.0	1/2 portion	Pork, Sweet and Sour, frozen, Chun King
2.0	1 portion	Turkey breast, frozen, Healthy Choice
2.0	6 ounces	Cod, smoked
2.0	6 ounces	Squid, raw
2.0	1 portion	Egg Rolls, Restaurant, frozen, Chun King
2.0	1/2 portion	Peppers, Sweet, Stuffed, frozen, Celentano
2.0	3 ounces	Beef ribs, baked
2.0	6 ounces	Haddock, smoked
2.0	1/2 piece	Taco, chicken
2.0	1 portion	Veal Parmigiana, frozen, Morton
2.0	1/2 piece	Wendy's Chicken Sandwich
2.0	1/2 portion	Chicken Parmigiana, frozen, Celentano
2.0	1/2 cup	Tuna, canned in oil
2.0	3 ounces	Beef brisket, lean, braised
2.0	3 ounces	Ham, baked, canned, 13-percent fat
2.0	1/2 portion	Beef Szechuan, frozen, Chun King
2.0	3 pieces	Chicken wing, baked, w/o skin
2.0	3 ounces	Veal roast, lean, braised
2.0	1/2 piece	Sandwich, BLT, whole wheat bread
2.0	3/4 cup	Beefaroni
2.0	1 portion	Chicken au Gratin, Slim, frozen, Budget Gourmet
2.0	3 ounces	Octopus, fried
2.0	1/2 portion	Pork, frozen dinner
1.5	1/2 piece	Sandwich, corned beef, rye bread

MEAT/FISH/POULTRY GROUP

Nutripoints	Serving Size	Food Name
1.5	½ piece	Meat loaf, frozen dinner
1.5	1 portion	Chicken Breast, Marsala, w/Vegetables, frozen, Stouffer's
1.5	3 ounces	Chicken leg, fried, w/o bread, w/skin
1.5	½ portion	Beef Steak, Chopped, frozen, Weight Watchers
1.5	½ portion	Chicken Chow Mein, frozen, Chun King
1.5	½ cup	Herring, canned
1.5	3 ounces	Duck, baked, w/o skin
1.5	3 ounces	Beef flank steak, medium fat, choice, broiled
1.5	½ piece	Sandwich, turkey, white bread
1.5	3 ounces	Barracuda, baked/broiled
1.5	1 portion	Chicken Breast, Glazed, frozen, Le Menu
1.5	3 pieces	Bacon, Canadian
1.5	½ portion	Sole, Stuffed, w/Newburg Sauce, frozen, Weight Watchers
1.5	1 cup	Soup, Chicken w/Noodles, Low-Sodium, Campbell's
1.5	3 ounces	Chicken breast, fried, w/o skin
1.5	3 ounces	Capon, baked, w/skin
1.5	1 portion	Chicken a l'Orange, w/Almonds and Rice, frozen, Stouffer's
1.5	½ piece	Carl's Jr. Charbroiler Barbeque Chicken Sandwich
1.5	½ serving	Jack in the Box Beef Fajita Pita
1.5	1 cup	Soup, chicken
1.5	½ portion	Chicken, frozen dinner
1.5	½ cup	Tuna, Chunk Light, in Oil, Star-Kist
1.5	1 piece	Fajita, beef
1.5	1 portion	Chicken Tenders, Sweet 'n Sour, frozen, Weight Watchers
1.5	½ piece	Hamburger w/bun, small, plain (fast-food)
1.5	3 ounces	Hamburger patty, lean, fried
1.5	¼ cup	Bacon bits, imitation
1.5	6 pieces	Sardines, canned in mustard sauce
1.5	1 cup	Chicken Chow Mein w/Rice, Dining Lite
1.5	1 portion	Fish Fillet, Divan, frozen, Stouffer's
1.5	3 ounces	Eel, smoked

MEAT/FISH/POULTRY GROUP

Nutripoints	Serving Size	Food Name
1.5	1/2 cup	Chicken, creamed
1.5	1/2 portion	Tortellini, Veal w/Tomato Sauce, frozen, Stouffer's
1.5	3 ounces	Eel
1.5	3 pieces	Oysters, fried
1.5	1 portion	Beef, Sliced, w/Gravy, frozen, Morton
1.5	1 portion	Chicken Imperial, frozen, Weight Watchers
1.5	1/2 serving	Wendy's New Beef Chili
1.5	1 portion	Beef Oriental Pepper Steak, frozen, Healthy Choice
1.5	1 portion	Sole au Gratin, frozen, Healthy Choice
1.5	1 portion	Chicken Italiano, frozen, Stouffer's Right Course
1.5	1 portion	Salisbury Steak, frozen, Healthy Choice
1.0	1 portion	Chicken, Mandarin, Slim, frozen, Budget Gourmet
1.0	3 ounces	Bonito, canned
1.0	1/2 piece	Dairy Queen Fish Fillet
1.0	1/4 cup	Hamburger Helper, Prepared
1.0	1/2 piece	Sandwich, BLT, white bread
1.0	1 cup	Soup, beef noodle
1.0	4 ounces	Turkey Breast, Roasted, No Salt Added, Mr. Turkey
1.0	4 ounces	Ham, canned, Armour Golden Star
1.0	3 ounces	Turkey Breast, Sliced, Mr. Turkey
1.0	3 1/2 ounces	Turkey, dark meat and skin, baked
1.0	3 ounces	Scallops, fried
1.0	1 portion	Chicken, Sesame, frozen, Stouffer's Right Course
1.0	1 portion	Turkey, sliced, frozen, Stouffer's Right Course
1.0	1 portion	Chicken Tenderloins in Peanut Sauce, frozen, Stouffer's Right Course
1.0	4 pieces	Turkey Ham, Louis Rich
1.0	6 ounces	Crab, canned
1.0	3 ounces	Chicken breast, fried, w/batter, w/skin
1.0	4 pieces	Salami, pork
1.0	3 ounces	Barracuda, breaded/floured, fried

MEAT/FISH/POULTRY GROUP

Nutripoints	Serving Size	Food Name
1.0	½ piece	Dairy Queen Fish Fillet w/Cheese Sandwich
1.0	½ cup	Ham salad
1.0	3 ounces	Beef Swiss steak
1.0	3 ounces	Perch, fried, w/breading
1.0	½ piece	Wendy's Small Hamburger
1.0	1 piece	Fajita, chicken
1.0	½ piece	Fish, sandwich (fast-food)
1.0	3 ounces	Chicken thigh, baked, w/o skin
1.0	½ piece	Sandwich, roast beef, hot
1.0	1 piece	Taco Bell Steak Fajita
1.0	½ piece	Wendy's Kids' Meal Hamburger
1.0	½ piece	Taco Bell Double Beef Burrito Supreme w/Red Sauce
1.0	½ piece	Sandwich, sloppy joe, w/bun
1.0	½ piece	Taco Bell Double Beef Burrito Supreme w/Green Sauce
1.0	½ piece	Arby's Super Roast Beef Sandwich
1.0	2 ounces	Veal patty, fried
1.0	1 piece	Chicken thigh, baked, w/o skin
1.0	3 ounces	Beef short ribs, lean, braised
1.0	½ piece	Wendy's Small Cheeseburger
1.0	1 portion	Veal Parmigiana Patty, frozen, Weight Watchers
1.0	½ portion	Lobster Newburg, frozen dinner
1.0	1 cup	Soup, chowder, fish
1.0	1 portion	Beef Sirloin, in Herb Sauce, Slim, frozen, Budget Gourmet
1.0	3 ounces	Veal cutlet, medium fat, braised
1.0	3 ounces	Swordfish fillet, breaded, fried
1.0	½ piece	Carl's Jr. California Roast Beef 'n Swiss Sandwich
1.0	1 portion	Beef Sirloin Salisbury Steak, Slim, frozen, Budget Gourmet
1.0	½ piece	Wendy's Kids' Meal Cheeseburger
1.0	3 pieces	Pastrami, turkey
1.0	1 portion	Enchiladas, Sirloin, Ranchero, Slim, frozen, Budget Gourmet

MEAT/FISH/POULTRY GROUP

Nutripoints	Serving Size	Food Name
1.0	1 portion	Turkey Breast, Sliced, w/Mushroom Sauce, frozen, Stouffer's
1.0	½ piece	Jack in the Box Grilled Chicken Fillet Sandwich
1.0	3 ounces	Beef tenderloin, medium fat, broiled
1.0	1 portion	Beef, Fiesta w/Corn Pasta, frozen, Stouffer's Right Course
1.0	3 ounces	Salmon patty, fried
1.0	½ portion	Chicken Cacciatore, frozen, Budget Gourmet
1.0	4 ounces	Turkey roll, light/dark meat
1.0	1 portion	Shrimp Primavera, frozen, Stouffer's Right Course
1.0	½ cup	Chicken, sweet and sour
1.0	½ cup	Chicken, canned
1.0	½ piece	Roy Rogers Roast Beef Sandwich
0.5	½ portion	Chicken Teriyaki, frozen, Budget Gourmet
0.5	1 portion	Enchiladas, Chicken, Suiza, Slim, frozen, Budget Gourmet
0.5	2 pieces	Herring, pickled
0.5	½ portion	Chicken, Sweet and Sour, w/Rice, frozen, Budget Gourmet
0.5	½ piece	Dairy Queen Double Hamburger
0.5	3 ounces	Carp, baked/broiled
0.5	½ piece	Arby's King Roast Beef Sandwich
0.5	2 ounces	Pâté, chicken liver, canned
0.5	1 piece	Arby's Junior Roast Beef Sandwich
0.5	1 piece	Fajita, Chicken, frozen, Weight Watchers
0.5	1 cup	Carl's Jr. Old-Fashioned Chicken Noodle Soup
0.5	½ piece	Carl's Jr. Charbroiler Chicken Club Sandwich
0.5	3 ounces	Veal roast, medium fat, braised
0.5	1 portion	Beef Dijon, w/Pasta and Vegetables, frozen, Stouffer's Right Course
0.5	½ piece	Arby's Regular Roast Beef Sandwich
0.5	1 portion	Chicken Oriental, frozen, Stouffer's
0.5	1 cup	Soup, Beef, Campbell's

MEAT/FISH/POULTRY GROUP

Nutripoints	Serving Size	Food Name
0.5	½ pie	Turkey pot pie
0.5	½ cup	Chop suey, beef/pork
0.5	½ portion	Beef Meatloaf Dinner, frozen, Morton
0.5	½ portion	Fajita, Beef, Weight Watchers
0.5	1 cup	Soup, Chunky Steak 'n Potato, Campbell's
0.5	1 portion	Turkey, Divan, frozen, Le Menu
0.5	1 cup	Soup, Chunky Chicken Noodle, Campbell's
0.5	1 portion	Beef Ragout w/Rice Pilaf, frozen, Stouffer's Right Course
0.5	1 portion	Fish Fillet au Gratin, frozen, Weight Watchers
0.5	3 ounces	Fish, fried
0.5	½ piece	Sandwich, ham/cheese, whole wheat bread
0.5	3 ounces	Lamb roast, leg, medium fat, baked
0.5	½ piece	Dairy Queen Single Hamburger
0.5	½ pie	Beef pot pie
0.5	1 portion	Chicken Cacciatore w/Vermicelli, frozen, Stouffer's
0.5	1 portion	Shrimp Creole, frozen, Healthy Choice
0.5	1 piece	Taco Bell Chicken Fajita
0.5	½ piece	Dairy Queen Double Hamburger w/Cheese
0.5	2 ounces	Beef chuck roast, medium fat, baked
0.5	½ piece	Roy Rogers Large Roast Beef Sandwich
0.5	½ portion	Beef Sirloin Tips, w/Burgundy Sauce, frozen, Budget Gourmet
0.5	1 piece	McDonald's Hamburger
0.5	2 pieces	Ham, chopped
0.5	½ piece	Chicken, Fried, w/Corn, frozen, Morton
0.5	½ portion	Beef Salisbury Steak Dinner, frozen, Morton
0.5	½ piece	Burger King Ham and Cheese Specialty Sandwich
0.5	6 pieces	Burger King Chicken Tenders
0.5	½ pie	Chicken pot pie
0.5	½ portion	Turkey Breast, Sliced, frozen, Budget Gourmet
0.5	4 pieces	Fish sticks
0.5	3 ounces	Beef top loin, medium fat, broiled
0.5	½ piece	Sandwich, ham/cheese, rye bread

MEAT/FISH/POULTRY GROUP

Nutripoints	Serving Size	Food Name
0.5	½ piece	Dairy Queen Single Hamburger w/Cheese
0.5	1 piece	Catfish, Fillets, Light, Mrs. Paul's
0.5	3 ounces	Pike fillet, breaded, fried
0.5	½ portion	Scallops and Shrimp Mariner, frozen, Budget Gourmet
0.5	½ piece	Wendy's Single Hamburger w/Everything
0.5	½ piece	Burger King Hamburger
0.5	2 pieces	Bologna, pork
0.5	2 ounces	Beef rump roast, baked
0.5	1 portion	Turkey, Glazed, Slim, frozen, Budget Gourmet
0.5	½ piece	Wendy's Single Cheese Hamburger w/Everything
0.5	3 ounces	Goat
0.5	1 cup	Soup, chicken noodle
0.5	½ piece	Wendy's Plain Single Hamburger
0.5	3 ounces	Pompano, baked/broiled
0.5	15 pieces	Shrimp, steamed
0.0	½ portion	Beef Pot Roast, Yankee, frozen, Budget Gourmet
0.0	1 portion	Beef Salisbury Steak, w/Potatoes, frozen, Morton
0.0	1 portion	Chicken a la King, frozen, Weight Watchers
0.0	2 ounces	Chicken-fried steak
0.0	¼ piece	Sandwich, submarine
0.0	3 ounces	Hamburger patty, broiled
0.0	¼ piece	Dairy Queen Triple Hamburger w/Cheese
0.0	½ piece	Cheeseburger w/bun, small, plain (fast-food)
0.0	½ piece	Wendy's Plain Single Hamburger w/Cheese
0.0	½ piece	Sandwich, ham/cheese, white bread
0.0	1 piece	Beef Stroganoff, Slim, frozen, Budget Gourmet
0.0	1 piece	Chicken thigh, meat and skin, baked
0.0	3 ounces	Shark, mixed species, batter-dipped, fried
0.0	3 ounces	Catfish, fried, w/breading
0.0	½ portion	Veal Parmigiana, frozen, Budget Gourmet
0.0	½ portion	Chicken, Fried, Dinner, frozen, Morton

MEAT/FISH/POULTRY GROUP

Nutripoints	Serving Size	Food Name
0.0	½ piece	Carl's Jr. Old-Time Star Hamburger
0.0	1 ounce	Wendy's Sliced Pepperoni
0.0	¼ piece	Dairy Queen Triple Hamburger
0.0	1 piece	Carl's Jr. Happy Star Hamburger
0.0	2 ounces	Pork roast, baked
0.0	½ cup	Beef Stroganoff
0.0	½ portion	Tuna Noodle Casserole, frozen, Stouffer's
0.0	½ piece	Jack in the Box Jumbo Jack
0.0	¾ cup	Pork, sweet and sour
0.0	½ piece	Chicken Kiev
0.0	2 pieces	Chicken wing, fried, w/o breading
0.0	1 portion	Egg Rolls, Chicken, frozen, Chun King
0.0	½ piece	Dairy Queen Chicken Breast Fillet
0.0	1 portion	Beef Oriental w/Vegetables and Rice, frozen, Stouffer's
0.0	½ piece	Dairy Queen Chicken Breast Fillet w/Cheese
0.0	3 ounces	Beef porterhouse steak, medium fat, choice, broiled
0.0	½ piece	Sandwich, ham salad, whole wheat bread
0.0	1 ounce	Pork skins
0.0	½ portion	Pepper Steak, w/Rice, frozen, Budget Gourmet
0.0	2 cups	Soup, clam chowder, Manhattan tomato base
0.0	4 ounces	Chicken, White and Dark, Premium Chunk, canned, Swanson
0.0	½ portion	Beef Salisbury Steak, Romana, frozen, Weight Watchers
0.0	4 ounces	Turkey, White and Dark, Premium Chunk, canned, Swanson
0.0	3 ounces	Squid, fried
0.0	1 portion	Ham, Asparagus au Gratin, Slim, frozen, Budget Gourmet
0.0	½ cup	Chicken a la king
0.0	1 portion	Egg Rolls, Shrimp, frozen, Chun King
0.0	½ piece	Fish Sandwich, Whaler, Burger King
0.0	½ piece	Taco Bell Beef Enchirito w/Red Sauce

MEAT/FISH/POULTRY GROUP

Nutripoints	Serving Size	Food Name
0.0	1/2 portion	Meatballs, Italian Style, w/Noodles and Peppers, frozen, Budget Gourmet
0.0	1/2 piece	Burger King Cheeseburger
0.0	2 pieces	Ham and cheese loaf/roll
0.0	1 portion	Chicken a la King, w/Rice, frozen, Stouffer's
0.0	1/2 piece	Burger King Whopper Jr. Sandwich
0.0	1 piece	Jack in the Box Hamburger
0.0	1 piece	Chicken thigh, meat and skin, batter-fried
0.0	1/2 piece	Arby's Beef 'n Cheddar Sandwich
0.0	1 piece	Taco Bell Soft Taco
0.0	1/2 piece	Wendy's Philly Swiss Hamburger
0.0	1 cup	Soup, cream of chicken
0.0	1 portion	Beef Szechwan, w/Noodles and Vegetables, frozen, Stouffer's
0.0	1 piece	Haddock Fillet, Light, Mrs. Paul's
0.0	3 ounces	Goose, meat and skin, baked
0.0	2 ounces	Sausage, Polish
0.0	1 portion	Western Dinner, frozen, Morton
0.0	1/2 portion	Enchiladas, Beef Ranchero, frozen, Weight Watchers
0.0	2 ounces	Salami, beef
0.0	1/2 piece	McDonald's Cheeseburger
0.0	1 portion	Beef Salisbury Steak, frozen, Le Menu
0.0	2 ounces	Ham, minced
0.0	1/2 piece	Taco Bell Beef Enchirito w/Green Sauce
0.0	1/3 piece	Wendy's Big Classic Hamburger
0.0	1/2 piece	Jack in the Box Cheeseburger
0.0	2 pieces	Chicken wing, meat and skin, baked
−0.5	3 ounces	Beef tongue, simmered
−0.5	1 piece	Egg Rolls, Shrimp/Meat, frozen, Chun King
−0.5	3 ounces	Veal chop, medium fat, fried
−0.5	1/2 cup	Hash
−0.5	1/2 piece	Carl's Jr. Country Fried Steak Sandwich
−0.5	4 ounces	Chicken, Chunk White, Premium, canned, Swanson
−0.5	2 ounces	Pork chop, broiled
−0.5	2 pieces	Meatballs

MEAT/FISH/POULTRY GROUP

Nutripoints	Serving Size	Food Name
−0.5	1 portion	Beef Stew, frozen, Stouffer's
−0.5	1 piece	Taco Bell Super Combo Taco
−0.5	1/3 piece	Wendy's Big Classic Hamburger w/Cheese
−0.5	4 ounces	Yellowtail, raw
−0.5	1 portion	Veal Primavera, frozen, Stouffer's
−0.5	1/2 piece	Burger King Whopper Jr. Sandwich w/Cheese
−0.5	1/2 portion	Turkey a la King, w/Rice, frozen, Budget Gourmet
−0.5	1/2 piece	Jack in the Box Hot Club Supreme
−0.5	1/2 portion	Enchiladas, Beef Dinner, frozen, Patio
−0.5	1 piece	Chicken wing, meat and skin, batter-fried
−0.5	3 ounces	Lobster, floured/breaded, fried
−0.5	1/2 portion	Chicken Pie, frozen, Stouffer's
−0.5	3 ounces	Meat loaf
−0.5	1 piece	Dairy Queen All-White Chicken Nuggets
−0.5	1/4 piece	Wendy's Bacon Swiss Hamburger
−0.5	3 ounces	Beef T-bone steak, medium fat, broiled
−0.5	1 portion	Veal Marsala, frozen, Le Menu
−0.5	2 ounces	Sausage, Italian
−0.5	1/2 piece	Roy Rogers Roast Beef Sandwich w/Cheese
−0.5	1 cup	Soup, New England Clam Chowder, w/milk, Campbell's
−0.5	1/2 pie	Beef Pie, frozen, Stouffer's
−0.5	3 ounces	Cod, floured/breaded, fried
−0.5	1/2 piece	Sandwich, ham salad, white
−0.5	1/2 portion	Enchiladas, Chicken, Suiza, frozen, Weight Watchers
−0.5	2 rolls	Jack in the Box Egg Rolls (5 rolls)
−0.5	1/2 portion	Seafood Newburg, frozen, Budget Gourmet
−0.5	4 ounces	Turkey Roll, White, Cooked, Mr. Turkey
−0.5	1/2 piece	Beef, Pie, frozen, Morton
−0.5	1/2 piece	Chicken Parmigiana Patty, frozen, Weight Watchers
−0.5	1 piece	Taco Bell Supreme Soft Taco
−0.5	1 piece	Cod Fillets, Light, Mrs. Paul's
−0.5	1/2 serving	Jack in the Box Taquitos (7 servings)
−0.5	1/2 piece	Burger King Chicken Specialty Sandwich

MEAT/FISH/POULTRY GROUP

Nutripoints	Serving Size	Food Name
−0.5	½ piece	Carl's Jr. Famous Star Hamburger
−0.5	3 ounces	Flounder, fillet, breaded, fried
−0.5	½ portion	Beef Sirloin Salisbury Steak, frozen, Budget Gourmet
−0.5	½ piece	McDonald's Quarter Pounder
−0.5	½ pie	Turkey, Pie, frozen, Morton
−0.5	1 portion	Green Pepper, Stuffed w/Beef and Tomato Sauce, frozen, Stouffer's
−0.5	½ piece	Roy Rogers Large Roast Beef w/Cheese Sandwich
−0.5	3 ounces	Carp, floured/breaded, fried
−0.5	½ pie	Chicken, Pie, frozen, Morton
−0.5	3 ounces	Pompano, floured/breaded, fried
−0.5	½ portion	McDonald's Sausage McMuffin
−0.5	1 piece	Kentucky Fried Chicken, Chicken Keel, Extra Crispy
−0.5	½ piece	Frankfurter, pork and beef, w/bun
−0.5	2 ounces	Lamb chop, loin, medium fat, baked
−0.5	1 portion	Fish Fillet, Florentine, frozen, Stouffer's
−0.5	½ piece	Burger King Whaler Fish Sandwich
−1.0	1 piece	Kentucky Fried Chicken, Chicken Keel
−1.0	1 portion	Turkey, w/Dressing and Potatoes, frozen, Swanson
−1.0	1 piece	Pork chop, pan-fried
−1.0	3 ounces	Haddock, floured/breaded, fried
−1.0	½ portion	Turkey Breast, Stuffed, frozen, Weight Watchers
−1.0	3 ounces	Pork feet, pickled
−1.0	½ cup	Beef, creamed chipped
−1.0	1 portion	Beef Salisbury Steak, in Gravy, frozen, Stouffer's
−1.0	4 ounces	Fish Sticks, Crunchy, frozen, Mrs. Paul's
−1.0	½ portion	Beef Stroganoff, frozen, Weight Watchers
−1.0	2 pieces	Luncheon Meat, Picnic Loaf, Oscar Mayer
−1.0	1 piece	Flounder Fillet, Light, Mrs. Paul's
−1.0	½ portion	Tortellini, Veal, Alfredo, frozen, Stouffer's
−1.0	1 piece	Fish Fillet, Batter-Dipped, frozen, Mrs. Paul's

MEAT/FISH/POULTRY GROUP

Nutripoints	Serving Size	Food Name
—1.0	1/2 portion	Chicken Divan, frozen, Stouffer's
—1.0	1 portion	Beef Salisbury Steak, w/Italian Sauce, frozen, Stouffer's
—1.0	1 piece	Wendy's Fish Fillet
—1.0	2 ounces	Luncheon meat, pimiento loaf
—1.0	1/2 piece	Burger King Whopper Sandwich w/Cheese
—1.0	1/2 piece	McDonald's Big Mac
—1.0	1/2 piece	Carl's Jr. Fillet of Fish Sandwich
—1.0	2 rolls	Jack in the Box Egg Rolls (3 rolls)
—1.0	3 pieces	Bacon, Low-Salt, Oscar Mayer
—1.0	2 pieces	Luncheon meat, pickle and pimiento loaf
—1.0	1/2 portion	Chicken, w/Fettucini, frozen, Budget Gourmet
—1.0	1/3 piece	McDonald's McD.L.T.
—1.0	3 ounces	Duck, meat and skin, baked
—1.0	3 ounces	Lamb shoulder, medium fat, baked
—1.0	4 ounces	Lobster, baked/broiled, w/butter
—1.0	1/2 serving	Jack in the Box Chicken Strips (6 pieces)
—1.0	1/2 pie	Turkey Pie, frozen, Stouffer's
—1.0	4 pieces	Turkey, Luncheon Loaf, Louis Rich
—1.0	1 piece	Dairy Queen Hot Dog
—1.0	1 ounce	Pâté, de foie gras, canned (goose liver)
—1.0	1/2 piece	Corn dog
—1.0	1/2 portion	Beef Sirloin Tips, w/Country Style Vegetables, frozen, Budget Gourmet
—1.0	3 pieces	Shrimp, fried
—1.0	1/2 piece	McDonald's Fillet-O-Fish
—1.0	1/2 piece	Dairy Queen Hot Dog w/Chili
—1.0	1 piece	Ocean Perch Fillet, Light, Mrs. Paul's
—1.0	3 ounces	Clams, Fried in Light Batter, Mrs. Paul's
—1.0	1/2 pie	Turkey Pot Pie, Swanson
—1.0	2 pieces	Sausage, summer
—1.0	2 ounces	Beef short ribs, medium fat, braised
—1.0	1/2 piece	Carl's Jr. Western Bacon Cheeseburger
—1.0	1/2 serving	Jack in the Box Chicken Strips (4 pieces)
—1.0	1/2 piece	Jack in the Box Fish Supreme
—1.0	1/2 pie	Chicken Pot Pie, frozen, Swanson

MEAT/FISH/POULTRY GROUP

Nutripoints	Serving Size	Food Name
−1.0	1 piece	Roy Rogers Chicken Drumstick/Leg
−1.0	1/2 cup	Crab salad
−1.0	1 piece	Frankfurter, chicken, w/bun
−1.0	2 ounces	Bratwurst
−1.0	1/2 piece	McDonald's Quarter Pounder w/Cheese
−1.0	1 piece	Enchiladas Suiza, Chicken, Van de Kamp's
−1.0	1/2 piece	Jack in the Box Bacon Cheeseburger
−1.0	1/2 piece	Roy Rogers Chicken Breast
−1.0	3 ounces	Crab, soft-shell, fried
−1.0	4 ounces	Fish Fillet, Light Recipe, frozen, Gorton's
−1.0	1/2 piece	Burger King Bacon Double Cheeseburger
−1.0	1 piece	Taco Bell Taco
−1.0	1 piece	Kentucky Fried Chicken
−1.0	1 piece	Kentucky Fried Chicken, Side Breast, Extra Crispy
−1.0	1/2 piece	Jack in the Box Double Cheeseburger
−1.0	1/2 portion	Chicken, Fried, Homestyle, frozen, Swanson
−1.0	1 piece	Sole Fillet, Light, Mrs. Paul's
−1.0	3 pieces	Bacon, fried
−1.5	1/2 piece	Dairy Queen Hot Dog w/Cheese
−1.5	1/2 piece	Roy Rogers Hamburger
−1.5	1/4 piece	Carl's Jr. Double Western Bacon Cheeseburger
−1.5	3 ounces	Sausage, Italian, 1 link
−1.5	2 ounces	Spam
−1.5	1 piece	Kentucky Fried Chicken, Side Breast
−1.5	1 cup	Soup, Chicken Noodle, Campbell's
−1.5	3 ounces	Kielbasa
−1.5	3 pieces	Pork spareribs
−1.5	1 serving	McDonald's Chicken McNuggets
−1.5	8 ounces	Soup, Oyster Stew, w/Milk, Campbell's
−1.5	1/2 piece	Roy Rogers Chicken Breast and Wing
−1.5	1/2 piece	Carl's Jr. Super Star Hamburger
−1.5	1 cup	Soup, chicken rice
−1.5	1 piece	Kentucky Fried Chicken, Drumstick, Extra Crispy
−1.5	1/2 piece	Taco Bell Taco Bellgrande
−1.5	3 pieces	Bacon, Low-Sodium, No Sugar, Bryan

MEAT/FISH/POULTRY GROUP

Nutripoints	Serving Size	Food Name
−1.5	1/2 pie	Beef Pot Pie, frozen, Swanson
−1.5	4 pieces	Wendy's Crispy Chicken Nuggets (fried in vegetable oil)
−1.5	3 ounces	Chicken, Smoked, Sliced, Buddig
−1.5	2 ounces	Luncheon meat, beef
−1.5	1 tablespoon	McDonald's Bacon Bits
−1.5	1/2 piece	Veal parmigiana
−1.5	1/2 portion	Beef Stroganoff, w/Parsley Noodles, frozen, Stouffer's
−1.5	2 pieces	Luncheon meat, head cheese
−1.5	1/2 piece	Roy Rogers Bar Burger
−1.5	1/2 piece	Jack in the Box Jumbo Jack w/Cheese
−1.5	1/2 piece	Jack in the Box Chicken Supreme
−1.5	1/2 piece	Dairy Queen Hounder w/Chili
−1.5	1/2 piece	Taco Bell Taco Light
−1.5	3 3/4 ounces	Fish Sticks, Crispy Crunchy, Mrs. Paul's
−1.5	1 portion	Fish amondine, frozen dinner
−1.5	1/2 piece	Roy Rogers Chicken Thigh and Leg
−1.5	1 cup	Carl's Jr. Boston Clam Chowder Soup
−1.5	2 ounces	Bologna, turkey
−1.5	1/2 piece	McDonald's Biscuit w/Sausage
−1.5	1 cup	Soup, Cream of Chicken, 1/3 Less Salt, Campbell's
−1.5	1 piece	Kentucky Fried Chicken, Drumstick
−1.5	1/2 piece	Roy Rogers Bacon Cheeseburger
−1.5	3 ounces	Halibut, smoked
−1.5	1 piece	Fish Fillet, Crispy Crunchy, frozen, Mrs. Paul's
−1.5	6 ounces	Squid, boiled
−2.0	3 pieces	Salami, Turkey Cotto, Louis Rich
−2.0	1/4 piece	Jack in the Box Ultimate Cheeseburger
−2.0	1/2 piece	Roy Rogers Cheeseburger
−2.0	2 pieces	Salami, Cotto, Oscar Mayer
−2.0	3 pieces	Bacon, Bryan
−2.0	4 pieces	Wendy's Crispy Chicken Nuggets (fried in animal oil)
−2.0	2 ounces	Knockwurst
−2.0	2 pieces	Frog legs, fried

MEAT/FISH/POULTRY GROUP

Nutripoints	Serving Size	Food Name
−2.0	½ dinner	Chicken Breast Portions, Fried, frozen, Swanson
−2.0	½ piece	Roy Rogers Chicken Thigh
−2.0	½ portion	Chicken and Egg Noodles, w/Broccoli, frozen, Budget Gourmet
−2.0	2 ounces	Beef sirloin steak, broiled
−2.0	3 ounces	Corned Beef, Smoked, Sliced, Buddig
−2.0	4 ounces	Pastrami, Land O' Frost
−2.0	½ portion	Chicken, Southern Fried Patty, frozen, Weight Watchers
−2.0	3 pieces	Bacon, Oscar Mayer
−2.0	1 piece	Roy Rogers Chicken Wing
−2.0	⅓ piece	Wendy's Chicken-fried Steak
−2.0	½ piece	Dairy Queen Hounder w/Cheese
−2.0	3 ounces	Corned Beef, Libby's
−2.0	1 piece	Kentucky Fried Chicken, Thigh, Extra Crispy
−2.0	3 ounces	Beef, smoked, sliced, Buddig
−2.0	½ piece	Dairy Queen Hounder
−2.0	1 piece	Kentucky Fried Chicken, Wing, Extra Crispy
−2.0	1 cup	Soup, Cream of Chicken, Campbell's
−2.0	4 ounces	Beef, Land O' Frost
−2.0	4 ounces	Ham, Turkey, Mr. Turkey
−2.0	2 pieces	Luncheon Meat, Olive Loaf, Oscar Mayer
−2.0	4 ounces	Sole Fillet, Fishmarket Fresh, frozen, Gorton's
−2.5	1 cup	Soup Mix, Chicken Noodle, w/Chicken Meat, Lipton
−2.5	1 cup	Soup Mix, Chicken Rice, Lipton
−2.5	4 pieces	Salami, Hard (Genoa), Oscar Mayer
−2.5	4 ounces	Scrod, Baked, Stuffed, frozen, Gorton's
−2.5	3 pieces	Bacon, West Virginia Brand, Hygrade's
−2.5	½ piece	Jack in the Box Swiss and Bacon Burger
−2.5	2 pieces	Bologna, Turkey, Louis Rich
−2.5	⅓ portion	Meatballs, Swedish, w/Noodles, frozen, Budget Gourmet
−2.5	1 piece	Carl's Jr. Sausage, 1 patty
−2.5	1 piece	Kentucky Fried Chicken, Chicken Wing
−2.5	1 piece	Frankfurter, beef

MEAT/FISH/POULTRY GROUP

Nutripoints	Serving Size	Food Name
−2.5	1 piece	Kentucky Fried Chicken, Thigh
−2.5	1 piece	McDonald's Shrimp Salad
−2.5	½ portion	Beef Salisbury Steak, Homestyle, frozen, Swanson
−2.5	2 pieces	Bologna, Bryan
−2.5	2 pieces	Sausage link, pork
−2.5	3 pieces	Beef, Breakfast Strip, Lean n'Tasty, Oscar Mayer
−2.5	2 ounces	Beef prime rib, baked
−2.5	2 ounces	Pastrami, beef
−2.5	3 pieces	Bacon, Sliced, Farmland
−2.5	5½ ounces	Enchiladas, Beef, Shredded, Van de Kamp's
−2.5	½ piece	Jack in the Box Breakfast Jack
−2.5	2 pieces	Bologna, Beef, Bryan
−2.5	½ piece	Jack in the Box Supreme Crescent Breakfast
−2.5	2 ounces	Luncheon Meat, Olive Loaf, Eckrich
−2.5	½ piece	Beef, barbecue, sandwich, w/bun
−2.5	1 piece	Frankfurter, Bryan
−2.5	3 ounces	Corned beef
−2.5	7 pieces	Jack in the Box Shrimp (10 pieces)
−3.0	1 piece	Frankfurter, Beef, Original Brown 'n Serve, Swift
−3.0	1 piece	Wendy's Sausage Patty
−3.0	2 ounces	Sausage, Little, Jones
−3.0	½ piece	Jack in the Box Sausage Crescent Breakfast
−3.0	1 piece	Frankfurter, Oscar Mayer
−3.0	2 ounces	Sandwich, Steak, frozen, Steak-Umm
−3.0	1 piece	Frankfurter, w/Cheese, Oscar Mayer
−3.0	2 ounces	Liverwurst, Original, Jones
−3.0	½ piece	Jack in the Box Canadian Crescent Breakfast
−3.5	1 piece	Frankfurter, Pork, Original Brown 'n Serve, Swift
−3.5	1 piece	Frankfurter, Beef, Eckrich
−3.5	1 cup	Soup, Mushroom, Beefy, Campbell's
−3.5	1 piece	Frankfurter, Beef, Oscar Mayer
−3.5	1 piece	Frankfurter, turkey

MEAT/FISH/POULTRY GROUP

Nutripoints	Serving Size	Food Name
−3.5	2 pieces	Luncheon Meat, Oscar Mayer
−3.5	2 ounces	Bologna, beef
−3.5	1 piece	McDonald's Pork Sausage
−3.5	2 ounces	Sausage, Pork, Jimmy Dean
−3.5	2 ounces	Ham, Deviled, Underwood
−3.5	2 pieces	Bologna, Oscar Mayer
−3.5	1 piece	Frankfurter, Eckrich
−3.5	2 pieces	Bologna, Garlic, Eckrich
−3.5	2 pieces	Bologna, Beef, Oscar Mayer
−3.5	3 ounces	Crab cake
−3.5	1 piece	Frankfurter, Chicken, Tyson
−3.5	3 ounces	Ham, Land O' Frost
−3.5	1 piece	Frankfurter, pork and beef
−3.5	3 pieces	Bacon, Premium Sizzlean, Swift
−3.5	3 pieces	Sausage, Vienna
−3.5	2 ounces	Pâté
−4.0	3 ounces	Shrimp, Fried, frozen, Mrs. Paul's
−4.0	1 piece	Frankfurter, Ball Park
−4.0	2 pieces	Bologna, Eckrich
−4.0	½ serving	McDonald's Sausage McMuffin w/Egg
−4.0	2 ounces	Salami, Cooked, Armour
−4.0	2 ounces	Frankfurter, Beef, Ball Park
−4.0	1 piece	Frankfurter, Beef, Armour
−4.0	1 ounce	Salami, Cotto Beef, Eckrich
−4.0	1 ounce	Salt pork, raw
−4.0	2 pieces	Bologna, Beef, Armour
−4.5	½ serving	McDonald's Biscuit w/Sausage and Egg
−4.5	2 ounces	Treet
−5.0	3 ounces	Chicken, Land O' Frost
−5.0	1 ounce	Pepperoni
−6.0	1 ounce	Pepperoni, Gallo
−52.0	3 ounces	Sweetbreads

OTHER GROUPS

FAT/OIL GROUP

Nutripoints	Serving Size	Food Name
8.0	1/4 cup	Dressing, Lite, Blue Cheese, Nutripoint
7.5	1/4 cup	Dip, Guacamole, Slim, Nutripoint
3.5	1/4 cup	Dressing, Lite, Ranch, Nutripoint
2.5	1/4 cup	Dressing, Lite, 16 Island, Nutripoint
2.5	2 tablespoons	Dressing, Vinaigrette, Orange, Nutripoint
2.0	2 tablespoons	Dressing, Caper, Nutripoint
1.5	1/4 cup	Sauce mix, Stroganoff, prepared w/milk and water
1.5	1/4 cup	Mayo Mix, Lite, Nutripoint
1.0	1/4 cup	Sauce mix, mushroom, prepared w/milk
1.0	1/4 cup	Gravy, beef, canned
0.0	1/4 cup	Gravy mix, chicken, prepared w/milk
0.0	1/4 cup	Sauce mix, curry, w/milk
0.0	1/4 cup	Sauce mix, sweet and sour, prepared
0.0	2 tablespoons	Mayonnaise, Light, Kraft
0.0	1/4 cup	Gravy, mushroom, canned
0.0	1/4 cup	Gravy, turkey, canned
−0.5	1 tablespoon	Sauce, Tartar, Sauce Works, Kraft
−0.5	2 tablespoons	Dip, clam
−0.5	1/4 cup	Gravy mix, turkey, prepared w/milk
−0.5	1/4 cup	Gravy mix, mushroom, prepared w/milk
−0.5	2 tablespoons	Dressing, Russian, low-cal.
−1.0	1/4 cup	Sauce, white
−1.0	2 tablespoons	Dressing, salad, low-cal.
−1.0	1 tablespoon	Margarine, low-cal.
−1.5	2 tablespoons	Dressing, low-cal., French

FAT/OIL GROUP

Nutripoints	Serving Size	Food Name
−1.5	1/4 cup	Gravy, chicken, canned
−1.5	2 tablespoons	Dressing, Vinaigrette, Lite, Nutripoint
−1.5	1/4 cup	Kentucky Fried Chicken, Gravy
−2.0	1/4 cup	Gravy mix, pork, prepared w/milk
−2.0	4 tablespoons	Margarine, Sweet Unsalted, Heart Beat
−2.0	2 tablespoons	Margarine, Reduced Calorie, Unsalted, Weight Watchers
−2.0	1 tablespoon	Margarine, Promise
−2.0	1 tablespoon	Margarine, Family Spread, Mrs. Filbert's
−2.0	1 tablespoon	Dressing, French, Catalina, Kraft
−2.5	1 tablespoon	Margarine, Safflower, Hain
−2.5	2 tablespoons	Margarine, Extra Light, Promise
−2.5	2 tablespoons	Dressing, Thousand Island, low-cal.
−2.5	1 tablespoon	Dressing, French, Kraft
−2.5	1 tablespoon	Margarine, Reduced Calorie, Spread, Blue Bonnet
−2.5	2 tablespoons	Dressing, Russian
−2.5	1 tablespoon	Margarine, Unsalted, Mazola
−2.5	2 tablespoons	Margarine, Corn Oil Spread, Light, Mazola
−2.5	2 tablespoons	Margarine, Diet, Imitation, Mazola
−2.5	2 tablespoons	Margarine, Diet, Soft, Parkay
−2.5	2 tablespoons	Margarine, Soft Spread, Touch of Butter, Kraft
−2.5	2 tablespoons	Margarine, Reduced Calorie, Weight Watchers
−2.5	1 tablespoon	Margarine, hard, coconut, safflower and palm
−2.5	1 tablespoon	Mayonnaise, Cholesterol Free, Kraft
−2.5	1 tablespoon	Oil, hazelnut
−2.5	2 tablespoons	Margarine, Diet, Fleischmann's
−2.5	1 tablespoon	Dressing, mayonnaise
−2.5	1 tablespoon	Oil, almond
−2.5	1 tablespoon	Oil, Canola, Puritan
−2.5	1 tablespoon	Margarine, Stick, Unsalted, Fleischmann's
−2.5	2 tablespoons	Margarine, Reduced Calorie, Diet, Mazola
−2.5	1 tablespoon	Oil, walnut
−2.5	2 tablespoons	McDonald's French Dressing
−2.5	1 tablespoon	Margarine, Parkay
−2.5	1 tablespoon	Oil, safflower

FAT/OIL GROUP

Nutripoints	Serving Size	Food Name
−2.5	1/4 cup	Sauce mix, teriyaki, prepared w/milk
−2.5	1 tablespoon	Oil, linseed
−2.5	1 tablespoon	Margarine, Whipped Spread, Parkay
−2.5	1 tablespoon	Margarine, Squeeze, Parkay
−2.5	1 tablespoon	Margarine, Cookery, Parkay
−2.5	1 tablespoon	Margarine, corn oil
−2.5	2 tablespoons	Mayonnaise, low-cal.
−2.5	1 tablespoon	Mayonnaise, Cholesterol Free, Miracle Whip
−2.5	1 tablespoon	Margarine, Mazola
−2.5	1 tablespoon	Oil, sunflower
−2.5	1 tablespoon	Margarine, Soft, Corn Oil, Mrs. Filbert's
−2.5	1 tablespoon	Margarine, Stick, Land O Lakes
−2.5	1/4 cup	Gravy mix, turkey, prepared w/milk and butter
−2.5	1/4 cup	Gravy
−2.5	1/4 cup	Gravy mix, chicken, prepared w/milk and butter
−2.5	2 tablespoons	Margarine, Whipped, Imperial
−2.5	2 tablespoons	Dressing, Italian
−2.5	1 tablespoon	Mayonnaise, Light, Reduced Calorie, Kraft
−2.5	1 tablespoon	Margarine, I Can't Believe It's Not Butter!
−2.5	1 tablespoon	Oil, Sunlite
−2.5	1 tablespoon	Oil, Puritan
−2.5	1 tablespoon	Oil, Safflower, Hollywood
−2.5	1 tablespoon	Mayonnaise
−3.0	1 tablespoon	Margarine, Stick, Fleischmann's
−3.0	1 tablespoon	Margarine, Stick, Blue Bonnet
−3.0	1 tablespoon	Margarine, Soft, Blue Bonnet
−3.0	2 tablespoons	Dressing, Thousand Island
−3.0	1 tablespoon	Margarine, Stick, Imperial
−3.0	1 tablespoon	Oil, soybean
−3.0	4 tablespoons	Margarine, Heart Beat
−3.0	2 tablespoons	Mayonnaise, Light, Reduced Calorie, Hellman's
−3.0	1 tablespoon	Margarine, County Crock Spread, Shedd's
−3.0	1 tablespoon	Margarine
−3.0	1 tablespoon	Oil, olive
−3.0	2 tablespoons	Dressing, Green Goddess

FAT/OIL GROUP

Nutripoints	Serving Size	Food Name
−3.0	1 tablespoon	Oil, Corn, Mazola
−3.0	1 tablespoon	Margarine, liquid, soybean and cottonseed
−3.0	1 tablespoon	Oil, sesame
−3.0	1 tablespoon	Oil, Olive, Bertolli
−3.0	1 tablespoon	Margarine, Soft, Chiffon
−3.0	1 tablespoon	Oil, Corn, Crisco
−3.0	1 tablespoon	Oil, Crisco
−3.0	1 tablespoon	Mayonnaise, imitation, soybean
−3.0	1 tablespoon	Margarine, Soft, Imperial
−3.0	2 tablespoons	McDonald's 1,000 Island Dressing
−3.0	1 tablespoon	Oil, Wesson
−3.0	1 tablespoon	Oil, peanut
−3.0	2 tablespoons	Mayonnaise, Light, Miracle Whip
−3.0	2 tablespoons	McDonald's Ranch Dressing
−3.0	1 tablespoon	Dressing, Salad, Miracle Whip, Kraft
−3.0	1 tablespoon	Dressing, oil and vinegar
−3.0	2 tablespoons	Dressing, French
−3.0	1 tablespoon	Dressing, French, home recipe
−3.0	1 tablespoon	Jack in the Box Bleu Cheese Dressing
−3.0	1 tablespoon	Crisco, Butter Flavored
−3.0	1 tablespoon	Mayonnaise, Real, Best Foods
−3.0	1 tablespoon	Mayonnaise, Blue Plate
−3.0	1 tablespoon	Oil, wheat germ
−3.0	1 tablespoon	Jack in the Box Buttermilk House Dressing
−3.0	2 tablespoons	Dressing, blue cheese
−3.0	3 ounces	Wendy's Sausage Gravy
−3.0	1 tablespoon	Oil
−3.5	2 tablespoons	Dressing, ranch/buttermilk
−3.5	1 tablespoon	Jack in the Box Thousand Island Dressing
−3.5	1 tablespoon	McDonald's Bleu Cheese Dressing
−3.5	1 tablespoon	Dressing, Oil and Vinegar, Kraft
−3.5	1 tablespoon	Shortening, Crisco
−3.5	1 tablespoon	Shortening, soybean and cottonseed
−3.5	2 tablespoons	Taco Bell Sour Cream
−3.5	2 tablespoons	Sauce, tartar
−3.5	1 tablespoon	Mayonnaise, Real, Kraft
−3.5	1 tablespoon	Mayonnaise, Real, Hellman's
−3.5	2 ounces	Wendy's Imitation Sour Topping

FAT/OIL GROUP

Nutripoints	Serving Size	Food Name
−3.5	1 tablespoon	Mayonnaise, imitation, milk cream
−3.5	1 tablespoon	Oil, cottonseed
−3.5	1 tablespoon	Dressing, Salad, Reduced-Calorie, Miracle Whip
−3.5	1/4 cup	Gravy, Mushroom, Franco-American
−3.5	2 tablespoons	Dressing, salad
−4.0	1 tablespoon	Taco Bell Ranch Dressing
−4.0	1 tablespoon	Shortening, soybean and palm
−4.0	1/4 cup	Gravy Mix, Brown, French's
−4.0	1 tablespoon	Margarine, Soft, Low-Sodium, Country Morning Blend, Land O Lakes
−4.0	1/4 cup	Gravy, Chicken, Franco-American
−4.0	1/4 cup	Gravy Mix, Mushroom, French's
−4.0	1 tablespoon	Fat, goose
−4.5	1 tablespoon	Fat, chicken
−4.5	2 tablespoons	Jack in the Box Reduced-Calorie French Dressing
−4.5	1 tablespoon	Fat, turkey
−4.5	1 tablespoon	Fat, duck
−4.5	1/4 cup	Gravy Mix, Chicken, McCormick's
−4.5	2 tablespoons	Dressing, low-cal., blue cheese
−4.5	1 tablespoon	Shortening, lard and vegetable oil
−5.0	1 tablespoon	Oil, palm
−5.0	1 tablespoon	Lard
−5.0	1 tablespoon	Dip, onion
−5.0	1/4 cup	Sauce, Hollandaise
−5.5	1/4 cup	Sauce mix, Béarnaise, w/milk and butter
−5.5	1 tablespoon	Fat, mutton tallow
−5.5	1 tablespoon	Oil, cocoa butter
−6.0	1 tablespoon	Wendy's Creamy Peppercorn Dressing
−6.5	1 tablespoon	Fat, beef tallow
−6.5	1 tablespoon	Butter, unsalted
−6.5	1 tablespoon	Butter, Sweet, Cream, Unsalted, Land O Lakes
−6.5	1 tablespoon	Oil, palm kernel
−7.0	1 tablespoon	Butter, Sweet, Lite Salt, Land O Lakes
−7.0	1 tablespoon	Oil, coconut
−7.5	1 tablespoon	Butter, salted

SUGAR GROUP

Nutripoints	Serving Size	Food Name
3.5	2 tablespoons	Molasses, blackstrap
3.0	6 fluid ounces	*Fruit Drink, Tang
−1.0	4 tablespoons	Jelly, low-cal., all flavors
−1.0	6 pieces	Gingersnaps
−2.0	1 ounce	Halvah, plain
−2.0	1 ounce	Candy bar, diet
−2.0	1 ounce	Candy, M&M's Peanut
−2.0	1 piece	Candy Bar, Kit Kat
−2.0	½ piece	Candy Bar, Baby Ruth
−2.5	½ piece	Pie, chocolate cream
−2.5	1 piece	Fudge, peanut butter
−2.5	1 piece	Candy Bar, Butterfinger
−3.0	1 piece	Candy, Peanut Butter Cups, Reese's
−3.0	2 tablespoons	Molasses
−3.0	1 ounce	Chocolate, Unsweetened, Baker's
−3.0	1 piece	Candy, pralines
−3.0	1 piece	Cake, Choco-Bake, Nestlé
−3.0	½ piece	Candy Bar, Snickers
−3.0	½ piece	Candy Bar, Mr. Goodbar
−3.0	10 pieces	Gum
−3.5	1 piece	Candy, Milk Chocolate w/Almonds, Hershey's
−3.5	½ piece	Candy Bar, Mars Bar
−3.5	1 piece	Fudge, divinity
−3.5	6 pieces	Candy, Kisses, Hershey's
−3.5	1 piece	Fudge, chocolate, w/nuts
−3.5	1 piece	Fudge, vanilla, w/nuts
−3.5	2 tablespoons	Jelly, all flavors
−3.5	2 teaspoons	Syrup, sorghum
−3.5	3 pieces	Candy, caramels
−3.5	2 tablespoons	Sauce, chocolate fudge
−4.0	2 pieces	Candy Bar, Twix Caramel
−4.0	1 ounce	Candy, Brach Toffees
−4.0	1 piece	Candy Bar, Chocolit
−4.0	2 tablespoons	Syrup, maple, low-cal.
−4.0	½ piece	Candy Bar, 3 Musketeers

*Fortified

SUGAR GROUP

Nutripoints	Serving Size	Food Name
−4.0	1 piece	Candy Bar, $100,000
−4.0	1 piece	Fudge, vanilla
−4.0	½ piece	Candy Bar, Milky Way
−4.0	1 ounce	Candy, Brach Royals
−4.0	1 piece	Frozen Dessert, Creamsicle
−4.0	1 ounce	Chocolate, baking
−4.0	8 fluid ounces	Drink Mix, Rainbow Punch, Sweetened, Kool-Aid
−4.5	1½ ounces	Candy Bar, Nestle Crunch
−4.5	3 tablespoons	Sugar, powdered
−4.5	1 ounce	Chocolate, Semi-Sweet, Baker's
−4.5	1 ounce	Candy, Semi-Sweet Morsels, Nestle
−4.5	10 pieces	Gum, Doublemint, Wrigley's
−4.5	2 tablespoons	Sauce, butterscotch
−4.5	5 pieces	Candy, Rolo
−4.5	2 tablespoons	Frosting
−4.5	½ piece	Pie, chiffon
−4.5	1 ounce	Chocolate, sweet or dark
−4.5	1 ounce	Candy, M&M's Chocolate
−4.5	1 ounce	Chocolate, semi-sweet
−4.5	2 tablespoons	Frosting, chocolate
−5.0	2 teaspoons	Syrup, cane
−5.0	2 tablespoons	Syrup, maple
−5.0	2 tablespoons	Marmalade
−5.0	8 fluid ounces	Drink mix, Strawberry, Sweetened, Kool-Aid
−5.0	2 tablespoons	Sugar, brown
−5.0	2 tablespoons	Syrup, corn
−5.0	2 tablespoons	Sauce, chocolate
−5.0	2 pieces	Frozen Dessert, Popsicle
−5.0	2 tablespoons	Sauce, Butterscotch, Smucker's
−5.0	2 tablespoons	Sugar, raw
−5.0	12 fluid ounces	Soft drink, ginger ale
−5.0	12 fluid ounces	Soft drink, w/o caffeine
−5.5	2 tablespoons	Sugar, cinnamon
−5.5	1 ounce	Fudge, chocolate
−5.5	½ cup	Mousse, chocolate
−5.5	12 fluid ounces	Soft drink, lemon-lime, w/o caffeine

SUGAR GROUP

Nutripoints	Serving Size	Food Name
−5.5	4 pieces	Marshmallows, Jet-Puffed, Kraft
−5.5	1 cup	Dairy Queen Mr. Misty Kiss (1/2 cup)
−5.5	2 tablespoons	Honey
−5.5	28 pieces	Candy, gum drop, small
−5.5	2 tablespoons	Topping, marshmallow cream
−5.5	12 fluid ounces	Tonic water, sweetened
−5.5	12 fluid ounces	Soft Drink, 7-Up
−5.5	12 fluid ounces	Soft drink, cream soda
−5.5	12 fluid ounces	Soft Drink, Dr Pepper
−5.5	1/2 cup	Dairy Queen Mr. Misty, medium (1 cup)
−5.5	8 fluid ounces	Quinine water
−5.5	15 pieces	Jelly beans
−5.5	3 tablespoons	Sugar, maple
−5.5	4 pieces	Candy, marshmallow
−5.5	1 ounce	Candy, taffy, plain
−5.5	4 tablespoons	Sugar, white confectioner's
−6.0	5 pieces	Gum, Bubble, Original, Hubba Bubba
−6.0	1 ounce	Candy, chocolate chips
−6.0	10 pieces	Candy, Wild Cherry, Life Savers
−6.0	10 pieces	Candy, Spear O Mint, Life Savers
−6.0	2 teaspoons	Syrup, butter blends
−6.0	2 tablespoons	Sugar, white
−6.0	1 ounce	Candy, hard
−6.0	12 fluid ounces	Soft drink, Coke w/caffeine
−6.0	12 fluid ounces	Root beer
−6.5	8 fluid ounces	Iced Tea Mix, Sugar and Lemonade Flavor, Nestea
−6.5	12 fluid ounces	Soft Drink, Mountain Dew
−7.0	12 fluid ounces	Soft drink, w/caffeine
−7.5	8 fluid ounces	Tea Mix, Iced, Lipton
−8.0	2 cups	Gatorade

ALCOHOL GROUP

Nutripoints	Serving Size	Food Name
5.0	12 fluid ounces	Beer, Alcohol-Free, Clark's
4.0	12 fluid ounces	Beer, near
1.0	12 fluid ounces	Beer, nonalcoholic
−5.5	12 fluid ounces	Beer, light
−7.5	3 fluid ounces	Piña colada
−8.0	12 fluid ounces	Beer
−8.5	1½ fluid ounces	Cordials/liqueurs
−8.5	2 fluid ounces	Grasshopper
−9.0	8 fluid ounces	Wine cooler
−9.0	8 fluid ounces	Screwdriver
−9.5	2 fluid ounces	Gold Cadillac
−10.0	6 fluid ounces	Tequila sunrise
−10.5	6 fluid ounces	Rum and carbonated beverage
−11.0	6 fluid ounces	Bloody Mary
−11.0	8 fluid ounces	Gin and tonic
−11.5	2 fluid ounces	Mai tai
−12.0	3 fluid ounces	Alexander
−12.5	2 fluid ounces	Stinger
−12.5	3 fluid ounces	Rum, hot buttered
−13.0	2 fluid ounces	Black Russian
−13.0	4 fluid ounces	Wine, sweet
−13.0	2 fluid ounces	White Russian
−13.0	2 fluid ounces	Bacardi
−13.5	6 fluid ounces	Singapore sling
−13.5	6 fluid ounces	Champagne
−13.5	3 fluid ounces	Manhattan
−13.5	3 fluid ounces	Margarita
−14.0	6 fluid ounces	Wine, table
−14.0	8 fluid ounces	Tom Collins
−14.0	6 fluid ounces	Wine, light
−14.5	6 fluid ounces	Wine spritzer
−14.5	3 fluid ounces	Daiquiri
−14.5	6 fluid ounces	Wine, Chinese
−14.5	8 fluid ounces	Sloe gin fizz
−15.0	2 fluid ounces	Mint julep
−15.5	2 fluid ounces	Old fashioned
−15.5	6 fluid ounces	Gin rickey
−15.5	3 fluid ounces	Martini

ALCOHOL GROUP

Nutripoints	Serving Size	Food Name
−16.5	2 fluid ounces	Whiskey
−16.5	2 fluid ounces	Vodka
−16.5	2 fluid ounces	Rum
−17.0	6 fluid ounces	Bourbon or scotch w/soda
−17.0	2 fluid ounces	Alcohol, 68 proof
−17.0	3 fluid ounces	Brandy
−17.5	2 fluid ounces	Gin
−19.0	3 fluid ounces	Whiskey sour

CONDIMENT GROUP

Nutripoints	Serving Size	Food Name
4.0	1/4 cup	Sauce, picante
3.5	1 cup	Soup, Chicken Broth, Low-Sodium, Campbell's
3.0	2 ounces	Wendy's Picante Sauce
2.5	1 tablespoon	Peppers, green, hot chili
2.5	1/4 lemon	Lemon
2.5	1 teaspoon	Paprika
2.0	1 teaspoon	Taco Bell Salsa
2.0	1 teaspoon	Chili powder
1.5	1 tablespoon	Sauce, steak
1.5	1 teaspoon	Pepper, cayenne/red
1.0	2 tablespoons	Taco Bell Pico De Gallo
1.0	2 stalks	Onion, green
1.0	1 tablespoon	Chives, raw
1.0	2 tablespoons	Dressing, Lite, Zero, Nutripoint
1.0	1 teaspoon	Sauce, Worcestershire
1.0	1 teaspoon	Cinnamon
1.0	1 teaspoon	Oregano
1.0	1 tablespoon	Juice, Lemon, ReaLemon
1.0	1 tablespoon	Sauce, chili
1.0	1/4 cup	Endive, raw
1.0	1 tablespoon	Juice, lemon
1.0	1/4 lime	Lime

CONDIMENT GROUP

Nutripoints	Serving Size	Food Name
0.5	1 teaspoon	Marjoram
0.5	1 teaspoon	Celery seed
0.5	1 teaspoon	Basil
0.5	1 teaspoon	Seasoning, poultry
0.5	1 teaspoon	Turmeric
0.5	1 teaspoon	Garlic powder
0.5	1 teaspoon	Thyme
0.5	1 teaspoon	Curry powder
0.5	2 tablespoons	Ketchup, Low-Sodium, Heinz
0.5	1 teaspoon	Poppy seed
0.5	1 teaspoon	Ginger
0.5	1 teaspoon	Chili Seasoning Mix, McCormick's
0.5	1 teaspoon	Dill weed
0.5	1 teaspoon	Mayonnaise, Reduced Calorie, Light n'Lively
0.5	1 teaspoon	Bouillon, Chicken, Low-Sodium, Lite-Line, Borden
0.5	1 teaspoon	Pepper, black
0.5	1 teaspoon	Caraway seed
0.5	1 teaspoon	Sage
0.5	1 tablespoon	Juice, lime
0.5	1 teaspoon	Bay leaves
0.5	1 teaspoon	Cloves
0.5	1 teaspoon	Tarragon
0.5	1 teaspoon	Rosemary
0.5	1 tablespoon	Dressing, Mustard, Spicy, Nutripoint
0.5	1 pepper	Pepper, jalapeño
0.5	1 teaspoon	Parsley, dried
0.5	1 teaspoon	Mustard, dry
0.5	1 teaspoon	Onion powder
0.5	1 teaspoon	Allspice, ground
0.5	1 piece	Garlic, raw
0.5	1/4 cup	Coriander, raw
0.0	1 packet	Equal
0.0	1 tablespoon	Sauce, barbecue
0.0	1 tablespoon	McDonald's Barbeque Sauce
0.0	1 teaspoon	Taco Bell Taco Hot Sauce
0.0	2 tablespoons	Sandwich, Manwich, Original, Hunt's
0.0	1 tablespoon	Vinegar

CONDIMENT GROUP

Nutripoints	Serving Size	Food Name
0.0	1 teaspoon	Taco Bell Taco Sauce
0.0	1 cup	Broth, beef
0.0	1 teaspoon	Vanilla extract
0.0	1 tablespoon	McDonald's Oriental Dressing
0.0	1 tablespoon	McDonald's Lite Vinaigrette Dressing
0.0	1 teaspoon	Salt, Iodized, Morton
0.0	1 teaspoon	Salt
0.0	1 teaspoon	Mustard
0.0	1 teaspoon	Salt, Lite, Morton
0.0	1 cup	Broth, chicken
0.0	1 tablespoon	Horseradish
0.0	1 tablespoon	Seasoning, Shake 'n Bake Original Chicken
0.0	1 tablespoon	McDonald's Sweet and Sour Sauce
0.0	2 tablespoons	Sauce, Juniper Berry, Nutripoint
0.0	1 teaspoon	Nutmeg
0.0	1 teaspoon	Sauce, soy
−0.5	0.3 gm or 1 spray	Oil, Pam Spray
−0.5	1 tablespoon	McDonald's Hot Mustard Sauce
−0.5	1 tablespoon	Mustard, Bold 'n Spicy, French's
−0.5	1 tablespoon	Sauce, teriyaki
−0.5	1 tablespoon	Dressing, Ranch, Free, Kraft
−0.5	1 tablespoon	Mustard, Yellow, Prepared, French's
−0.5	1 teaspoon	Sauce, Soy, Kikkoman
−0.5	1 tablespoon	Mustard, w/Horseradish, French's
−0.5	1 tablespoon	Dressing, Italian, Light, Bernstein's
−0.5	1 tablespoon	Sauce, Barbecue, All-Natural Original Flavor, Hunt's
−0.5	1 tablespoon	Dressing, Italian, Free, Kraft
−0.5	2 tablespoons	Butter Mix, Imitation, Butter Buds
−1.0	1 tablespoon	Dressing, French, Free, Kraft
−1.0	1 ounce	Pickles, Sweet Butter Chips, Vlasic
−1.0	1 tablespoon	Seasoning, Shake 'N Bake for Pork
−1.0	1 tablespoon	Dressing, Ranch, Take Heart, Hidden Valley
−1.0	1 tablespoon	Sauce, Barbecue, Hickory Smoke Flavor, Open Pit
−1.0	1 tablespoon	Sauce, Heinz 57
−1.5	1 tablespoon	Sauce, Barbecue, All-Natural Hot and Zesty, Hunt's

CONDIMENT GROUP

Nutripoints	Serving Size	Food Name
−1.5	1 tablespoon	Sauce, Barbecue, w/Onion Bits, Kraft
−1.5	2 tablespoons	Taco Bell Jalapeño Peppers
−1.5	1 tablespoon	Sauce, Barbecue, Original Flavor, Open Pit
−1.5	1 tablespoon	Sauce, sweet and sour
−2.0	1 teaspoon	Bouillon, Beef, Wyler's, Borden
−2.0	1 cup	Bouillon, Chicken Flavor, Wyler's, Borden
−2.5	1 tablespoon	Sauce, Barbecue, Kraft

MISCELLANEOUS GROUP

Nutripoints	Serving Size	Food Name
5.5	6 fluid ounces	Postum
3.5	1 tablespoon	Yeast, Brewer's
2.0	1 tablespoon	Protein powder
2.0	8 fluid ounces	Drink Mix, Grape, Sugar-Free, Kool-Aid
1.5	8 fluid ounces	Drink Mix, Tropical Punch, Sugar-Free, Kool-Aid
1.0	8 fluid ounces	Drink Mix, Orange, Sugar-Free, Crystal Light
1.0	8 fluid ounces	Lemonade Mix, Sugar-Free, Country Time
1.0	8 fluid ounces	Fruit Drink Mix, Wild Grape, Sugar-Free, Wyler's, Borden
1.0	1 tablespoon	Carob powder
0.5	1 cup	Coffee, decaffeinated
0.5	1 teaspoon	Baking powder
0.5	6 fluid ounces	Tea, herb
0.5	1 cup	Consommé
0.5	1 tablespoon	Cocoa powder
0.5	1/4 ounce	Yeast, Active Dry, Fleischmann's
0.0	1 cup	Tea, decaffeinated
0.0	1 package	Yeast, active dry
0.0	1 tablespoon	Cornstarch
0.0	12 fluid ounces	Soft drink, diet, w/o caffeine
0.0	8 fluid ounces	Perrier Mineral Water
0.0	6 fluid ounces	Club soda
0.0	1 teaspoon	Baking soda
−1.0	1 piece	Bouillon cube

MISCELLANEOUS GROUP

Nutripoints	Serving Size	Food Name
−1.0	1 cup	Soup, wonton
−1.5	1 serving	Soup mix, chicken noodle, dehydrated
−1.5	2 tablespoons	Soup mix, onion, dehydrated
−2.5	8 fluid ounces	Tea Mix, Iced, Lemon, Sugar-Free, Lipton
−2.5	12 fluid ounces	Soft drink, diet, w/caffeine
−3.0	1 cup	Tea, American black
−3.0	1 tablespoon	Gravy, dehydrated
−3.5	1 cup	Coffee
−10.0	1 tablespoon	Coffee, International
−11.5	1 tablespoon	Caviar

ALPHABETICAL RATINGS

Food Name	Nutrigroup	Serving Size	Nutripoints
Abalone	Meat/Fish/Poultry	3 ounces	6.5
Abalone, Floured, Fried	Meat/Fish/Poultry	3 ounces	4.5
Alcohol, 68 proof	Alcohol	2 fluid ounces	−17.0
Alexander	Alcohol	3 fluid ounces	−12.0
Alfalfa Sprouts, Arrowhead Mills	Vegetable	1 cup	13.0
Alfalfa sprouts, raw	Vegetable	2 cups	17.5
Allspice, ground	Condiment	1 teaspoon	0.5
Almond butter, salted	Legume/Nut/Seed	1 tablespoon	0.5
Almonds, Blanched, Blue Diamond	Legume/Nut/Seed	1 ounce	0.5
Almonds, chocolate-covered	Legume/Nut/Seed	6 pieces	−1.0
Almonds, oil roasted, salted	Legume/Nut/Seed	12 pieces	0.5
Almonds, raw	Legume/Nut/Seed	18 pieces	1.5
Almonds, sugar-coated	Legume/Nut/Seed	6 pieces	−1.5
Amaranth, dry, Arrowhead Mills	Grain	1 ounce	5.0
Anchovy, canned	Meat/Fish/Poultry	3 ounces	4.0
Apple crisp	Fruit	¼ cup	−1.0
Apple, fresh	Fruit	1 apple	4.5
Apples, Dried, Chunks, Sun-Maid	Fruit	2 ounces	2.5

Food Name	Nutrigroup	Serving Size	Nutripoints
Apples, Escalloped, frozen, Stouffer's	Fruit	½ portion	−0.5
Apples, Glazed, Raspberry Sauce, frozen, Budget Gourmet	Fruit	½ piece	10.5
Applesauce, Natural Style, Mott's	Fruit	½ cup	3.0
Applesauce, no sugar	Fruit	½ cup	3.5
Applesauce, Nutripoint	Fruit	½ cup	3.0
Applesauce, Unsweetened, Musselman	Fruit	½ cup	2.0
Applesauce, w/sugar	Fruit	½ cup	−0.5
Apricot nectar, canned	Fruit	4 fluid ounces	4.5
Apricot, fresh	Fruit	3 pieces	13.5
Apricots, canned in heavy syrup	Fruit	½ cup	2.5
Apricots, canned, unsweetened	Fruit	½ cup	11.0
Apricots, dried	Fruit	6 pieces	11.0
Apricots, Dried, Del Monte	Fruit	6 pieces	7.5
Apricots, Dried, Sun-Maid	Fruit	6 pieces	8.0
Arby's Beef 'n Cheddar Sandwich	Meat/Fish/Poultry	½ piece	0.0
Arby's Junior Roast Beef Sandwich	Meat/Fish/Poultry	1 piece	0.5
Arby's King Roast Beef Sandwich	Meat/Fish/Poultry	½ piece	0.5
Arby's Regular Roast Beef Sandwich	Meat/Fish/Poultry	½ piece	0.5
Arby's Super Roast Beef Sandwich	Meat/Fish/Poultry	½ piece	1.0
Artichoke hearts, marinated	Vegetable	¼ cup	3.0
Artichoke, cooked	Vegetable	1 whole	12.5

Food Name	Nutrigroup	Serving Size	Nutripoints
Asparagus, 50-Percent Less Salt, canned, Green Giant	Vegetable	1 cup	14.5
Asparagus, canned	Vegetable	8 stalks	32.5
Asparagus, Cuts, canned, Green Giant	Vegetable	½ cup	14.0
Asparagus, fresh	Vegetable	8 stalks	44.0
Asparagus, frozen, cooked	Vegetable	8 stalks	27.0
Asparagus, Marinated, Nutripoint	Vegetable	8 stalks	38.5
Avocado, California	Fruit	¼ avocado	2.5
Avocado, Florida	Fruit	¼ avocado	4.0
Bacardi	Alcohol	2 fluid ounces	−13.0
Bacon bits, imitation	Meat/Fish/Poultry	¼ cup	1.5
Bacon, Breakfast Strip, frozen, Morningstar Farms	Meat/Fish/Poultry	3 pieces	3.5
Bacon, Bryan	Meat/Fish/Poultry	3 pieces	−2.0
Bacon, Canadian	Meat/Fish/Poultry	3 pieces	1.5
Bacon, Canadian Style, Oscar Mayer	Meat/Fish/Poultry	3 pieces	4.5
Bacon, fried	Meat/Fish/Poultry	3 pieces	−1.0
Bacon, Low-Sodium, No Sugar, Bryan	Meat/Fish/Poultry	3 pieces	−1.5
Bacon, Low-Salt, Oscar Mayer	Meat/Fish/Poultry	3 pieces	−1.0
Bacon, Oscar Mayer	Meat/Fish/Poultry	3 pieces	−2.0
Bacon, Premium Sizzlean, Swift	Meat/Fish/Poultry	3 pieces	−3.5
Bacon, Sliced, Farmland	Meat/Fish/Poultry	3 pieces	−2.5
Bacon, West Virginia Brand, Hygrade's	Meat/Fish/Poultry	3 pieces	−2.5
Bagel	Grain	1 whole	2.0
Bagel, plain, Lender's	Grain	1 whole	2.0
Bagel, pumpernickel	Grain	1 whole	3.5
Bagel, Raisin 'n Honey, Lender's	Grain	1 whole	2.0

Food Name	Nutrigroup	Serving Size		Nutripoints
Bagel, whole wheat	Grain	1	whole	4.0
Baking powder	Miscellaneous	1	teaspoon	0.5
Baking soda	Miscellaneous	1	teaspoon	0.0
Bamboo shoots, canned	Vegetable	1	cup	16.5
Bamboo shoots, raw	Vegetable	½	cup	17.0
Banana	Fruit	½	piece	7.5
Banana Flambé, Nutripoint	Milk/Dairy	⅓	cup	2.5
Banana Gladje, Nutripoint	Fruit	⅓	cup	6.0
Banana split	Fruit	¼	serving	−1.5
Barley, uncooked	Grain	¼	cup	4.0
Barracuda, baked/broiled	Meat/Fish/Poultry	3	ounces	1.5
Barracuda, breaded/floured, fried	Meat/Fish/Poultry	3	ounces	1.0
Basil	Condiment	1	teaspoon	0.5
Bass, freshwater, baked	Meat/Fish/Poultry	6	ounces	7.0
Bay leaves	Condiment	1	teaspoon	0.5
Bean Sprouts, Mung, Arrowhead Mills	Legume/Nut/Seed	2	cups	10.5
Bean sprouts, mung, fresh	Legume/Nut/Seed	2	cups	18.0
Beans, Adzuki, Dry, Arrowhead Mills	Legume/Nut/Seed	1	ounce	5.5
Beans, Baked, Barbecue, B&M	Legume/Nut/Seed	½	cup	0.5
Beans, baked, w/tomato sauce	Legume/Nut/Seed	½	cup	7.5
Beans, Boston baked	Legume/Nut/Seed	½	cup	3.5
Beans, Chili, Loma Linda	Legume/Nut/Seed	½	cup	3.0
Beans, cooked	Legume/Nut/Seed	¾	cup	8.5
Beans, garbanzo, cooked	Legume/Nut/Seed	½	cup	8.0

Food Name	Nutrigroup	Serving Size	Nutripoints
Beans, Green Cut, No Salt Added, canned, Del Monte	Vegetable	1 cup	13.5
Beans, Green, 50-Percent Less Salt, canned, Green Giant	Vegetable	1 cup	8.0
Beans, green, cooked	Vegetable	1 cup	24.5
Beans, Green, Cut, frozen, Birds Eye	Vegetable	1 cup	15.5
Beans, Green, French Cut, in Butter, Green Giant	Vegetable	½ cup	3.0
Beans, Green, French Style Cut, canned, Green Giant	Vegetable	1 cup	3.5
Beans, Green, Kitchen Cut, canned, Green Giant	Vegetable	1 cup	4.5
Beans, Green, Whole, canned, Del Monte	Vegetable	1 cup	13.0
Beans, Home Style, Campbell's	Legume/Nut/Seed	½ cup	1.0
Beans, Kidney, Best Light, canned, Bush's	Legume/Nut/Seed	½ cup	4.0
Beans, kidney, cooked	Legume/Nut/Seed	½ cup	8.5
Beans, Lima, Baby, w/Butter, frozen, Green Giant	Legume/Nut/Seed	½ cup	2.0
Beans, lima, cooked	Legume/Nut/Seed	¾ cup	9.5
Beans, navy, cooked	Legume/Nut/Seed	1 cup	13.5
Beans, pinto, cooked	Legume/Nut/Seed	½ cup	6.5
Beans, refried	Legume/Nut/Seed	½ cup	2.0
Beans, Refried, Old El Paso	Legume/Nut/Seed	1 cup	3.5

Food Name	Nutrigroup	Serving Size	Nutripoints
Beans, Refried, w/Sausage, Old El Paso	Legume/Nut/Seed	1/2 cup	−1.0
Beans, Vegetarian Style, Van Camp's	Legume/Nut/Seed	1/2 cup	2.5
Beans, w/Frankfurters Dinner, frozen, Morton	Legume/Nut/Seed	1/2 portion	2.0
Beans, w/pork	Legume/Nut/Seed	1/2 cup	3.0
Beans, w/Pork in Tomato Sauce, Campbell's	Legume/Nut/Seed	1/2 cup	1.5
Beans, w/Pork, Showboat, Bush's	Legume/Nut/Seed	1/2 cup	1.5
Beans, w/Pork, Van Camp's	Legume/Nut/Seed	1/2 cup	2.0
Beans, yellow snap, cooked	Vegetable	1/2 cup	13.5
Beef brisket, lean, braised	Meat/Fish/Poultry	3 ounces	2.0
Beef chuck roast, lean, braised	Meat/Fish/Poultry	3 ounces	3.5
Beef chuck roast, medium fat, baked	Meat/Fish/Poultry	2 ounces	0.5
Beef Dijon, w/Pasta and Vegetables, frozen, Stouffer's Right Course	Meat/Fish/Poultry	1 portion	0.5
Beef flank steak, lean, broiled	Meat/Fish/Poultry	3 ounces	4.0
Beef flank steak, medium fat, choice, broiled	Meat/Fish/Poultry	3 ounces	1.5
Beef heart, braised	Meat/Fish/Poultry	3 ounces	4.0
Beef jerky	Meat/Fish/Poultry	3 pieces	2.5
Beef liver, fried	Meat/Fish/Poultry	3 ounces	7.0
Beef Meatloaf Dinner, frozen, Morton	Meat/Fish/Poultry	1/2 portion	0.5
Beef Pie, frozen, Stouffer's	Meat/Fish/Poultry	1/2 portion	−0.5

Food Name	Nutrigroup	Serving Size	Nutripoints
Beef porterhouse steak, lean, broiled	Meat/Fish/Poultry	3 ounces	2.5
Beef porterhouse steak, medium fat, choice, broiled	Meat/Fish/Poultry	3 ounces	0.0
Beef pot pie	Meat/Fish/Poultry	½ pie	0.5
Beef Pot Pie, frozen, Swanson	Meat/Fish/Poultry	½ pie	−1.5
Beef, Pot Roast, Homestyle, frozen, Stouffer's Right Course	Meat/Fish/Poultry	1 portion	2.0
Beef Pot Roast, Yankee, frozen, Budget Gourmet	Meat/Fish/Poultry	½ portion	0.0
Beef prime rib, baked	Meat/Fish/Poultry	2 ounces	−2.5
Beef Ragout w/Rice Pilaf, frozen, Stouffer's Right Course	Meat/Fish/Poultry	1 portion	0.5
Beef rib eye, lean, broiled	Meat/Fish/Poultry	3 ounces	2.5
Beef ribs, baked	Meat/Fish/Poultry	3 ounces	2.0
Beef round steak, lean, broiled	Meat/Fish/Poultry	3 ounces	4.0
Beef round steak, medium fat, broiled	Meat/Fish/Poultry	3 ounces	2.0
Beef rump roast, baked	Meat/Fish/Poultry	2 ounces	0.5
Beef Salisbury Steak Dinner, frozen, Morton	Meat/Fish/Poultry	½ portion	0.5
Beef Salisbury steak, frozen dinner	Meat/Fish/Poultry	½ portion	2.0
Beef Salisbury Steak, frozen, Healthy Choice	Meat/Fish/Poultry	1 piece	1.5
Beef Salisbury Steak, frozen, Le Menu	Meat/Fish/Poultry	1 portion	0.0

Food Name	Nutrigroup	Serving Size	Nutripoints
Beef Salisbury Steak, Homestyle, frozen, Swanson	Meat/Fish/Poultry	½ portion	−2.5
Beef Salisbury Steak, in gravy, frozen, Stouffer's	Meat/Fish/Poultry	1 piece	−1.0
Beef Salisbury Steak, Romana, frozen, Weight Watchers	Meat/Fish/Poultry	½ portion	0.0
Beef Salisbury Steak, w/Italian Sauce, frozen, Stouffer's	Meat/Fish/Poultry	1 piece	−1.0
Beef Salisbury Steak, w/Potatoes, frozen, Morton	Meat/Fish/Poultry	1 portion	0.0
Beef short ribs, lean, braised	Meat/Fish/Poultry	3 ounces	1.0
Beef short ribs, medium fat, braised	Meat/Fish/Poultry	2 ounces	−1.0
Beef Sirloin Salisbury Steak, frozen, Budget Gourmet	Meat/Fish/Poultry	½ piece	−0.5
Beef Sirloin Salisbury Steak, Slim, frozen, Budget Gourmet	Meat/Fish/Poultry	1 portion	1.0
Beef sirloin steak, broiled	Meat/Fish/Poultry	2 ounces	−2.0
Beef Sirloin Tips, frozen, Healthy Choice	Meat/Fish/Poultry	1 portion	3.0
Beef Sirloin Tips, w/Burgundy Sauce, frozen, Budget Gourmet	Meat/Fish/Poultry	½ portion	0.5
Beef Sirloin Tips, w/Country Style Vegetables, frozen, Budget Gourmet	Meat/Fish/Poultry	½ portion	−1.0

Food Name	Nutrigroup	Serving Size		Nutripoints
Beef Sirloin, w/Herb Sauce, Slim, frozen, Budget Gourmet	Meat/Fish/Poultry	1	piece	1.0
Beef Steak, Chopped, frozen, Weight Watchers	Meat/Fish/Poultry	½	portion	1.5
Beef stew	Meat/Fish/Poultry	1	cup	3.5
Beef Stew, frozen, Stouffer's	Meat/Fish/Poultry	1	portion	−0.5
Beef Stroganoff	Meat/Fish/Poultry	½	cup	0.0
Beef Stroganoff, frozen, Weight Watchers	Meat/Fish/Poultry	½	piece	−1.0
Beef Stroganoff, Slim, frozen, Budget Gourmet	Meat/Fish/Poultry	1	piece	0.0
Beef Stroganoff, w/Parsley Noodles, frozen, Stouffer's	Meat/Fish/Poultry	½	portion	−1.5
Beef Swiss steak	Meat/Fish/Poultry	3	ounces	1.0
Beef Szechuan, frozen, Chun King	Meat/Fish/Poultry	½	portion	2.0
Beef Szechwan, w/Noodles and Vegetables, frozen, Stouffer's	Meat/Fish/Poultry	1	portion	0.0
Beef T-bone steak, lean, choice, broiled	Meat/Fish/Poultry	3	ounces	2.5
Beef T-bone steak, medium fat, broiled	Meat/Fish/Poultry	3	ounces	−0.5
Beef tenderloin fillet, lean, broiled	Meat/Fish/Poultry	3	ounces	3.5
Beef tenderloin, medium fat, broiled	Meat/Fish/Poultry	3	ounces	1.0
Beef Teriyaki, frozen, Chun King	Meat/Fish/Poultry	½	portion	5.0
Beef tongue, simmered	Meat/Fish/Poultry	3	ounces	−0.5

Food Name	Nutrigroup	Serving Size	Nutripoints
Beef top loin, lean, broiled	Meat/Fish/Poultry	3 ounces	4.0
Beef top loin, medium fat, broiled	Meat/Fish/Poultry	3 ounces	0.5
Beef, Asada, Nutripoint	Meat/Fish/Poultry	1 piece	7.0
Beef, barbecue, sandwich, w/bun	Meat/Fish/Poultry	½ piece	−2.5
Beef, Breakfast Strip, Lean n' Tasty, Oscar Mayer	Meat/Fish/Poultry	3 pieces	−2.5
Beef, creamed chipped	Meat/Fish/Poultry	½ cup	−1.0
Beef, Fiesta w/Corn Pasta, frozen, Stouffer's Right Course	Meat/Fish/Poultry	1 portion	1.0
Beef, frozen dinner	Meat/Fish/Poultry	½ portion	3.5
Beef, Land O' Frost	Meat/Fish/Poultry	4 ounces	−2.0
Beef, macaroni and tomato sauce	Meat/Fish/Poultry	1 cup	3.0
Beef Oriental, w/Vegetables and Rice, frozen, Stouffer's	Meat/Fish/Poultry	1 portion	0.0
Beef Oriental Pepper Steak, frozen, Healthy Choice	Meat/Fish/Poultry	1 portion	1.5
Beef Pepper Oriental, frozen, Chun King	Meat/Fish/Poultry	½ portion	3.0
Beef Pie, frozen, Morton	Meat/Fish/Poultry	½ piece	−0.5
Beef, Roast, Slices, frozen, Loma Linda	Legume/Nut/Seed	2 ounces	6.5
Beef, Sliced, frozen, Morton	Meat/Fish/Poultry	1 piece	4.0
Beef, Sliced, w/Gravy, frozen, Morton	Meat/Fish/Poultry	1 portion	1.5

Food Name	Nutrigroup	Serving Size		Nutripoints
Beef, Smoked, Sliced, Buddig	Meat/Fish/Poultry	3	ounces	−2.0
Beefaroni	Meat/Fish/Poultry	3/4	cup	2.0
Beer	Alcohol	12	fluid ounces	−8.0
Beer, Alcohol-Free, Clark's	Alcohol	12	fluid ounces	5.0
Beer, light	Alcohol	12	fluid ounces	−5.5
Beer, near	Alcohol	12	fluid ounces	4.0
Beer, nonalcoholic	Alcohol	12	fluid ounces	1.0
Beer, root	Sugar	12	fluid ounces	−6.0
Beet greens, cooked	Vegetable	1	cup	56.5
Beets, canned, cooked	Vegetable	1/2	cup	7.5
Beets, cooked	Vegetable	1/2	cup	11.0
Beets, pickled, canned	Vegetable	1/2	cup	3.5
Biscuit	Grain	1	biscuit	1.0
Biscuit Mix, Multigrain, Arrowhead Mills	Grain	1	piece	3.5
Biscuit, buttermilk, from mix	Grain	1	biscuit	1.0
Biscuit, Butter, Pillsbury	Grain	2	whole	2.0
Biscuit, Buttermilk, Big Country, Pillsbury	Grain	2	biscuits	1.0
Biscuit, Country Style, Pillsbury	Grain	2	whole	1.5
Biscuit, Extra Rich Buttermilk, Hungry Jack	Grain	2	whole	3.0
Biscuit, Flaky, Hungry Jack	Grain	2	biscuits	0.5
Biscuit, Uneeda	Grain	6	pieces	1.5
Black Russian	Alcohol	2	fluid ounces	−13.0
Blackberries, fresh	Fruit	1/2	cup	13.0
Blackberries, frozen, unsweetened	Fruit	1/2	cup	7.5
Blackberry Freeze, Nutripoint	Fruit	3/4	cup	8.5
Bloody Mary	Alcohol	6	fluid ounces	−11.0
Blueberries, fresh	Fruit	1/2	cup	7.0

Food Name	Nutrigroup	Serving Size	Nutripoints
Blueberries, frozen, unsweetened	Fruit	½ cup	4.5
Bok choy, raw, shredded	Vegetable	1 cup	72.5
Bologna, beef	Meat/Fish/Poultry	2 ounces	−3.5
Bologna, Beef, Armour	Meat/Fish/Poultry	2 pieces	−4.0
Bologna, Beef, Bryan	Meat/Fish/Poultry	2 pieces	2.5
Bologna, Beef, Oscar Mayer	Meat/Fish/Poultry	2 pieces	−3.5
Bologna, Bryan	Meat/Fish/Poultry	2 pieces	−2.5
Bologna, Eckrich	Meat/Fish/Poultry	2 pieces	−4.0
Bologna, Garlic, Eckrich	Meat/Fish/Poultry	2 pieces	−3.5
Bologna, Oscar Mayer	Meat/Fish/Poultry	2 pieces	−3.5
Bologna, pork	Meat/Fish/Poultry	2 pieces	0.5
Bologna, Slices, frozen, Loma Linda	Legume/Nut/Seed	2 ounces	7.0
Bologna, turkey	Meat/Fish/Poultry	2 ounces	−1.5
Bologna, Turkey, Louis Rich	Meat/Fish/Poultry	2 pieces	−2.5
Bonito, canned	Meat/Fish/Poultry	3 ounces	1.0
Bouillon cube	Miscellaneous	1 piece	−1.0
Bouillon, Beef, Wyler's, Borden	Condiment	1 teaspoon	−2.0
Bouillon, Chicken, Wyler's, Borden	Condiment	1 cup	−2.0
Bouillon, Chicken, Low-Sodium, Lite-Line, Borden	Condiment	1 teaspoon	0.5
Bourbon or scotch w/soda	Alcohol	6 fluid ounces	−17.0
Boysenberries, frozen	Fruit	½ cup	9.0
Bran, oat, Arrowhead Mills	Grain	⅓ cup	9.0
Bran, Rice	Grain	2 ounces	9.0
Bran, wheat	Grain	½ cup	26.5
Bran, wheat, toasted, Kretschmer	Grain	1 ounce	27.5
Brandy	Alcohol	3 fluid ounces	−17.0
Bratwurst	Meat/Fish/Poultry	2 ounces	−1.0

Food Name	Nutrigroup	Serving Size	Nutripoints
Braunschweiger	Meat/Fish/Poultry	2 ounces	4.0
Brazil nuts, unsalted	Legume/Nut/Seed	6 pieces	0.0
Bread crumbs	Grain	½ cup	2.0
Bread Crumbs, plain, Progresso	Grain	½ cup	1.5
Bread, 100% Whole Wheat, Home Pride	Grain	2 slices	3.5
Bread, 100% Whole Wheat, Wonder	Grain	2 slices	4.0
Bread, 7 Grain, Home Pride	Grain	2 slices	3.0
Bread, banana	Grain	1 piece	−0.5
Bread, bran	Grain	2 slices	3.5
Bread, Bran'nola, Oroweat	Grain	2 slices	3.5
Bread, Bran'nola Multi-Bran, Oroweat	Grain	2 slices	2.0
Bread, Bran'nola Rice Bran, Oroweat	Grain	2 slices	2.5
Bread, Carrot, Nut, Pillsbury	Grain	1 piece	−2.0
Bread, cracked wheat	Grain	2 slices	4.5
Bread, Date, Pillsbury	Grain	1 piece	−1.5
Bread, diet 40 cal/slice	Grain	3 slices	5.5
Bread, 5 Bran, Home Pride	Grain	2 slices	5.0
Bread, French	Grain	2 slices	3.0
Bread, garlic	Grain	1 piece	0.0
Bread, gluten	Grain	2 slices	1.5
Bread, Grape-Nuts, Oroweat	Grain	2 slices	3.0
Bread, Health Nut, Oroweat	Grain	1 slice	3.0
Bread, Hi-Fiber, Wonder	Grain	3 slices	6.5
Bread, Honey Nut and Oat Bran, Roman Meal	Grain	2 slices	3.5

Food Name	Nutrigroup	Serving Size	Nutripoints
Bread, Honey Wheat Berry, Arnold	Grain	2 slices	3.5
Bread, Honey Wheat Berry, Oroweat	Grain	2 slices	2.5
Bread, Honey Wheat Berry, Pepperidge Farm	Grain	2 slices	3.0
Bread, Italian	Grain	2 slices	2.5
Bread, Less, Mrs. Baird's	Grain	3 slices	6.0
Bread, Light Bran & Oat, Oatmeal Goodness	Grain	3 slices	5.5
Bread, low-sodium	Grain	2 slices	3.5
Bread, mixed grain	Grain	2 slices	5.0
Bread, Oat Bran n' Honey, Light, Roman Meal	Grain	3 slices	5.5
Bread, Oat Bran, Honey, Earth Grains	Grain	2 slices	3.0
Bread, oatmeal	Grain	2 slices	2.0
Bread, Oatmeal and Bran, Oatmeal Goodness	Grain	2 slices	3.5
Bread, Oatmeal and Sunflower Seeds, Oatmeal Goodness	Grain	2 slices	3.5
Bread, Oatmeal, Pepperidge Farm	Grain	2 slices	3.0
Bread, Oatnut, Oroweat	Grain	2 slices	2.5
Bread, Old-Fashioned Buttermilk, Country Hearth	Grain	2 slices	3.0
Bread, Original Bran'nola, Arnold	Grain	2 slices	3.5
Bread, pita	Grain	1 whole	3.5
Bread, pita, whole wheat	Grain	1 whole	4.0

Food Name	Nutrigroup	Serving Size	Nutripoints
Bread, potato	Grain	2 slices	2.0
Bread, Protogen Protein, Thomas'	Grain	2 slices	3.5
Bread, pumpernickel	Grain	2 pieces	4.5
Bread, Pumpernickel, Arnold	Grain	2 slices	2.0
Bread, raisin	Grain	2 slices	4.0
Bread, Roman Meal	Grain	2 slices	4.5
Bread, Rye, Family, Pepperidge Farm	Grain	2 slices	3.0
Bread, Rye, Jewish, Real Unseeded, Levy's	Grain	2 slices	2.5
Bread, Rye, Light, Earth Grains	Grain	2 slices	3.0
Bread, Sandwich, Salt-Free, Earth Grains	Grain	2 slices	3.5
Bread, sourdough	Grain	2 slices	2.5
Bread, sprouted wheat	Grain	2 slices	5.0
Bread, Sprouted Wheat, Pepperidge Farm	Grain	2 slices	3.0
Bread, stuffing	Grain	½ cup	0.5
Bread, triticale	Grain	2 slices	4.5
Bread, Wheat and Oatmeal, Oatmeal Goodness	Grain	2 slices	3.0
Bread, Wheat Berry, Home Pride	Grain	2 slices	3.0
Bread, Wheat Berry, Honey, Earth Grains	Grain	2 slices	4.0
Bread, wheat germ	Grain	2 slices	4.0
Bread, Wheat, Fresh Horizons	Grain	2 slices	5.0
Bread, Wheat, Lite 35, Earth Grains	Grain	2 slices	4.5

Food Name	Nutrigroup	Serving Size	Nutripoints
Bread, Wheat, Stone-Ground, Earth Grains	Grain	2 slices	3.5
Bread, white	Grain	2 slices	2.5
Bread, White, Brick Oven, Arnold	Grain	2 slices	3.0
Bread, White, butter-top, Home Pride	Grain	2 slices	3.0
Bread, White, Wonder	Grain	2 slices	2.5
Bread, whole rye	Grain	2 slices	4.0
Bread, whole wheat	Grain	2 slices	6.0
Bread, Whole Wheat, Brick Oven, Arnold	Grain	2 slices	2.5
Bread, Whole Wheat, Stone-ground, The Sourdough	Grain	2 slices	6.0
Bread, Whole Wheat, Stone-ground, Country Hearth	Grain	2 slices	4.5
Bread, Whole Wheat, Thin, Pepperidge Farm	Grain	2 slices	4.5
Breadsticks	Grain	6 pieces	3.5
Breadsticks, Garlic, Keebler	Grain	6 pieces	1.0
Breadsticks, Onion, Keebler	Grain	6 pieces	2.0
Breadsticks, Plain, Keebler	Grain	6 pieces	2.5
Breadsticks, Sesame, Keebler	Grain	6 pieces	1.5
Breakfast bar	Grain	1 bar	2.0
Breakfast Bar, Chocolate, Carnation	Grain	1 bar	4.0
Breakfast Bar, Honey Nut, Carnation	Grain	1 bar	4.5

Food Name	Nutrigroup	Serving Size	Nutripoints
Broccoli Spears, frozen, Birds Eye	Vegetable	½ cup	46.0
Broccoli Spears, w/Butter Sauce, frozen, Green Giant	Vegetable	½ cup	6.0
Broccoli w/Cheddar Cheese Sauce, frozen, Stouffer's	Vegetable	½ piece	2.0
Broccoli, Baby Carrots, and Water Chestnuts, frozen, Birds Eye	Vegetable	½ cup	31.0
Broccoli, Carrots, and Cauliflower, frozen, Pictsweet	Vegetable	1 cup	36.0
Broccoli, Carrots, and Red Peppers, frozen, Birds Eye	Vegetable	¾ cup	17.0
Broccoli, Cauliflower, and Carrots w/Cheese Sauce, Green Giant	Vegetable	½ cup	13.0
Broccoli, Cauliflower and Carrots w/Cheese Sauce, frozen, Birds Eye	Vegetable	½ cup	13.0
Broccoli, Cauliflower and Carrots, frozen, Birds Eye	Vegetable	1 cup	30.5
Broccoli, Cauliflower and Carrots, frozen, Green Giant	Vegetable	1 cup	33.0
Broccoli, Cauliflower and Red Peppers, frozen, Birds Eye	Vegetable	1 cup	41.5
Broccoli, cooked	Vegetable	1 cup	38.5

Food Name	Nutrigroup	Serving Size	Nutripoints
Broccoli, Corn, and Red Peppers, frozen, Birds Eye	Vegetable	½ cup	17.0
Broccoli, fried, w/breading	Vegetable	¼ cup	1.5
Broccoli, raw	Vegetable	1 cup	53.0
Broccoli, Sweet Peas, and Carrots, frozen, Green Giant	Vegetable	½ cup	24.5
Broth, beef	Condiment	1 cup	0.0
Broth, chicken	Condiment	1 cup	0.0
Brownie, Chocolate, frozen, Weight Watchers	Grain	1 piece	−3.0
Brownie, w/frosting	Grain	1 piece	−3.5
Brownie, w/o frosting	Grain	1 piece	−3.5
Brownie, Walnut, Betty Crocker	Grain	1 piece	−3.0
Brussels Sprouts, Baby, frozen, Seabrook Farms	Vegetable	½ cup	25.0
Brussels sprouts, cooked	Vegetable	½ cup	40.0
Brussels sprouts, frozen, cooked	Vegetable	½ cup	27.0
Brussels Sprouts w/Butter, frozen, Green Giant	Vegetable	½ cup	12.0
Bulgar, dry	Grain	¼ cup	3.0
Bun, cinnamon	Grain	1 bun	0.0
Bun, Hot Dog, Arnold	Grain	1 whole	1.5
Bun, submarine/hoagie	Grain	½ bun	3.0
Bun, white, hamburger	Grain	1 piece	2.0
Burger King Apple Pie	Fruit	¼ piece	−1.0
Burger King Bacon Double Cheeseburger	Meat/Fish/Poultry	½ piece	−1.0

Food Name	Nutrigroup	Serving Size	Nutripoints
Burger King Breakfast Croissan'wich w/Bacon	Milk/Dairy	½ piece	−4.0
Burger King Breakfast Croissan'wich w/Ham	Milk/Dairy	½ serving	−3.5
Burger King Breakfast Croissan'wich w/Sausage	Milk/Dairy	½ serving	−5.5
Burger King Cheeseburger	Meat/Fish/Poultry	½ piece	0.0
Burger King Chicken Specialty Sandwich	Meat/Fish/Poultry	½ piece	−0.5
Burger King Chicken Tenders	Meat/Fish/Poultry	6 pieces	0.5
Burger King Chocolate Shake	Milk/Dairy	½ serving	−1.0
Burger King French Toast Sticks	Grain	¼ piece	−1.0
Burger King Great Danish	Grain	¼ Danish	−3.0
Burger King Ham and Cheese Specialty Sandwich	Meat/Fish/Poultry	½ piece	0.5
Burger King Hamburger	Meat/Fish/Poultry	½ piece	0.5
Burger King Scrambled Egg Platter	Milk/Dairy	½ serving	−4.5
Burger King Scrambled Egg Platter w/Bacon	Milk/Dairy	½ serving	−4.0
Burger King Scrambled Egg Platter w/Sausage	Milk/Dairy	¼ serving	−4.0
Burger King Vanilla Shake	Milk/Dairy	½ serving	−2.5
Burger King Whaler Fish Sandwich	Meat/Fish/Poultry	½ piece	−0.5
Burger King Whopper Jr. Sandwich	Meat/Fish/Poultry	½ piece	0.0

Food Name	Nutrigroup	Serving Size	Nutripoints
Burger King Whopper Jr. Sandwich w/Cheese	Meat/Fish/Poultry	½ piece	−0.5
Burger King Whopper Sandwich w/Cheese	Meat/Fish/Poultry	½ piece	−1.0
Burrito Dinner, frozen, Patio	Legume/Nut/Seed	¼ piece	1.0
Burrito, Bean/Beef, frozen, Patio	Legume/Nut/Seed	½ portion	0.0
Burrito, Bean/Beef, Green, frozen, Patio	Legume/Nut/Seed	½ portion	0.5
Burrito, Bean/Beef, Red Chili, frozen, Patio	Legume/Nut/Seed	½ portion	0.5
Burrito, bean/cheese	Legume/Nut/Seed	½ piece	2.5
Burrito, Beef/Bean, Patio	Legume/Nut/Seed	5 ounces	−1.0
Burrito, beef/cheese	Legume/Nut/Seed	½ portion	0.0
Burrito, Beefsteak, frozen, Weight Watchers	Legume/Nut/Seed	½ portion	0.0
Burrito, chicken	Meat/Fish/Poultry	½ piece	3.5
Burrito, Chicken, frozen, Weight Watchers	Legume/Nut/Seed	½ portion	0.0
Burrito, Red Hot, frozen, Patio	Legume/Nut/Seed	½ portion	0.0
Butter Beans, frozen, Pictsweet	Legume/Nut/Seed	½ cup	4.0
Butter Mix, Imitation, Butter Buds	Condiment	2 tablespoons	−0.5
Butter, salted	Fat/Oil	1 tablespoon	−7.5
Butter, Sweet, Cream, Unsalted, Land O Lakes	Fat/Oil	1 tablespoon	−6.5
Butter, Sweet, Light Salt, Land O Lakes	Fat/Oil	1 tablespoon	−7.0
Butter, unsalted	Fat/Oil	1 tablespoon	−6.5

Food Name	Nutrigroup	Serving Size	Nutripoints
Buttermilk, regular	Milk/Dairy	1 cup	5.0
Buttermilk, skim	Milk/Dairy	1 cup	9.5
Butternuts	Legume/Nut/Seed	1 ounce	1.0
Cabbage roll, frozen dinner	Vegetable	½ piece	1.5
Cabbage, common, chopped, cooked	Vegetable	1 cup	31.5
Cabbage, common, raw, shredded	Vegetable	1 cup	39.0
Cabbage, red, raw, shredded	Vegetable	1 cup	29.5
Cabbage, savoy, raw, shredded	Vegetable	1 cup	24.5
Cake, Angel Food, Duncan Hines	Grain	1 piece	−1.5
Cake, angel food, plain	Grain	1 piece	−2.5
Cake, angel food, w/glaze	Grain	½ piece	−3.5
Cake, Banana, Sara Lee	Grain	1 piece	−2.0
Cake, banana, w/frosting	Grain	1 piece	−2.0
Cake, Black Forest, frozen, Weight Watchers	Grain	1 piece	−2.5
Cake, Boston Cream, Supreme, Pepperidge Farm	Grain	½ piece	−3.0
Cake, Bundt Pound Supreme, Pillsbury	Grain	½ piece	−3.0
Cake, Carrot, frozen, Weight Watchers	Grain	1 piece	−0.5
Cake, carrot, w/cream cheese frosting	Grain	½ piece	−2.5
Cake, cheese, plain	Milk/Dairy	½ piece	−3.0
Cake, cheese, w/fruit topping	Milk/Dairy	½ piece	−2.0
Cake, Choco-Bake, Nestlé	Sugar	1 piece	−3.0

Food Name	Nutrigroup	Serving Size	Nutripoints
Cake, Chocolate Fudge Snack, Sara Lee	Grain	1 piece	−3.5
Cake, Chocolate Mint Plus, Pillsbury	Grain	½ piece	−4.0
Cake, chocolate w/frosting (12 pieces/cake)	Grain	½ piece	−3.0
Cake, chocolate w/o frost (12 pieces/cake)	Grain	½ piece	−3.0
Cake, Chocolate, frozen, Weight Watchers	Grain	1 piece	−2.0
Cake, coffee	Grain	½ piece	−2.0
Cake, crumb	Grain	1 piece	−2.0
Cake, Crumb, Hostess	Grain	1 piece	−2.0
Cake, Devil's Food, Deluxe, Streusel Swirl, Duncan Hines	Grain	½ piece	−3.0
Cake, Dutch Apple Pillsbury	Grain	½ piece	−3.5
Cake, Elfin Loaves, Apple Cinnamon, frozen, Keebler	Grain	1 cake	0.5
Cake, Elfin Loaves, Banana, frozen, Keebler	Grain	1 piece	0.5
Cake, Elfin Loaves, Blueberry, frozen, Keebler	Grain	1 cake	1.0
Cake, German chocolate	Grain	½ piece	−3.0
Cake, German Chocolate, frozen, Weight Watchers	Grain	1 piece	−2.0

Food Name	Nutrigroup	Serving Size	Nutripoints
Cake, German Chocolate, Moist, Betty Crocker	Grain	½ piece	−3.5
Cake, Golden Layer, Pepperidge Farm	Grain	1 piece	−3.5
Cake, pound	Grain	1 piece	−5.0
Cake, Pound, Blueberry Topping, frozen, Weight Watchers	Grain	1 piece	−2.5
Cake, Pound, Original, Sara Lee	Grain	1 piece	−4.0
Cake, sponge	Grain	1 piece	−4.5
Cake, sponge, w/icing	Grain	½ piece	−3.5
Cake, sponge, w/whipped cream and fruit	Grain	½ piece	−2.0
Cake, torte	Grain	½ piece	−3.0
Cake, upside down, pineapple	Grain	½ piece	−0.5
Cake, white	Grain	1 piece	−0.5
Candy bar, $100,000	Sugar	1 piece	−4.0
Candy Bar, 3 Musketeers	Sugar	½ piece	−4.0
Candy Bar, Baby Ruth	Sugar	½ piece	−2.0
Candy Bar, Butterfinger	Sugar	1 piece	−2.5
Candy Bar, Chocolit	Sugar	1 piece	−4.0
Candy Bar, Coconut Almond Joy	Fruit	½ bar	−4.0
Candy bar, diet	Sugar	1 ounce	−2.0
Candy Bar, Ideal Green Apple, Thompson Foods	Grain	2 bars	13.5
Candy Bar, Kit Kat	Sugar	1 piece	−2.0
Candy Bar, Mars Bar	Sugar	½ piece	−3.5
Candy bar, milk chocolate	Milk/Dairy	1 ounce	−3.5

Food Name	Nutrigroup	Serving Size	Nutripoints
Candy bar, milk chocolate w/almonds	Legume/Nut/Seed	1 ounce	−3.5
Candy bar, milk chocolate w/peanuts	Legume/Nut/Seed	1 ounce	−3.0
Candy Bar, Milky Way	Sugar	½ piece	−4.0
Candy Bar, Mr. Goodbar	Sugar	½ piece	−3.0
Candy Bar, Nestlé Crunch	Sugar	1½ ounces	−4.5
Candy Bar, Peanut, Planters	Legume/Nut/Seed	1 piece	0.0
Candy Bar, Rice Krispies, Kellogg's	Grain	1 bar	0.5
Candy Bar, Slim-Fast	Grain	1 bar	17.0
Candy Bar, Snickers	Sugar	½ piece	−3.0
Candy Bar, Tiger's Milk Nutrition	Grain	1 bar	5.0
Candy Bar, Twix Caramel	Sugar	2 pieces	−4.0
Candy Bar, Twix Peanut Butter	Legume/Nut/Seed	2 pieces	−1.5
Candy, Brach Royals	Sugar	1 ounce	−4.0
Candy, Brach Toffees	Sugar	1 ounce	−4.0
Candy, caramel w/nuts, chocolate-covered	Legume/Nut/Seed	1 ounce	−2.5
Candy, caramels	Sugar	3 pieces	−3.5
Candy, chocolate chips	Sugar	1 ounce	−6.0
Candy, Cracker Jacks	Grain	1 ounce	−3.0
Candy, gum drop, small	Sugar	28 pieces	−5.5
Candy, hard	Sugar	1 ounce	−6.0
Candy, Kisses, Hershey's	Sugar	6 pieces	−3.5
Candy, M&M's Chocolate	Sugar	1 ounce	−4.5

Food Name	Nutrigroup	Serving Size	Nutripoints
Candy, M&M's Peanut	Sugar	1 ounce	−2.0
Candy, marshmallow	Sugar	4 pieces	−5.5
Candy, Milk Chocolate w/Almonds, Hershey's	Sugar	1 piece	−3.5
Candy, peanut brittle	Legume/Nut/Seed	1 ounce	−3.0
Candy, peanut butter cup	Legume/Nut/Seed	1 piece	−3.5
Candy, Peanut Butter Cups, Reese's	Sugar	1 piece	−3.0
Candy, peanut butter morsels	Legume/Nut/Seed	1 ounce	−0.5
Candy, pralines	Sugar	1 piece	−3.0
Candy, Reese's Pieces	Legume/Nut/Seed	1 ounce	−2.0
Candy, Rolo	Sugar	5 pieces	−4.5
Candy, Semi-Sweet Morsels, Nestlé	Sugar	1 ounce	−4.5
Candy, Spear O Mint, Life Savers	Sugar	10 pieces	−6.0
Candy, taffy, plain	Sugar	1 ounce	−5.5
Candy, Wild Cherry, Life Savers	Sugar	10 pieces	−6.0
Cannelloni, Cheese, Lean Cuisine, frozen, Stouffer's	Milk/Dairy	½ portion	0.5
Cannelloni, Florentine, frozen, Celentano	Milk/Dairy	½ portion	5.5
Capon, baked, w/skin	Meat/Fish/Poultry	3 ounces	1.5
Carambola (starfruit)	Fruit	1 piece	12.5
Caraway seed	Condiment	1 teaspoon	0.5
Carl's Jr. Bacon and Cheese Potato	Vegetable	¼ piece	−0.5
Carl's Jr. Blueberry Muffin	Grain	½ muffin	−1.5
Carl's Jr. Boston Clam Chowder Soups	Meat/Fish/Poultry	1 cup	−1.5
Carl's Jr. Bran Muffin	Grain	1 muffin	−1.0
Carl's Jr. Broccoli and Cheese Potato	Vegetable	¼ piece	2.0

Food Name	Nutrigroup	Serving Size	Nutripoints
Carl's Jr. California Roast Beef 'n Swiss Sandwich	Meat/Fish/Poultry	½ piece	1.0
Carl's Jr. Charbroiler Barbeque Chicken Sandwich	Meat/Fish/Poultry	½ piece	1.5
Carl's Jr. Charbroiler Chicken Club Sandwich	Meat/Fish/Poultry	½ piece	0.5
Carl's Jr. Cheese Potato	Vegetable	¼ serving	0.5
Carl's Jr. Chef Salad (take-out)	Vegetable	½ serving	4.0
Carl's Jr. Chicken Salad (take-out)	Meat/Fish/Poultry	1 serving	3.5
Carl's Jr. Chocolate Cake	Grain	½ piece	−3.5
Carl's Jr. Chocolate Chip Cookie	Grain	½ cookie	−3.0
Carl's Jr. Country Fried Steak Sandwich	Meat/Fish/Poultry	½ piece	−0.5
Carl's Jr. Cream of Broccoli Soup	Vegetable	½ cup	1.0
Carl's Jr. Danish (all varieties)	Grain	½ Danish	−0.5
Carl's Jr. Double Western Bacon Cheeseburger	Meat/Fish/Poultry	¼ piece	−1.5
Carl's Jr. English Muffin w/Margarine	Grain	1 whole	1.0
Carl's Jr. Famous Star Hamburger	Meat/Fish/Poultry	½ piece	−0.5
Carl's Jr. Fiesta Potato	Vegetable	¼ serving	0.5
Carl's Jr. Fillet of Fish Sandwich	Meat/Fish/Poultry	½ piece	−1.0
Carl's Jr. French Toast Dips	Grain	1 piece	−1.5

Food Name	Nutrigroup	Serving Size	Nutripoints
Carl's Jr. Fried Zucchini	Vegetable	1 piece	−1.0
Carl's Jr. Garden Salad (take-out)	Vegetable	1 serving	8.5
Carl's Jr. Happy Star Hamburger	Meat/Fish/Poultry	1 piece	0.0
Carl's Jr. Hash Browns Nuggets	Vegetable	2 piece	−1.5
Carl's Jr. Hot Cakes w/Margarine	Grain	1 serving	0.0
Carl's Jr. Lite Potato	Vegetable	½ piece	3.0
Carl's Jr. Lumber Jack Mixed Vegetable Soup	Vegetable	1 cup	2.5
Carl's Jr. Old Fashioned Chicken Noodle Soup	Meat/Fish/Poultry	1 cup	0.5
Carl's Jr. Old-Time Star Hamburger	Meat/Fish/Poultry	½ piece	0.0
Carl's Jr. Onion Rings	Vegetable	1 piece	−1.0
Carl's Jr. Sausage, 1 patty	Meat/Fish/Poultry	1 piece	−2.5
Carl's Jr. Scrambled Eggs	Milk/Dairy	2 eggs	−11.0
Carl's Jr. Shakes, regular size	Milk/Dairy	½ cup	−1.5
Carl's Jr. Sour Cream and Chive Potato	Vegetable	¼ serving	1.0
Carl's Jr. Sunrise Sandwich w/Bacon	Milk/Dairy	½ serving	−2.0
Carl's Jr. Sunrise Sandwich w/Sausage	Milk/Dairy	¼ serving	−2.5
Carl's Jr. Super Star Hamburger	Meat/Fish/Poultry	½ piece	−1.5
Carl's Jr. Taco Salad (take-out)	Vegetable	¼ piece	1.5
Carl's Jr. Western Bacon Cheeseburger	Meat/Fish/Poultry	⅕ piece	−1.0

Food Name	Nutrigroup	Serving Size	Nutripoints
Carob powder	Miscellaneous	1 tablespoon	1.0
Carp, baked/broiled	Meat/Fish/Poultry	3 ounces	0.5
Carp, floured/breaded, fried	Meat/Fish/Poultry	3 ounces	−0.5
Carp, smoked	Meat/Fish/Poultry	3 ounces	2.5
Carrots, raw	Vegetable	1 whole	35.5
Carrots, sliced, cooked	Vegetable	½ cup	30.0
Cashew butter, salted	Legume/Nut/Seed	1 ounce	0.5
Cashews, dry roasted, salted	Legume/Nut/Seed	1 ounce	0.5
Cashews, dry roasted, unsalted	Legume/Nut/Seed	12 pieces	1.5
Cashews, Dry Roasted, Unsalted, Planters	Legume/Nut/Seed	1 ounce	1.5
Cashews, oil roasted, salted	Legume/Nut/Seed	1 ounce	0.5
Cashews, oil roasted, unsalted	Legume/Nut/Seed	1 ounce	0.5
Casserole, Five-Cheese, Nutripoint	Milk/Dairy	½ cup	5.5
Catfish, baked	Meat/Fish/Poultry	5 ounces	3.0
Catfish, Fillets, Light, Mrs. Paul's	Meat/Fish/Poultry	1 piece	0.5
Catfish, fried, w/breading	Meat/Fish/Poultry	3 ounces	0.0
Catsup	Vegetable	2 tablespoons	1.0
Catsup, low-sodium, low-sugar	Vegetable	2 tablespoons	0.5
Catsup, tomato, Del Monte	Vegetable	2 tablespoons	0.5
Cauliflower, w/Cheddar Cheese Sauce, frozen, Budget Gourmet	Vegetable	½ piece	2.0
Cauliflower, w/Cheese Sauce, frozen, Green Giant	Vegetable	½ cup	6.0

Food Name	Nutrigroup	Serving Size	Nutripoints
Cauliflower, cooked	Vegetable	1 cup	37.5
Cauliflower, fried, w/breading	Vegetable	¼ cup	−0.5
Cauliflower, frozen, Birds Eye	Vegetable	1 cup	23.0
Cauliflower, raw	Vegetable	1 cup	40.5
Cavatelli, frozen, Celentano	Grain	½ portion	3.0
Caviar	Miscellaneous	1 tablespoon	−11.5
Celeriac, raw	Vegetable	½ cup	8.0
Celery seed	Condiment	1 teaspoon	0.5
Celery, raw	Vegetable	8 stalks	20.0
Cereal, 100% Bran with Oat Bran, Nabisco	Grain	½ cup	23.5
Cereal, 100% Bran, Nabisco	Grain	½ cup	31.0
Cereal, 100% Natural, Quaker	Grain	¼ cup	1.0
Cereal, 100% Natural, Raisin and Date, Quaker	Grain	¼ cup	0.0
Cereal, 40+ Bran Flakes, Kellogg's	Grain	⅔ cup	21.0
Cereal, 7 Grain, Stone-Buhr	Grain	1 ounce	4.0
Cereal, All Bran Extra Fiber, Kellogg's	Grain	½ cup	43.5
Cereal, All Bran, Kellogg's	Grain	⅓ cup	27.0
Cereal, Almond Delight, Ralston	Grain	¾ cup	7.0
Cereal, Alpen	Grain	¼ cup	3.5
Cereal, Alpha-Bits, Post	Grain	1 cup	8.5
Cereal, Apple Cinnamon Cheerios, General Mills	Grain	¾ cup	8.0

Food Name	Nutrigroup	Serving Size	Nutripoints
Cereal, Apple Cinnamon Oh's, Quaker	Grain	1 cup	9.0
Cereal, Apple Jacks, Kellogg's	Grain	1 cup	9.5
Cereal, Apple Raisin Crisp, Kellogg's	Grain	2/3 cup	8.5
Cereal, Blueberry Fruit Wheats, Nabisco	Grain	1/2 cup	13.0
Cereal, Bran Buds, Kellogg's	Grain	1/3 cup	25.5
Cereal, Bran Chex, Ralston	Grain	3/4 cup	15.5
Cereal, Bran Flakes, Kellogg's	Grain	2/3 cup	21.0
Cereal, Bran News, Ralston	Grain	3/4 cup	9.5
Cereal, C.W. Post, Post	Grain	1/4 cup	7.0
Cereal, C.W. Post, w/Raisins, Post	Grain	1/2 cup	7.5
Cereal, Cap'n Crunch, Peanut Butter, Quaker	Grain	3/4 cup	9.0
Cereal, Cap'n Crunch, Quaker	Grain	3/4 cup	8.5
Cereal, Cheerios, General Mills	Grain	1 1/4 cups	13.0
Cereal, Cinnamon Toast Crunch, General Mills	Grain	3/4 cup	7.5
Cereal, Clusters, General Mills	Grain	1/2 cup	10.5
Cereal, Cocoa Krispies, Kellogg's	Grain	3/4 cup	7.0
Cereal, Cocoa Pebbles, Post	Grain	7/8 cup	7.5
Cereal, Cocoa Puffs, General Mills	Grain	1 cup	6.5

Food Name	Nutrigroup	Serving Size	Nutripoints
Cereal, Common Sense Oat Bran, Kellogg's	Grain	⅔ cup	13.5
Cereal, Common Sense Oat Bran w/Raisins, Kellogg's	Grain	⅔ cup	14.0
Cereal, Cookie-Crisp, Ralston	Grain	1 cup	7.5
Cereal, Corn Chex, Ralston	Grain	1 cup	10.0
Cereal, Corn Flakes, Kellogg's	Grain	1 cup	18.0
Cereal, Corn Pops, Kellogg's	Grain	1 cup	8.0
Cereal, Country Morning	Grain	¼ cup	0.5
Cereal, Cracklin' Oat Bran, Kellogg's	Grain	½ cup	14.0
Cereal, cream of rice, cooked	Grain	¾ cup	2.5
Cereal, Cream of Wheat, Quick, Nabisco	Grain	1 cup	4.5
Cereal, Crispix, Kellogg's	Grain	1 cup	10.0
Cereal, Crispy Wheat 'n Raisins, General Mills	Grain	¾ cup	9.5
Cereal, Crunch Berries, Quaker	Grain	¾ cup	9.0
Cereal, Crunchy Bran, Quaker	Grain	½ cup	16.0
Cereal, Dinersaurs, Ralston	Grain	1 cup	7.5
Cereal, Familia, w/Fruit and Nuts	Grain	¼ cup	2.5
Cereal, Fiber One, General Mills	Grain	½ cup	31.5

Food Name	Nutrigroup	Serving Size	Nutripoints
Cereal, Frosted Flakes, Kellogg's	Grain	3/4 cup	7.0
Cereal, Frosted Mini-Wheats, Kellogg's	Grain	1/2 cup	12.5
Cereal, Frosted Wheat Squares, Nabisco	Grain	1/2 cup	11.5
Cereal, Fruit Loops, Kellogg's	Grain	1 cup	13.0
Cereal, Fruit and Fibre, w/Cinnamon/Apple Crisp, Post	Grain	1/2 cup	16.0
Cereal, Fruit and Fibre, w/Dates/ Raisins/Walnuts, Post	Grain	1/2 cup	15.5
Cereal, Fruit and Fibre, w/ Pineapple/Banana/ Coconut, Post	Grain	1/2 cup	15.0
Cereal, Fruit and Fibre, w/Raisins/ Peaches/Almonds, Post	Grain	1/2 cup	15.5
Cereal, Fruitful Bran, Kellogg's	Grain	2/3 cup	28.5
Cereal, Fruity Pebbles, Post	Grain	7/8 cup	7.5
Cereal, Fruity Yummy Mummy, General Mills	Grain	1 cup	8.0
Cereal, Golden Grahams, General Mills	Grain	3/4 cup	9.0
Cereal, Grape-Nuts Flakes, Post	Grain	7/8 cup	18.0
Cereal, Grape-Nuts, Post	Grain	1/4 cup	13.5

Food Name	Nutrigroup	Serving Size	Nutripoints
Cereal, Heartwise, Kellogg's	Grain	1 cup	12.0
Cereal, Honey Buc-Wheat Crisp, General Mills	Grain	3/4 cup	18.0
Cereal, Honey Graham Chex, Ralston	Grain	2/3 cup	6.5
Cereal, Honey Graham Oh's, Quaker	Grain	1 cup	11.5
Cereal, Honey Nut Cheerios, General Mills	Grain	3/4 cup	10.0
Cereal, Honey-Comb, Ralston	Grain	1 1/3 cup	8.5
Cereal, Honeybunches of Oats w/Almonds, Post	Grain	2/3 cup	7.5
Cereal, Horizon Trail Mix, Post	Grain	1/3 cup	10.0
Cereal, Hot, High-Fiber, Ralston	Grain	1/4 cup	8.5
Cereal, Hot, High-Fiber, w/milk, Ralston	Grain	1/4 cup	6.0
Cereal, Instant Cream of Wheat, w/low-fat milk, Nabisco	Grain	1/2 cup	4.5
Cereal, Instant Oatmeal w/Apples/Cinnam-on, Quaker	Grain	1 1/4 ounces	3.5
Cereal, Instant Oatmeal w/Maple and Brown Sugar, Quaker	Grain	1 1/4 ounces	1.5

Food Name	Nutrigroup	Serving Size	Nutripoints
Cereal, Instant Oatmeal w/Peaches/Cream, Quaker	Grain	1 cup	5.5
Cereal, Instant Total Oatmeal, w/skim milk, General Mills	Grain	½ cup	51.0
Cereal, Just Right w/Fruit and Nuts, Kellogg's	Grain	¾ cup	36.5
Cereal, Just Right, Kellogg's	Grain	⅔ cup	51.0
Cereal, Kenmei Rice Bran, Kellogg's	Grain	¾ cup	9.5
Cereal, Kix, General Mills	Grain	1½ cups	10.0
Cereal, Life, Cinnamon, Quaker	Grain	⅔ cup	11.0
Cereal, Life, Quaker	Grain	⅔ cup	9.5
Cereal, Lucky Charms, General Mills	Grain	1 cup	10.5
Cereal, Malt-O Meal, w/water, cooked	Grain	1 cup	7.5
Cereal, Malt-O Meal, Quick, w/whole milk	Grain	½ cup	4.5
Cereal, Muesli w/Raisins/Dates/ Almonds, Ralston	Grain	½ cup	9.0
Cereal, Muesli w/Raisins/Peaches /Pecans, Ralston	Grain	½ cup	8.0
Cereal, Müeslix, 5 Grain Muesli, Kellogg's	Grain	½ cup	10.0
Cereal, Müeslix, Bran Muesli, Kellogg's	Grain	½ cup	12.5
Cereal, Natural Bran Flakes, Post	Grain	⅔ cup	17.5

Food Name	Nutrigroup	Serving Size	Nutripoints
Cereal, Natural Raisin Bran, Post	Grain	½ cup	17.0
Cereal, Natural, Heartland	Grain	¼ cup	0.5
Cereal, Natural, w/Raisins, Heartland	Grain	¼ cup	0.0
Cereal, Nut and Honey Crunch Biscuits, Kellogg's	Grain	½ cup	13.0
Cereal, Nutri-Grain, Biscuits, Kellogg's	Grain	⅔ cup	15.0
Cereal, Nutri-Grain, w/Almonds and Raisins, Kellogg's	Grain	⅔ cup	9.5
Cereal, Nutri-Grain, w/Wheat and Raisins, Kellogg's	Grain	⅔ cup	11.5
Cereal, Nutri-Grain, Wheat, Kellogg's	Grain	⅔ cup	15.5
Cereal, Nutrific Oatmeal, Kellogg's	Grain	1 cup	10.5
Cereal, Oat Bran, prepared w/low-fat milk, Nabisco	Grain	½ cup	12.0
Cereal, Oat Bran, Instant, w/skim milk, 3 Minute Brand	Grain	½ cup	6.5
Cereal, Oat Bran, Instant, w/water, 3 Minute Brand	Grain	1 ounce	6.0
Cereal, Oat Bran, Instant, w/whole milk, 3 Minute Brand	Grain	1 cup	5.5
Cereal, Oat Bran, Quaker	Grain	½ cup	7.0
Cereal, Oat Flakes, Post	Grain	⅔ cup	13.0

Food Name	Nutrigroup	Serving Size	Nutripoints
Cereal, Oat Squares, Quaker	Grain	1/2 cup	17.0
Cereal, Oatbake, Kellogg's	Grain	1/3 cup	10.0
Cereal, Oatmeal Raisin Crisp, General Mills	Grain	1/2 cup	9.5
Cereal, oatmeal, cooked, prepared w/water	Grain	1 cup	2.0
Cereal, oatmeal, dry	Grain	1/2 cup	5.5
Cereal, Oatmeal, Fruited Cinnamon, Nutripoint	Grain	1 cup	5.0
Cereal, Oats, Instant, w/Bran, w/low-fat milk, 3 Minute Brand	Grain	1/2 cup	9.5
Cereal, Oats, Old-Fashioned, Quaker	Grain	3/4 cup	4.5
Cereal, Oats, Quick, prepared w/low-fat milk, Quaker	Grain	1/2 cup	3.0
Cereal, Oats, Steel-Cut, Arrowhead Mills	Grain	1 ounce	4.0
Cereal, Orangeola w/Bran and Whole Fruit, Health Valley	Grain	1/4 cup	2.0
Cereal, Product 19, Kellogg's	Grain	1 cup	56.0
Cereal, puffed rice	Grain	2 cups	2.0
Cereal, Puffed Rice, Quaker	Grain	1 cup	2.5
Cereal, puffed wheat	Grain	2 cups	4.5
Cereal, Puffed Wheat, Quaker	Grain	1 cup	5.5

Food Name	Nutrigroup	Serving Size	Nutripoints
Cereal, Puffed, Seven Whole Grains and Sesame Seeds, Kashi	Grain	2 cups	3.0
Cereal, Raisin Bran, Kellogg's	Grain	¾ cup	15.5
Cereal, Raisin Nut Bran, General Mills	Grain	½ cup	10.0
Cereal, Raspberry Fruit Wheats, Nabisco	Grain	½ cup	13.0
Cereal, Rice Chex, Ralston	Grain	1⅛ cups	9.0
Cereal, Rice Krispies, Kellogg's	Grain	1 cup	11.5
Cereal, S.W. Graham Shredded Biscuits, Kellogg's	Grain	½ cup	10.0
Cereal, S.W. Graham w/Cinnamon, Kellogg's	Grain	½ cup	9.0
Cereal, Shredded Wheat 'n Bran, Nabisco	Grain	1 ounce	6.0
Cereal, Shredded Wheat (Large Biscuit), Nabisco	Grain	1 piece	5.0
Cereal, Shredded Wheat, Spoon-Size, Nabisco	Grain	⅔ cup	5.0
Cereal, Shredded Wheat Squares w/Raisins, Kellogg's	Grain	½ cup	14.0
Cereal, Smurf Magic Berries, Post	Grain	1 cup	8.0
Cereal, Special K, Kellogg's	Grain	1 cup	14.0
Cereal, Sun Flakes, Ralston	Grain	1 cup	10.5

Food Name	Nutrigroup	Serving Size	Nutripoints
Cereal, Super Golden Crisp, Post	Grain	7/8 cup	8.0
Cereal, Team Flakes, Nabisco	Grain	1 cup	11.5
Cereal, Toasties Corn Flakes, Post	Grain	1¼ cups	9.0
Cereal, Total Corn Flakes, General Mills	Grain	1 cup	57.5
Cereal, Total Raisin Bran, General Mills	Grain	½ cup	40.5
Cereal, Trix, General Mills	Grain	1 cup	8.0
Cereal, Wheat Chex, Ralston	Grain	2/3 cup	13.0
Cereal, Wheaties, General Mills	Grain	1 cup	12.0
Cereal, Whole Wheat Total, General Mills	Grain	1 cup	64.5
Cereal, whole wheat, cooked	Grain	½ cup	4.5
Cereal, Whole Wheat, Weetabix	Grain	2 pieces	4.0
Champagne	Alcohol	6 fluid ounces	−13.5
Cheese fondue	Milk/Dairy	¼ cup	−4.5
Cheese Food Substitute, Low Cholesterol, Lite-Line	Milk/Dairy	1 ounce	−1.5
Cheese Puffs, Cheetos	Grain	25 pieces	−1.5
Cheese spread	Milk/Dairy	1 ounce	−1.5
Cheese Spread, Cheez Whiz, Kraft	Milk/Dairy	1 ounce	−3.5
Cheese Spread, Pasteurized Process, Velveeta	Milk/Dairy	1 ounce	−3.0

Food Name	Nutrigroup	Serving Size	Nutripoints
Cheese Spread, Pasteurized Process, Slices, Velveeta	Milk/Dairy	1 ounce	−2.5
Cheese Substitute, Pasteurized Process, Formagg	Milk/Dairy	1 piece	10.5
Cheese, American, Borden	Milk/Dairy	1 ounce	−2.5
Cheese, American, Light n' Lively, Kraft	Milk/Dairy	1 ounce	−1.0
Cheese, American, Pasteurized Process, Kraft	Milk/Dairy	1 ounce	−1.5
Cheese, American, Pasteurized Process, Lipton	Milk/Dairy	2 ounces	0.0
Cheese, American, processed	Milk/Dairy	1 ounce	−3.0
Cheese, blue	Milk/Dairy	1 ounce	−2.0
Cheese, brick	Milk/Dairy	1 ounce	−1.5
Cheese, Brie	Milk/Dairy	1 ounce	−2.0
Cheese, Camembert	Milk/Dairy	1 ounce	−1.0
Cheese, cheddar	Milk/Dairy	1 ounce	−2.0
Cheese, Cheddar Flavor, Sharp, Borden	Milk/Dairy	1 ounce	1.0
Cheese, Cheddar, Low-Sodium, Tillamook	Milk/Dairy	1 ounce	−3.0
Cheese, Cheddar, Mild, Reduced Fat, Kraft	Milk/Dairy	1 ounce	−1.0
Cheese, Cheddar, Naturally Mild, Kraft	Milk/Dairy	1 ounce	−3.0
Cheese, Cheddar, Sharp, Cracker Barrel	Milk/Dairy	1 ounce	−3.5

Food Name	Nutrigroup	Serving Size	Nutripoints
Cheese, Cheddar, Tillamook	Milk/Dairy	1 ounce	−3.0
Cheese, Colby	Milk/Dairy	1 ounce	−2.0
Cheese, cottage	Milk/Dairy	½ cup	1.5
Cheese, cottage, dry	Milk/Dairy	½ cup	5.5
Cheese, cottage, low-fat (1-percent)	Milk/Dairy	½ cup	4.5
Cheese, cottage, low-fat (2-percent)	Milk/Dairy	4 ounces	3.0
Cheese, Cottage, Low-Fat, Weight Watchers	Milk/Dairy	½ cup	1.5
Cheese, cream	Milk/Dairy	2 tablespoons	−5.0
Cheese, Cream, Honey, Nutripoint	Milk/Dairy	¼ cup	5.5
Cheese, Edam	Milk/Dairy	1 ounce	−1.0
Cheese, feta	Milk/Dairy	1 ounce	−2.5
Cheese, Gjetost	Milk/Dairy	1 ounce	−0.5
Cheese, Gouda	Milk/Dairy	1 ounce	−1.5
Cheese, Gouda, Kraft	Milk/Dairy	1 ounce	−3.5
Cheese, Gruyère	Milk/Dairy	1 ounce	−1.0
Cheese, Laughing Cow	Milk/Dairy	2 pieces	0.0
Cheese, Limburger	Milk/Dairy	1 ounce	−3.0
Cheese, low-cal.	Milk/Dairy	2 ounces	3.5
Cheese, Monterey Jack	Milk/Dairy	1 ounce	−1.5
Cheese, Monterey Jack, Casino Brand	Milk/Dairy	1 ounce	−4.0
Cheese, Monterey Jack, Kraft	Milk/Dairy	1 ounce	−3.5
Cheese, Monterey Jack, Low Fat, Alpine Lace	Milk/Dairy	2 ounces	−1.5
Cheese, Monterey Jack, Reduced Fat, Kraft	Milk/Dairy	1 ounce	−1.0
Cheese, mozzarella	Milk/Dairy	1 ounce	−1.5
Cheese, Mozzarella, Casino, Kraft	Milk/Dairy	1 ounce	−3.5

Food Name	Nutrigroup	Serving Size	Nutripoints
Cheese, mozzarella, low-fat	Milk/Dairy	1 ounce	0.5
Cheese, Mozzarella, Low Fat, Alpine Lace	Milk/Dairy	2 ounces	−1.5
Cheese, Mozzarella, Low-Fat, Borden	Milk/Dairy	1 ounce	0.0
Cheese, Mozzarella, Skim, Kraft	Milk/Dairy	1 ounce	−1.5
Cheese, Mozzarella, Skim, Land O Lakes	Milk/Dairy	1 ounce	0.5
Cheese, Muenster	Milk/Dairy	1 ounce	−1.5
Cheese, Muenster, Land O Lakes	Milk/Dairy	1 ounce	−2.5
Cheese, Natural Colby, Kraft	Milk/Dairy	1 ounce	−3.0
Cheese, Neufchâtel	Milk/Dairy	1 ounce	−4.0
Cheese, Neufchâtel, Philadelphia Brand	Milk/Dairy	1 ounce	−3.0
Cheese, Parmesan	Milk/Dairy	1 ounce	0.5
Cheese, Parmesan, Grated, Kraft	Milk/Dairy	1 ounce	−1.5
Cheese, Parmesan, Imitation, Grated, Formagg	Milk/Dairy	1 ounce	0.0
Cheese, Pasteurized Process, Reduced Sodium, Lite-Line	Milk/Dairy	1 ounce	−0.5
Cheese, Pimiento	Milk/Dairy	1 ounce	−2.0
Cheese, provolone	Milk/Dairy	1 ounce	−1.0
Cheese, Reduced Calorie, Laughing Cow	Milk/Dairy	2 ounces	2.5
Cheese, ricotta	Milk/Dairy	2 ounces	−2.0
Cheese, ricotta, low-fat	Milk/Dairy	2 ounces	0.5
Cheese, Romano	Milk/Dairy	1 ounce	−2.0
Cheese, Roquefort	Milk/Dairy	1 ounce	−3.0
Cheese, Swiss	Milk/Dairy	1 ounce	−0.5

Food Name	Nutrigroup	Serving Size	Nutripoints
Cheese, Swiss, Borden	Milk/Dairy	1 ounce	−1.5
Cheese, Swiss, Light n' Lively, Kraft	Milk/Dairy	1 ounce	−1.0
Cheese, Swiss, Low fat, Alpine Lace	Milk/Dairy	1 ounce	−2.0
Cheese, Swiss, Low-Sodium, Kraft	Milk/Dairy	1 ounce	−2.5
Cheese, Swiss, Natural, Kraft	Milk/Dairy	1 ounce	−2.0
Cheese, Swiss, Pasteurized Process, Kraft	Milk/Dairy	1 ounce	−4.0
Cheese, Swiss, processed	Milk/Dairy	1 ounce	−2.5
Cheese, Swiss, Reduced Fat, Kraft	Milk/Dairy	1 ounce	0.5
Cheese, Swiss, Sargento	Milk/Dairy	1 ounce	−2.5
Cheeseburger w/bun, fast-food, small, plain	Meat/Fish/Poultry	½ piece	0.0
Cheesecake, Classic Snack, Sara Lee	Grain	½ piece	−5.5
Cheesecake, frozen, Weight Watchers	Milk/Dairy	½ piece	−2.0
Cheesecake, Strawberry, frozen, Weight Watchers	Milk/Dairy	½ piece	−2.0
Cheetos	Grain	1 ounce	−1.0
Cherries, chocolate-covered	Fruit	2 pieces	−3.5
Cherries, sour, canned in heavy syrup	Fruit	½ cup	1.0
Cherries, sour, canned, unsweetened	Fruit	½ cup	7.5
Cherries, sour, raw	Fruit	10 pieces	7.5
Cherries, sweet, canned, heavy syrup	Fruit	½ cup	0.0

Food Name	Nutrigroup	Serving Size	Nutripoints
Cherries, sweet, canned, water	Fruit	½ cup	5.5
Cherries, sweet, fresh	Fruit	10 whole	5.5
Cherries, sweet, frozen, sweetened	Fruit	½ cup	2.0
Chicken and Egg Noodles, w/Broccoli, frozen, Budget Gourmet	Meat/Fish/Poultry	½ portion	−2.0
Chicken a l'Orange, w/Almonds and Rice, frozen, Stouffer's	Meat/Fish/Poultry	1 portion	1.5
Chicken a la king	Meat/Fish/Poultry	½ cup	0.0
Chicken a la King w/Rice, Dining Lite	Meat/Fish/Poultry	1 cup	3.0
Chicken a la King, frozen, Weight Watchers	Meat/Fish/Poultry	1 portion	0.0
Chicken a la King, w/Rice, frozen, Stouffer's	Meat/Fish/Poultry	1 portion	0.0
Chicken and Pasta Divan, frozen, Healthy Choice	Meat/Fish/Poultry	1 portion	2.5
Chicken au Gratin, Slim, frozen, Budget Gourmet	Meat/Fish/Poultry	1 portion	2.0
Chicken Breast Portions, Fried, frozen, Swanson	Meat/Fish/Poultry	½ dinner	−2.0
Chicken breast, baked, w/o skin	Meat/Fish/Poultry	3 ounces	4.0
Chicken breast, batter-fried, w/skin	Meat/Fish/Poultry	3 ounces	1.0
Chicken breast, fried, w/o bread, w/skin	Meat/Fish/Poultry	3 ounces	2.5

Food Name	Nutrigroup	Serving Size	Nutripoints
Chicken breast, fried, w/o skin	Meat/Fish/Poultry	3 ounces	1.5
Chicken Breast, Glazed, frozen, Le Menu	Meat/Fish/Poultry	1 portion	1.5
Chicken Breast, Marsala w/Vegetables, frozen, Stouffer's	Meat/Fish/Poultry	1 portion	1.5
Chicken Cacciatore w/Vermicelli, frozen, Stouffer's	Meat/Fish/Poultry	1 portion	0.5
Chicken Cacciatore, frozen, Budget Gourmet	Meat/Fish/Poultry	½ portion	1.0
Chicken Chow Mein w/Rice, Dining Lite	Meat/Fish/Poultry	1 cup	1.5
Chicken Chow Mein, frozen, Chun King	Meat/Fish/Poultry	½ portion	1.5
Chicken Divan, frozen, Stouffer's	Meat/Fish/Poultry	½ piece	−1.0
Chicken fricassee	Meat/Fish/Poultry	½ cup	2.5
Chicken-fried steak	Meat/Fish/Poultry	2 ounces	0.0
Chicken Imperial, frozen, Chun King	Meat/Fish/Poultry	½ portion	3.0
Chicken Imperial, frozen, Weight Watchers	Meat/Fish/Poultry	1 portion	1.5
Chicken Italiano, frozen, Stouffer's Right Course	Meat/Fish/Poultry	1 portion	1.5
Chicken Kiev	Meat/Fish/Poultry	½ piece	0.0
Chicken leg, baked, w/o skin	Meat/Fish/Poultry	3 ounces	2.5
Chicken leg, fried, w/o bread, w/skin	Meat/Fish/Poultry	3 ounces	1.5
Chicken liver, stewed	Meat/Fish/Poultry	3 ounces	2.0
Chicken Oriental, frozen, Healthy Choice	Meat/Fish/Poultry	1 portion	3.5

Food Name	Nutrigroup	Serving Size	Nutripoints
Chicken Oriental, frozen, Stouffer's	Meat/Fish/Poultry	1 portion	0.5
Chicken Parmigiana Patty, frozen, Weight Watchers	Meat/Fish/Poultry	½ piece	−0.5
Chicken Parmigiana, frozen, Celentano	Meat/Fish/Poultry	½ portion	2.0
Chicken Parmigiana, frozen, Healthy Choice	Meat/Fish/Poultry	1 portion	3.5
Chicken Pie, frozen, Stouffer's	Meat/Fish/Poultry	½ piece	−0.5
Chicken pot pie	Meat/Fish/Poultry	½ pie	0.5
Chicken Pot Pie, frozen, Swanson	Meat/Fish/Poultry	½ pie	−1.0
Chicken Primavera, frozen, Celentano	Meat/Fish/Poultry	½ portion	6.0
Chicken salad	Meat/Fish/Poultry	½ cup	2.0
Chicken Salad, Nutripoint	Meat/Fish/Poultry	¾ cup	6.5
Chicken Stir-Fry, Nutripoint	Meat/Fish/Poultry	1 cup	8.5
Chicken Tenderloins in Barbecue Sauce, frozen, Stouffer's Right Course	Meat/Fish/Poultry	1 portion	2.5
Chicken Tenderloins in Peanut Sauce, frozen, Stouffer's Right Course	Meat/Fish/Poultry	1 portion	1.0
Chicken Tenders, Sweet 'n Sour, frozen, Weight Watchers	Meat/Fish/Poultry	1 portion	1.5
Chicken Teriyaki, frozen, Budget Gourmet	Meat/Fish/Poultry	½ portion	0.5

Food Name	Nutrigroup	Serving Size	Nutripoints
Chicken thigh, baked, w/o skin	Meat/Fish/Poultry	1 piece	1.0
Chicken thigh, fried, w/o breading	Meat/Fish/Poultry	3 ounces	2.0
Chicken thigh, meat and skin, baked	Meat/Fish/Poultry	1 piece	0.0
Chicken thigh, meat and skin, batter-fried	Meat/Fish/Poultry	1 piece	0.0
Chicken w/dumplings	Meat/Fish/Poultry	3/4 cup	2.0
Chicken wing, baked, w/o skin	Meat/Fish/Poultry	3 pieces	2.0
Chicken wing, fried, w/o breading	Meat/Fish/Poultry	2 pieces	0.0
Chicken wing, meat and skin, baked	Meat/Fish/Poultry	2 pieces	0.0
Chicken wing, meat and skin, batter-fried	Meat/Fish/Poultry	1 piece	−0.5
Chicken, Cajun, Nutripoint	Meat/Fish/Poultry	3 ounces	5.5
Chicken, canned	Meat/Fish/Poultry	1/2 cup	1.0
Chicken, Chunk White, Premium, canned, Swanson	Meat/Fish/Poultry	4 ounces	−0.5
Chicken, creamed	Meat/Fish/Poultry	1/2 cup	1.5
Chicken, Fried, Dinner, frozen, Morton	Meat/Fish/Poultry	1/2 portion	0.0
Chicken, Fried, Homestyle, frozen, Swanson	Meat/Fish/Poultry	1/2 portion	−1.0
Chicken, Fried, Low-Fat, Nutripoint	Meat/Fish/Poultry	4 ounces	3.0
Chicken, Fried, w/Corn, frozen, Morton	Meat/Fish/Poultry	1/2 piece	0.5
Chicken, frozen dinner	Meat/Fish/Poultry	1/2 portion	1.5
Chicken, Grilled, w/Mango Sauce, Nutripoint	Meat/Fish/Poultry	4 ounces	4.5

Food Name	Nutrigroup	Serving Size	Nutripoints
Chicken, Land O' Frost	Meat/Fish/Poultry	3 ounces	−5.0
Chicken, Lemon, Nutripoint	Meat/Fish/Poultry	4 ounces	3.5
Chicken, low-cal., frozen dinner	Meat/Fish/Poultry	½ portion	2.5
Chicken, Mandarin, Slim, frozen, Budget Gourmet	Meat/Fish/Poultry	1 portion	1.0
Chicken, Marinated, Hawaiian, Nutripoint	Meat/Fish/Poultry	4 ounces	3.5
Chicken, Pie, frozen, Morton	Meat/Fish/Poultry	½ portion	−0.5
Chicken, Sesame, frozen, Stouffer's Right Course	Meat/Fish/Poultry	1 portion	1.0
Chicken, Slices, frozen, Loma Linda	Legume/Nut/Seed	2 ounces	5.5
Chicken, Smoked, Sliced, Buddig	Meat/Fish/Poultry	3 ounces	−1.5
Chicken, Southern Fried Patty, frozen, Weight Watchers	Meat/Fish/Poultry	½ portion	−2.0
Chicken, sweet and sour	Meat/Fish/Poultry	½ cup	1.0
Chicken, Sweet and Sour, w/Rice, frozen Budget Gourmet	Meat/Fish/Poultry	½ portion	0.5
Chicken, Sweet and Sour, frozen, Healthy Choice	Meat/Fish/Poultry	1 portion	3.0
Chicken, White and Dark, Premium Chunk, canned, Swanson	Meat/Fish/Poultry	4 ounces	0.0

Food Name	Nutrigroup	Serving Size	Nutripoints
Chicken, w/Fettucini, frozen, Budget Gourmet	Meat/Fish/Poultry	½ piece	−1.0
Chicken, w/Vegetables and Vermicelli, frozen, Stouffer's	Meat/Fish/Poultry	1 portion	2.0
Chicory greens, raw	Vegetable	1 cup	35.5
Chili powder	Condiment	1 teaspoon	2.0
Chili Seasoning Mix, McCormick's	Condiment	1 teaspoon	0.5
Chili w/Beans, Spicy Vegetarian, Health Valley	Legume/Nut/Seed	1 cup	3.0
Chili w/Lentils, Vegetarian, Health Valley	Legume/Nut/Seed	½ cup	3.0
Chili, bean	Legume/Nut/Seed	½ cup	5.0
Chili, bean/beef	Legume/Nut/Seed	½ cup	1.0
Chili, South-of-the-Border Vegetarian, Nutripoint	Legume/Nut/Seed	¾ cup	13.0
Chili, Vegetarian, canned, Worthington	Legume/Nut/Seed	½ cup	4.0
Chili, Vegetarian, w/Rice, frozen, Stouffer's Right Course	Legume/Nut/Seed	½ portion	2.0
Chives, raw	Condiment	1 tablespoon	1.0
Chocolate eclair	Grain	½ piece	−2.0
Chocolate Eclair, Good Humor	Grain	1 piece	−3.5
Chocolate, baking	Sugar	1 ounce	−4.0
Chocolate, hot	Milk/Dairy	1 cup	0.0
Chocolate, semi-sweet	Sugar	1 ounce	−4.5
Chocolate, Semi-Sweet, Baker's	Sugar	1 ounce	−4.5

Food Name	Nutrigroup	Serving Size	Nutripoints
Chocolate, sweet or dark	Sugar	1 ounce	−4.5
Chocolate, Unsweetened, Baker's	Sugar	1 ounce	−3.0
Chop suey, beef/pork	Meat/Fish/Poultry	½ cup	0.5
Cinnamon	Condiment	1 teaspoon	1.0
Clams, breaded, fried	Meat/Fish/Poultry	3 ounces	4.5
Clams, canned	Meat/Fish/Poultry	1 cup	8.0
Clams, Fried in Light Batter, Mrs. Paul's	Meat/Fish/Poultry	3 ounces	−1.0
Clams, mixed species, raw	Meat/Fish/Poultry	6 ounces	13.5
Clams, smoked, canned in oil	Meat/Fish/Poultry	3 ounces	5.0
Clams, steamed/boiled	Meat/Fish/Poultry	6 ounces	6.0
Cloves	Condiment	1 teaspoon	0.5
Club soda	Miscellaneous	6 fluid ounces	0.0
Cocoa Mix, Chocolate, Quik, Nestlé	Milk/Dairy	½ cup	−2.0
Cocoa Mix, Hot, 70 Calorie, Carnation	Milk/Dairy	1 cup	1.0
Cocoa Mix, Hot, Regular, Swiss Miss	Milk/Dairy	1 cup	−1.5
Cocoa Mix, Hot, Sugar-Free, Carnation	Milk/Dairy	2 cups	3.0
Cocoa Mix, Hot, Sugar-Free, Swiss Miss	Milk/Dairy	1 ounce	4.0
Cocoa Mix, Chocolate Flavor Ovaltine	Milk/Dairy	½ cup	4.0
Cocoa Mix, Sugar-Free, Quik, Nestlé	Milk/Dairy	1 cup	2.5
Cocoa powder	Miscellaneous	1 tablespoon	0.5
Coconut	Fruit	1 tablespoon	−2.0
Coconut, chocolate-covered	Fruit	1 piece	−2.0

Food Name	Nutrigroup	Serving Size	Nutripoints
Coconut, dried, sweetened, shredded	Fruit	1 tablespoon	−4.0
Coconut, raw	Fruit	1 ounce	−3.5
Coconut, Shredded Premium, Baker's	Fruit	1 tablespoon	−3.5
Cod Fillets, Light, Mrs. Paul's	Meat/Fish/Poultry	1 piece	−0.5
Cod, baked	Meat/Fish/Poultry	4 ounces	3.5
Cod, floured/breaded, fried	Meat/Fish/Poultry	3 ounces	−0.5
Cod, smoked	Meat/Fish/Poultry	6 ounces	2.0
Coffee	Miscellaneous	1 cup	−3.5
Coffee, decaffeinated	Miscellaneous	1 cup	0.5
Coffee, International	Miscellaneous	1 tablespoon	−10.0
Coleslaw	Vegetable	½ cup	3.0
Coleslaw, Nutripoint	Vegetable	½ cup	10.0
Collard greens, fresh, cooked	Vegetable	1 cup	42.0
Collard greens, frozen, cooked	Vegetable	½ cup	40.0
Collard greens, raw, chopped	Vegetable	1 cup	42.5
Combination Dinner, frozen, Patio	Legume/Nut/Seed	½ portion	−0.5
Consommé	Miscellaneous	1 cup	0.5
Cookie Dough, Chocolate Chip, Pillsbury	Grain	2 cookies	−3.5
Cookies	Grain	2 cookies	−4.0
Cookies, Animal, Oat Bran, Health Valley	Grain	10 pieces	4.0
Cookies, applesauce	Grain	2 cookies	−2.0
Cookies, Bordeaux, Pepperidge Farm	Grain	3 cookies	−4.0
Cookies, Buttercup, Keebler	Grain	4 cookies	−2.0
Cookies, Chessmen, Pepperidge Farm	Grain	3 cookies	−4.0

Food Name	Nutrigroup	Serving Size	Nutripoints
Cookies, Chips Deluxe, Keebler	Grain	2 cookies	−3.0
Cookies, chocolate chip	Grain	2 cookies	−4.0
Cookies, Chocolate Chip Oatmeal, Pillsbury	Grain	1 cookie	−3.5
Cookies, Chocolate Chip, Duncan Hines	Grain	2 cookies	−3.5
Cookies, Chocolate Chip, Pepperidge Farm	Grain	3 cookies	−4.0
Cookies, Chocolate Fudge Sandwich, Keebler	Grain	2 cookies	−1.5
Cookies, Commodore, Keebler	Grain	2 cookies	0.0
Cookies, French Vanilla Creme, Keebler	Grain	2 cookies	−1.5
Cookies, Fruit Chunks, Health Valley	Grain	3 cookies	3.0
Cookies, Gingersnaps	Grain	6 pieces	−1.0
Cookies, Homeplate, Keebler	Grain	2 cookies	−2.0
Cookies, Keebies, Keebler	Grain	2 cookies	−1.5
Cookies, Lemon Creme, Keebler	Grain	4 cookies	−1.5
Cookies, macaroon	Grain	2 cookies	−2.0
Cookies, Milano Distinctive, Pepperidge Farm	Grain	3 cookies	−3.5
Cookies, molasses	Grain	2 cookies	−2.0
Cookies, Nilla Wafers, Nabisco	Grain	7 cookies	−1.5
Cookies, O.F. Chocolate Chip, Keebler	Grain	2 cookies	−2.0

Food Name	Nutrigroup	Serving Size	Nutripoints
Cookies, O.F. Double Fudge, Keebler	Grain	2 cookies	−2.0
Cookies, O.F. Granola, large, Pepperidge Farm	Grain	1 cookie	−3.0
Cookies, O.F. Oatmeal, Keebler	Grain	2 cookies	−1.5
Cookies, O.F. Sugar, Keebler	Grain	2 cookies	−1.5
Cookies, oatmeal	Grain	2 cookies	−1.5
Cookies, Oatmeal Creme Sandwich, Keebler	Grain	2 cookies	−2.5
Cookies, Oatmeal Raisin, Pepperidge Farm	Grain	3 cookies	−3.0
Cookies, Oreo, Nabisco	Grain	2 cookies	−2.5
Cookies, peanut butter	Legume/Nut/Seed	2 pieces	−1.0
Cookies, Peanut Butter 'n Fudge, Duncan Hines	Grain	2 cookies	−3.5
Cookies, Pirouettes, Chocolate-Laced, Pepperidge Farm	Grain	3 cookies	−4.5
Cookies, Pitter Patter, Keebler	Grain	2 cookies	−1.5
Cookies, sandwich, chocolate/vanilla	Grain	2 cookies	−2.5
Cookies, Sandwich, Mystic Mint, Nabisco	Grain	2 cookies	−4.0
Cookies, sugar	Grain	1 cookie	−1.0
Cookies, vanilla wafers	Grain	6 cookies	−3.0
Cookies, Vanilla Wafers, Keebler	Grain	5 cookies	−1.5
Cordials/Liqueurs	Alcohol	1½ fluid ounces	−8.5
Coriander, raw	Condiment	¼ cup	0.5

Food Name	Nutrigroup	Serving Size	Nutripoints
Corn chips	Grain	15 pieces	−0.5
Corn Chips, Fritos	Vegetable	17 pieces	−1.0
Corn dog	Meat/Fish/Poultry	½ piece	−1.0
Corn meal, dry	Grain	¼ cup	3.5
Corn Meal, Yellow Enriched, Aunt Jemima	Grain	¼ cup	3.5
Corn on cob, fresh, cooked	Vegetable	½ piece	6.0
Corn Puffs, Cheese, Cheez Doodles, Borden	Grain	1 ounce	−1.5
Corn w/red and green peppers, canned	Vegetable	½ cup	5.0
Corn, 50-Percent Less Salt, canned, Green Giant	Vegetable	½ cup	3.0
Corn, canned	Vegetable	½ cup	4.5
Corn, Cream Style, canned, Green Giant	Vegetable	½ cup	−0.5
Corn, Cream Style, Golden Sweet, canned, Del Monte	Vegetable	½ cup	0.0
Corn, creamed, canned	Vegetable	½ cup	4.5
Corn, fried, w/breading	Vegetable	¼ piece	−0.5
Corn, frozen, cooked	Vegetable	½ cup	8.0
Corn, Golden, Family Style, No Salt, canned, Del Monte	Vegetable	½ cup	6.0
Corn, Little Ears, frozen, Birds Eye	Vegetable	1 package	7.0
Corn, Niblets, in butter, frozen, Green Giant	Vegetable	½ cup	1.5
Corn, Sweet, frozen, Birds Eye	Vegetable	½ cup	6.0

Food Name	Nutrigroup	Serving Size	Nutripoints
Corn, Sweet, in Butter Sauce, frozen, Budget Gourmet	Vegetable	1/3 piece	−0.5
Corn, Whole Kernel, canned, Del Monte	Vegetable	1/2 cup	2.0
Corn, Whole Kernel, canned, Green Giant	Vegetable	1/2 cup	2.5
Cornbread	Grain	1 piece	1.0
Cornbread, Southern, Nutripoint	Grain	1 piece	2.0
Corned beef	Meat/Fish/Poultry	3 ounces	−2.5
Corned Beef, Libby's	Meat/Fish/Poultry	3 ounces	−2.0
Corned Beef, Smoked, Sliced, Buddig	Meat/Fish/Poultry	3 ounces	−2.0
Cornstarch	Miscellaneous	1 tablespoon	0.0
Cowpeas, cooked	Legume/Nut/Seed	1 cup	8.0
Crab cake	Meat/Fish/Poultry	3 ounces	−3.5
Crab salad	Meat/Fish/Poultry	1/2 cup	−1.0
Crab, canned	Meat/Fish/Poultry	6 ounces	1.0
Crab, hard-shell, steamed	Meat/Fish/Poultry	6 ounces	4.5
Crab, soft-shell, fried	Meat/Fish/Poultry	3 ounces	−1.0
Cracker Meal, Keebler	Grain	1/4 cup	2.5
Cracker, 7 Grain Vegetable, Stone-Ground Wheat, Health Valley	Grain	6 pieces	1.0
Cracker, Amaranth Graham, Health Valley	Grain	4 pieces	1.0
Cracker, Cheese and Peanut Butter, Keebler	Grain	3 pieces	−0.5
Cracker, Crispbread Breakfast, Wasa	Grain	2 pieces	2.5
Cracker, Crispbread Dark Rye, Ryvita	Grain	4 pieces	3.0

Food Name	Nutrigroup	Serving Size	Nutripoints
Cracker, Crispbread Dark, Finn	Grain	6 pieces	2.5
Cracker, Crispbread Fiber Plus, Wasa	Grain	3 pieces	7.5
Cracker, Crispbread Golden Rye, Wasa	Grain	3 pieces	4.0
Cracker, Crispbread Hearty Rye, Wasa	Grain	3 pieces	3.5
Cracker, Crispbread Light and Natural, Krispen	Grain	8 pieces	2.5
Cracker, Crispbread Lite Rye, Wasa	Grain	4 pieces	2.0
Cracker, Graham, Honey Maid	Grain	4 pieces	0.5
Cracker, graham, plain	Grain	2 pieces	0.0
Cracker, Harvest Wheat, Keebler	Grain	6 pieces	0.0
Cracker, Hearty Wheat, Pepperidge Farm	Grain	4 pieces	−1.0
Cracker, Honey Graham, Health Valley	Grain	2 pieces	1.5
Cracker, matzo	Grain	1 piece	2.5
Cracker, melba toast	Grain	4 pieces	1.0
Cracker, Melba Toast, Garlic, Keebler	Grain	10 pieces	1.0
Cracker, Melba Toast, Onion, Keebler	Grain	10 pieces	1.0
Cracker, Melba Toast, plain, Keebler	Grain	10 pieces	1.0
Cracker, Melba Toast, Sesame, Keebler	Grain	10 pieces	0.5
Cracker, Melba Toast, White, Old London	Grain	6 pieces	2.0
Cracker, Norwegian Crispbread, Thick Style, Kavli	Grain	3 pieces	2.5

Food Name	Nutrigroup	Serving Size	Nutripoints
Cracker, Oat Bran Graham, Health Valley	Grain	7 pieces	0.5
Cracker, Oat Bran Krisp, Ralston	Grain	4 pieces	1.0
Cracker, Original Tiny Goldfish, Pepperidge Farm	Grain	45 pieces	−1.0
Cracker, peanut butter sandwich	Legume/Nut/Seed	2 pieces	0.0
Cracker, Petite Butter Crescents, Pepperidge Farm	Grain	1 piece	−0.5
Cracker, rice cake	Grain	4 pieces	1.5
Cracker, rice, small	Grain	10 pieces	0.5
Cracker, Ritz	Grain	8 pieces	−1.0
Cracker, Rykrisp, Ralston	Grain	6 pieces	5.0
Cracker, Saltine	Grain	8 pieces	1.0
Cracker, Saltine, Low-Sodium	Grain	10 pieces	1.0
Cracker, Saltine, Premium	Grain	10 pieces	0.5
Cracker, Sea Toast, Keebler	Grain	2 pieces	1.0
Cracker, Seasoned, Rykrisp	Grain	6 pieces	3.0
Cracker, Snackbread, High-Fiber, Ryvita	Grain	8 pieces	9.0
Cracker, soda	Grain	10 pieces	0.5
Cracker, Toast and Peanut Butter, Keebler	Grain	4 pieces	−1.0
Cracker, Triscuit	Grain	6 pieces	−0.5
Cracker, Wheat Thins	Grain	16 pieces	−0.5
Cracker, Wheat Vegetable, Stone-Ground, Hain	Grain	11 pieces	1.0
Cracker, whole wheat	Grain	8 pieces	3.0

Food Name	Nutrigroup	Serving Size	Nutripoints
Crackers, animal	Grain	10 pieces	−1.5
Crackers, Animal, Barnum's	Grain	10 pieces	−1.5
Crackers, Cheese Nips, Nabisco	Grain	20 pieces	0.5
Crackers, Oat Thins, Nabisco	Grain	12 pieces	0.5
Crackers, Oyster, Large, Keebler	Grain	26 pieces	0.5
Crackers, Oyster, small	Grain	50 pieces	1.0
Crackers, Oyster, Small, Keebler	Grain	50 pieces	1.0
Cranberries, raw	Fruit	1 cup	10.0
Cream, coffee, light	Milk/Dairy	2 tablespoons	−6.0
Cream, half-and-half	Milk/Dairy	¼ cup	−3.0
Cream, heavy	Milk/Dairy	2 tablespoons	−7.0
Cream, Nondairy, Coffee Mate, Carnation	Milk/Dairy	2 tablespoons	−3.5
Cream, Nondairy, Cremora	Milk/Dairy	2 tablespoons	−4.5
Cream, nondairy, imitation, liquid	Milk/Dairy	2 tablespoons	−4.0
Cream, nondairy, imitation, liquid (vegetable oil)	Milk/Dairy	2 tablespoons	−1.5
Cream, nondairy, imitation, powder	Milk/Dairy	2 tablespoons	−3.0
Cream, Nondairy, Mocha Mix	Milk/Dairy	¼ cup	−2.0
Cream, sour	Milk/Dairy	¼ cup	−3.5
Cream, Sour, Blend, Weight Watchers	Milk/Dairy	¼ cup	1.0
Cream, sour, imitation	Milk/Dairy	2 tablespoons	−5.5
Cream, Sour, Light, Dairy Blend, Land O Lakes	Milk/Dairy	¼ cup	−1.5

Food Name	Nutrigroup	Serving Size	Nutripoints
Cream, Sour, New Way, Nutripoint	Milk/Dairy	¼ cup	6.5
Cream, Sour, Slender Choice	Milk/Dairy	¼ cup	−1.0
Cream, Soy, Solait, Miller Farms	Legume/Nut/Seed	4 fluid ounces	−1.0
Cream, whipped	Milk/Dairy	¼ cup	−6.5
Cream, whipping, light	Milk/Dairy	2 tablespoons	−6.5
Cress, garden, cooked	Vegetable	1 cup	39.5
Crisco, Butter Flavored	Fat/Oil	1 tablespoon	−3.0
Croissant	Grain	1 croissant	−2.5
Croutons	Grain	½ cup	2.0
Croutons, Cheddar and Romano Cheese, Pepperidge Farm	Grain	½ cup	1.0
Cucumber, raw	Vegetable	1 piece	20.0
Cupcake, Chocolate, Hostess	Grain	1 piece	−3.0
Cupcake, w/frosting	Grain	1 piece	−4.0
Cupcake, w/o frosting	Grain	1 piece	−3.5
Currants, black	Fruit	¾ cup	19.0
Currants, zante	Fruit	¼ cup	4.5
Currants, Zante, Sun-Maid	Fruit	¼ cup	3.5
Curry powder	Condiment	1 teaspoon	0.5
Custard	Milk/Dairy	½ cup	−4.0
Daiquiri	Alcohol	3 fluid ounces	−14.5
Dairy Queen All-White Chicken Nuggets	Meat/Fish/Poultry	1 piece	−0.5
Dairy Queen Buster Bar	Milk/Dairy	¼ piece	−3.5
Dairy Queen Chicken Breast Fillet	Meat/Fish/Poultry	½ piece	0.0
Dairy Queen Chicken Breast Fillet w/Cheese	Meat/Fish/Poultry	½ piece	0.0
Dairy Queen Chipper Sandwich	Milk/Dairy	¼ serving	−1.5

Food Name	Nutrigroup	Serving Size	Nutripoints
Dairy Queen Cone, medium	Milk/Dairy	½ piece	−1.0
Dairy Queen Dilly Bar	Milk/Dairy	½ piece	−3.5
Dairy Queen Dipped Cone, medium	Milk/Dairy	½ piece	−3.5
Dairy Queen Double Hamburger	Meat/Fish/Poultry	½ piece	0.5
Dairy Queen Double Hamburger w/Cheese	Meat/Fish/Poultry	½ piece	0.5
Dairy Queen DQ Sandwich	Milk/Dairy	1 piece	−2.5
Dairy Queen Fish Fillet Sandwich	Meat/Fish/Poultry	½ piece	1.0
Dairy Queen Fish Fillet w/Cheese Sandwich	Meat/Fish/Poultry	½ piece	1.0
Dairy Queen Float	Milk/Dairy	½ cup	−4.0
Dairy Queen Freeze (1 cup)	Milk/Dairy	¼ cup	−1.5
Dairy Queen Frozen Dessert	Milk/Dairy	4 ounces	0.0
Dairy Queen Fudge Nut Bar	Grain	¼ bar	−2.0
Dairy Queen Heath Blizzard	Milk/Dairy	¼ serving	−1.5
Dairy Queen Hot Dog	Meat/Fish/Poultry	1 piece	−1.0
Dairy Queen Hot Dog w/Cheese	Meat/Fish/Poultry	½ piece	−1.5
Dairy Queen Hot Dog w/Chili	Meat/Fish/Poultry	½ piece	−1.0
Dairy Queen Hounder	Meat/Fish/Poultry	½ piece	−2.0
Dairy Queen Hounder w/Cheese	Meat/Fish/Poultry	½ piece	−2.0
Dairy Queen Hounder w/Chili	Meat/Fish/Poultry	½ piece	−1.5
Dairy Queen Malt, medium	Milk/Dairy	¼ cup	−1.5

Food Name	Nutrigroup	Serving Size	Nutripoints
Dairy Queen Mr. Misty, medium (1 cup)	Sugar	1/2 cup	−5.5
Dairy Queen Mr. Misty Float	Milk/Dairy	1/2 cup	−3.5
Dairy Queen Mr. Misty Freeze	Milk/Dairy	1/4 cup	−3.5
Dairy Queen Mr. Misty Kiss (1/2 cup)	Sugar	1 cup	−5.5
Dairy Queen Parfait	Milk/Dairy	1/4 cup	−1.5
Dairy Queen Peanut Buster Parfait	Milk/Dairy	1/4 cup	−3.5
Dairy Queen Shake, medium	Milk/Dairy	1/4 cup	−2.5
Dairy Queen Single Hamburger	Meat/Fish/Poultry	1/2 piece	0.5
Dairy Queen Single Hamburger w/Cheese	Meat/Fish/Poultry	1/2 piece	0.5
Dairy Queen Sundae, medium	Milk/Dairy	1/2 serving	−2.5
Dairy Queen Triple Hamburger	Meat/Fish/Poultry	1/4 piece	0.0
Dairy Queen Triple Hamburger w/Cheese	Meat/Fish/Poultry	1/4 piece	0.0
Dandelion greens, cooked	Vegetable	3/4 cup	40.0
Dandelion greens, raw	Vegetable	1 cup	44.5
Danish pastry	Grain	1/2 pastry	−2.5
Danish, Apple, Pillsbury	Grain	1/2 Danish	−2.0
Danish, Swiss Cheese, Borden	Grain	2 whole	0.5
Dates	Fruit	5 pieces	4.0
Dill weed	Condiment	1 teaspoon	0.5
Dip, bean	Legume/Nut/Seed	2 tablespoons	3.5

Food Name	Nutrigroup	Serving Size	Nutripoints
Dip, Black Bean, Nutripoint	Legume/Nut/Seed	¼ cup	8.0
Dip, clam	Fat/Oil	2 tablespoons	−0.5
Dip, Guacamole, Slim, Nutripoint	Fat/Oil	¼ cup	7.5
Dip, onion	Fat/Oil	1 tablespoon	−5.0
Domino's Large 16-Inch Cheese Pizza	Grain	1 piece	1.5
Domino's Large 16-Inch Deluxe Pizza	Grain	½ piece	0.5
Domino's Large 16-Inch Double Cheese and Pepperoni Pizza	Grain	½ piece	0.5
Domino's Large 16-Inch Ham Pizza	Grain	½ piece	1.0
Domino's Large 16-Inch Pepperoni Pizza	Grain	½ piece	1.0
Domino's Large 16-Inch Sausage and Mushroom Pizza	Grain	½ piece	1.5
Domino's Large 16-Inch Veggie Pizza	Grain	½ piece	1.0
Doughnut, cake w/frosting	Grain	1 doughnut	−2.5
Doughnut, cake w/o frosting	Grain	1 doughnut	−2.0
Doughnut, chocolate creme filled	Grain	½ doughnut	−3.0
Doughnut, chocolate, w/chocolate icing	Grain	½ doughnut	−2.5
Doughnut, custard filled	Grain	½ doughnut	−3.0
Doughnut, Devil's Food, Earth Grains	Grain	½ doughnut	−3.0

Food Name	Nutrigroup	Serving Size	Nutripoints
Doughnut, glazed	Grain	1 doughnut	−2.5
Doughnut, jelly	Grain	½ doughnut	−3.0
Doughnut, Old-Fashioned, Glazed, Earth Grains	Grain	½ doughnut	−3.0
Doughnut, whole wheat	Grain	1 doughnut	−1.5
Dressing, blue cheese	Fat/Oil	2 tablespoons	−3.0
Dressing, Caper, Nutripoint	Fat/Oil	2 tablespoons	2.0
Dressing, French	Fat/Oil	2 tablespoons	−3.0
Dressing, French, Catalina, Kraft	Fat/Oil	1 tablespoon	−2.0
Dressing, French, Free Kraft	Condiment	1 tablespoon	−1.0
Dressing, French, home recipe	Fat/Oil	1 tablespoon	−3.0
Dressing, French, Kraft	Fat/Oil	1 tablespoon	−2.5
Dressing, Green Goddess	Fat/Oil	2 tablespoons	−3.0
Dressing, Honey Yogurt, Nutripoint	Milk/Dairy	¼ cup	2.0
Dressing, Italian	Fat/Oil	2 tablespoons	−2.5
Dressing, Italian, Free, Kraft	Condiment	1 tablespoon	−0.5
Dressing, Italian, Light, Bernstein's	Condiment	1 tablespoon	−0.5
Dressing, Lite, 16-Island, Nutripoint	Fat/Oil	¼ cup	2.5
Dressing, Lite, Blue Cheese, Nutripoint	Fat/Oil	¼ cup	8.0
Dressing, Lite, Ranch, Nutripoint	Fat/Oil	¼ cup	3.5
Dressing, Lite, Zero, Nutripoint	Condiment	2 tablespoons	1.0
Dressing, low-cal., blue cheese	Fat/Oil	2 tablespoons	−4.5

Food Name	Nutrigroup	Serving Size	Nutripoints
Dressing, low-cal., French	Fat/Oil	2 tablespoons	−1.5
Dressing, mayonnaise type	Fat/Oil	1 tablespoon	−2.5
Dressing, Mustard, Spicy, Nutripoint	Condiment	1 tablespoon	0.5
Dressing, oil and vinegar	Fat/Oil	1 tablespoon	−3.0
Dressing, Oil and Vinegar, Kraft	Fat/Oil	1 tablespoon	−3.5
Dressing, Ranch, Free, Kraft	Condiment	1 tablespoon	−0.5
Dressing, Ranch, Take Heart, Hidden Valley	Condiment	1 tablespoon	−1.0
Dressing, ranch/buttermilk	Fat/Oil	2 tablespoons	−3.5
Dressing, Russian	Fat/Oil	2 tablespoons	−2.5
Dressing, Russian, low-cal.	Fat/Oil	2 tablespoons	−0.5
Dressing, salad	Fat/Oil	2 tablespoons	−3.5
Dressing, salad, low-cal.	Fat/Oil	2 tablespoons	−1.0
Dressing, Salad, Miracle Whip, Kraft	Fat/Oil	1 tablespoon	−3.0
Dressing, Salad, Reduced Calorie, Miracle Whip	Fat/Oil	1 tablespoon	−3.5
Dressing, Thousand Island	Fat/Oil	2 tablespoons	−3.0
Dressing, Thousand Island, low-cal.	Fat/Oil	2 tablespoons	−2.5
Dressing, Vinaigrette, Lite, Nutripoint	Fat/Oil	2 tablespoons	−1.5
Dressing, Vinaigrette, Orange, Nutripoint	Fat/Oil	2 tablespoons	2.5
Dressing, yogurt	Milk/Dairy	2 tablespoons	0.5

Food Name	Nutrigroup	Serving Size	Nutripoints
Drink Mix, Grape, Sugar-Free, Kool-Aid	Miscellaneous	8 fluid ounces	2.0
Drink Mix, Orange, Sugar-Free, Crystal Light	Miscellaneous	8 fluid ounces	1.0
Drink Mix, Rainbow Punch, Sweetened, Kool-Aid	Sugar	8 fluid ounces	−4.0
Drink Mix, Strawberry, Sweetened, Kool-Aid	Sugar	8 fluid ounces	−5.0
Drink Mix, Tropical Punch, Sugar-Free, Kool-Aid	Miscellaneous	8 fluid ounces	1.5
Duck, baked, w/o skin	Meat/Fish/Poultry	3 ounces	1.5
Duck, meat and skin, baked	Meat/Fish/Poultry	3 ounces	−1.0
Eel	Meat/Fish/Poultry	3 ounces	1.5
Eel, smoked	Meat/Fish/Poultry	3 ounces	1.5
Egg foo young	Milk/Dairy	½ cup	−7.0
Egg McMuffin, McDonald's	Milk/Dairy	½ serving	−1.5
Egg McMuffin, w/Sausage, McDonald's	Milk/Dairy	¼ serving	−1.5
Egg noodles, cooked (1⅛ cups = 2 ounces dry)	Grain	½ cup	1.5
Egg Noodles, Creamette, Borden	Grain	½ cup	−2.0
Egg roll	Grain	½ piece	−1.5
Egg Rolls, Chicken, frozen, Chun King	Meat/Fish/Poultry	1 portion	0.0
Egg Rolls, Restaurant, frozen, Chun King	Meat/Fish/Poultry	1 portion	2.0
Egg Rolls, Shrimp, frozen, Chun King	Meat/Fish/Poultry	1 portion	0.0

Food Name	Nutrigroup	Serving Size	Nutripoints
Egg Rolls, Shrimp/Meat, frozen, Chun King	Meat/Fish/Poultry	1 piece	−0.5
Egg salad	Milk/Dairy	¼ cup	−9.0
Egg Substitute, Egg Beaters w/Cheez, Fleischmann's	Milk/Dairy	4 ounces	6.0
Egg Substitute, Egg Beaters, Fleischmann's	Milk/Dairy	½ cup	17.5
Egg Substitue, Egg Beaters, Vegetable Omelette Mix, Fleischmanns	Milk/Dairy	½ cup	13.0
Egg Substitute, Egg Watchers, Tofutti	Milk/Dairy	½ serving	10.0
Egg Substitute, Scramblers	Milk/Dairy	½ cup	10.0
Egg Substitute, Second Nature	Milk/Dairy	½ cup	4.5
Egg white	Milk/Dairy	6 whites	6.0
Egg yolk	Milk/Dairy	2 yolks	−15.0
Egg, boiled	Milk/Dairy	2 eggs	−11.5
Egg, deviled (1 piece = whole egg)	Milk/Dairy	1 egg	−10.5
Egg, fried	Milk/Dairy	1 egg	−12.5
Egg, hard	Milk/Dairy	2 eggs	−11.5
Egg, omelet, w/ham/cheese (1 piece = 3 eggs)	Milk/Dairy	½ serving	−8.0
Egg, poached	Milk/Dairy	2 eggs	−11.5
Egg, scrambled	Milk/Dairy	1 egg	−13.5
Egg, Scrambled, Garden, Egg Beaters, Nutripoint	Milk/Dairy	¾ cup	23.5
Egg, Scrambled, Garden, Nutripoint	Milk/Dairy	¾ cup	5.5
Eggnog	Milk/Dairy	½ cup	−2.0

Food Name	Nutrigroup	Serving Size	Nutripoints
Eggplant Parmigiana, frozen, Celentano	Vegetable	1/4 portion	3.0
Eggplant Rollettes, frozen, Celentano	Vegetable	1/4 portion	4.0
Eggplant, cooked	Vegetable	1/2 cup	17.0
Enchiladas Ranchero, Cheese, frozen, Weight Watchers	Milk/Dairy	1/2 portion	−1.0
Enchiladas, Suiza, Chicken, Van de Kamp's	Meat/Fish/Poultry	1 piece	−1.0
Enchiladas, bean/cheese	Legume/Nut/Seed	1/2 piece	0.0
Enchiladas, beef/cheese	Legume/Nut/Seed	1/2 portion	4.0
Enchiladas, Beef Dinner, frozen, Patio	Meat/Fish/Poultry	1/2 portion	−0.5
Enchiladas, Beef Ranchero, frozen, Weight Watchers	Meat/Fish/Poultry	1/2 portion	0.0
Enchiladas, Beef, Shredded, Van de Kamp's	Meat/Fish/Poultry	5 1/2 ounces	−2.5
Enchiladas, Cheese Dinner, frozen, Patio	Milk/Dairy	1/2 portion	1.0
Enchiladas, Cheese Ranchero, frozen, Weight Watchers	Milk/Dairy	1/2 portion	−0.5
Enchiladas, Cheese Ranchero, Van de Kamp's	Legume/Nut/Seed	1/3 portion	−1.0
Enchiladas, chicken w/sour cream sauce	Legume/Nut/Seed	1/2 portion	0.5
Enchiladas, Chicken, Nutripoint	Meat/Fish/Poultry	2 pieces	5.0

Food Name	Nutrigroup	Serving Size	Nutripoints
Enchiladas, Chicken, Suiza, frozen, Weight Watchers	Meat/Fish/Poultry	½ portion	−0.5
Enchiladas, Chicken, Suiza, Slim, frozen, Budget Gourmet	Meat/Fish/Poultry	1 portion	0.5
Enchiladas, Mexican, legume	Legume/Nut/Seed	½ portion	5.5
Enchiladas, Sirloin, Ranchero, slim, frozen, Budget Gourmet	Meat/Fish/Poultry	1 portion	1.0
Endive, raw	Condiment	¼ cup	1.0
Ensure	Milk/Dairy	6 fluid ounces	5.5
Ensure Plus	Milk/Dairy	4 fluid ounces	6.0
Equal	Condiment	1 packet	0.0
Fajita, beef	Meat/Fish/Poultry	1 piece	1.5
Fajita, Beef, Weight Watchers	Meat/Fish/Poultry	½ portion	0.5
Fajita, chicken	Meat/Fish/Poultry	1 piece	1.0
Fajita, Chicken, frozen, Weight Watchers	Meat/Fish/Poultry	1 piece	0.5
Farina, cooked	Grain	1 cup	2.5
Fat, beef tallow	Fat/Oil	1 tablespoon	−6.5
Fat, chicken	Fat/Oil	1 tablespoon	−4.5
Fat, duck	Fat/Oil	1 tablespoon	−4.5
Fat, goose	Fat/Oil	1 tablespoon	−4.0
Fat, mutton tallow	Fat/Oil	1 tablespoon	−5.5
Fat, turkey	Fat/Oil	1 tablespoon	−4.5
Fettucini Primavera, frozen, Stouffer's	Grain	½ portion	−2.0
Fettucini w/Meat Sauce, Slim, frozen, Budget Gourmet	Grain	½ portion	1.5
Fettucini, Chicken, frozen, Weight Watchers	Grain	½ portion	−1.0

Food Name	Nutrigroup	Serving Size	Nutripoints
Fettucini, cooked (1 cup = 2 ounces dry)	Grain	½ cup	1.0
Fettucini, Garden Gourmet, frozen, Green Giant	Grain	½ cup	2.5
Fiesta Dinner, frozen, Patio	Legume/Nut/Seed	½ portion	−0.5
Fig Newton, Nabisco	Grain	2 pieces	−2.0
Figs, Calimyrna, Sun-Maid	Fruit	2 pieces	4.0
Figs, dried	Fruit	2 pieces	5.0
Figs, fresh	Fruit	1 whole	4.0
Figs, Mission, Sun-Maid	Fruit	2 pieces	4.5
Filberts, dry roasted, salted	Legume/Nut/Seed	1 ounce	−1.5
Filberts, oil roasted, salted	Legume/Nut/Seed	1 ounce	0.5
Fish amondine, frozen dinner	Meat/Fish/Poultry	1 portion	−1.5
Fish Dinner, frozen, Morton	Meat/Fish/Poultry	½ portion	2.0
Fish Fillet au Gratin, frozen, Weight Watchers	Meat/Fish/Poultry	1 portion	0.5
Fish Fillet, Batter-Dipped, frozen, Mrs. Paul's	Meat/Fish/Poultry	1 piece	−1.0
Fish Fillet, Crispy Crunchy, frozen, Mrs. Paul's	Meat/Fish/Poultry	1 piece	−1.5
Fish Fillet, Divan, frozen, Stouffer's	Meat/Fish/Poultry	1 portion	1.5
Fish Fillet, Florentine, frozen, Stouffer's	Meat/Fish/Poultry	1 piece	−0.5
Fish Fillet, Light Recipe, frozen, Gorton's	Meat/Fish/Poultry	4 ounces	−1.0

Food Name	Nutrigroup	Serving Size	Nutripoints
Fish Sandwich, Whaler, Burger King	Meat/Fish/Poultry	½ piece	0.0
Fish sticks	Meat/Fish/Poultry	4 pieces	0.5
Fish Sticks, Crispy Crunchy, Mrs. Paul's	Meat/Fish/Poultry	3¾ ounces	−1.5
Fish Sticks, Crunchy, frozen, Mrs. Paul's	Meat/Fish/Poultry	4 ounces	−1.0
Fish, Crunchy, Nutripoint	Meat/Fish/Poultry	3 ounces	6.5
Fish, fried	Meat/Fish/Poultry	3 ounces	0.5
Fish, sandwich (fast-food)	Meat/Fish/Poultry	½ piece	1.0
Fish, smoked	Meat/Fish/Poultry	3 ounces	3.5
Fish, w/Chips, frozen, Morton	Meat/Fish/Poultry	½ portion	2.0
Flounder Fillet, Light, Mrs. Paul's	Meat/Fish/Poultry	1 piece	−1.0
Flounder, baked	Meat/Fish/Poultry	3 ounces	3.5
Flounder, fillet, breaded, fried	Meat/Fish/Poultry	3 ounces	−0.5
Flour, All-Purpose Enriched, Pillsbury	Grain	¼ cup	3.0
Flour, All-Purpose, Gold Medal	Grain	¼ cup	3.0
Flour, Ezekiel, Arrowhead Mills	Grain	¼ cup	4.0
Flour, potato	Vegetable	¼ cup	5.5
Flour, Rye, Medium, Pillsbury	Grain	¼ cup	2.5
Flour, rye, whole grain	Grain	¼ cup	4.0
Flour, soybean	Grain	¼ cup	2.5
Flour, Triticale, Whole, Arrowhead Mills	Grain	¼ cup	4.0
Flour, white	Grain	¼ cup	3.0
Flour, White, All-Purpose Plain, Martha	Grain	¼ cup	3.0

Food Name	Nutrigroup	Serving Size	Nutripoints
Flour, whole buckwheat	Grain	¼ cup	3.5
Flour, whole wheat	Grain	¼ cup	6.0
Flour, Whole Wheat, Gold Medal	Grain	¼ cup	5.5
Flour, Whole Wheat, Pillsbury	Grain	¼ cup	3.5
Frankfurter, Ball Park	Meat/Fish/Poultry	1 piece	−4.0
Frankfurter, beef	Meat/Fish/Poultry	1 piece	−2.5
Frankfurter, Beef, Armour	Meat/Fish/Poultry	1 piece	−4.0
Frankfurter, Beef, Ball Park	Meat/Fish/Poultry	1 piece	−4.0
Frankfurter, Beef, Eckrich	Meat/Fish/Poultry	1 piece	−3.5
Frankfurter, Beef, Original Brown and Serve, Swift	Meat/Fish/Poultry	1 piece	−3.0
Frankfurter, Beef, Oscar Mayer	Meat/Fish/Poultry	1 piece	−3.5
Frankfurter, Bryan	Meat/Fish/Poultry	1 piece	−2.5
Frankfurter, Chicken, Tyson	Meat/Fish/Poultry	1 piece	−3.5
Frankfurter, chicken, w/bun	Meat/Fish/Poultry	1 piece	−1.0
Frankfurter, Eckrich	Meat/Fish/Poultry	1 piece	−3.5
Frankfurter, Linketts, Loma Linda	Legume/Nut/Seed	1 piece	5.0
Frankfurter, Oscar Mayer	Meat/Fish/Poultry	1 piece	−3.0
Frankfurter, Pork, Original Brown and Serve, Swift	Meat/Fish/Poultry	1 piece	−3.5
Frankfurter, pork and beef	Meat/Fish/Poultry	1 piece	−3.5
Frankfurter, pork and beef, w/bun	Meat/Fish/Poultry	½ piece	−0.5
Frankfurter, turkey	Meat/Fish/Poultry	1 piece	−3.5
Frankfurter, w/Cheese, Oscar Mayer	Meat/Fish/Poultry	1 piece	−3.0

Food Name	Nutrigroup	Serving Size	Nutripoints
French fries (18 pieces = ½ cup)	Vegetable	4 pieces	1.0
French toast	Grain	1 slice	−2.5
French Toast, Nutripoint	Grain	1½ slices	0.5
Fried cheese sticks	Milk/Dairy	4 pieces	−4.5
Frog legs, fried	Meat/Fish/Poultry	2 pieces	−2.0
Frosting	Sugar	2 tablespoons	−4.5
Frosting, chocolate	Sugar	2 tablespoons	−4.5
Frozen Dessert, Banana, Creamy, Frozfruit	Fruit	½ cup	−1.5
Frozen Dessert, Banana, Pudding Pops, Jell-O	Fruit	1 bar	−3.0
Frozen Dessert, Chocolate Pudding Pops, Jell-O	Milk/Dairy	1 piece	−1.5
Frozen Dessert, Creamsicle	Sugar	1 piece	−4.0
Frozen Dessert, Chunky Strawberry, Frozfruit	Fruit	½ cup	1.0
Frozen dessert, fruit bar	Fruit	1 bar	1.5
Frozen Dessert, Fudgesicle	Fruit	1 bar	0.5
Frozen Dessert, Low-Fat, Tofutti	Legume/Nut/Seed	½ cup	−2.0
Frozen Dessert, Orange, Vitari Soft Serve	Fruit	½ cup	4.5
Frozen Dessert, Peach, Vitari Soft Serve	Fruit	½ cup	6.5
Frozen Dessert, Pineapple, Frozfruit	Fruit	1 bar	−0.5
Frozen Dessert, Popsicle	Sugar	2 pieces	−5.0

Food Name	Nutrigroup	Serving Size	Nutripoints
Frozen Dessert, Strawberry, Vitari Soft Serve	Fruit	½ cup	3.0
Frozen Dessert, Vanilla, Lite Bar, Dove	Milk/Dairy	1 piece	−2.0
Frozen Dessert, Wildberry, Vitari Soft Serve	Fruit	½ cup	3.5
Fruit Bits, Dried, Sun-Maid	Fruit	1 ounce	3.5
Fruit cocktail, canned in heavy syrup	Fruit	½ cup	1.0
Fruit cocktail, canned, unsweetened	Fruit	½ cup	10.0
Fruit Cocktail, Hot, Nutripoint	Fruit	½ cup	5.0
Fruit Cocktail, in Light Syrup, Del Monte	Fruit	½ cup	2.5
Fruit Cocktail, in Light Syrup, Libby's	Fruit	½ cup	2.5
Fruit Drink, Citrus Punch, Sunny Delite	Fruit	6 fluid ounces	3.5
Fruit Drink, Crangrape, Ocean Spray	Fruit	6 fluid ounces	2.5
Fruit Drink, Cranicot, Ocean Spray	Fruit	6 fluid ounces	−1.5
Fruit Drink, Fruit Juicy Red, Hawaiian Punch	Fruit	6 fluid ounces	1.5
Fruit Drink, Grape, frozen, Welchade	Fruit	6 fluid ounces	0.0
Fruit Drink, Grape, Hi-C	Fruit	6 fluid ounces	1.5
Fruit Drink, Guava, Ocean Spray	Fruit	6 fluid ounces	3.0
Fruit Drink, Hawaiian Punch	Fruit	6 fluid ounces	−1.5

Food Name	Nutrigroup	Serving Size	Nutripoints
Fruit Drink, Hawaiian Punch, Low-Cal.	Fruit	8 fluid ounces	4.5
Fruit drink, lemonade	Fruit	6 fluid ounces	−4.5
Fruit drink, limeade	Fruit	1 cup	−3.0
Fruit Drink, Orange, Capri Sun	Fruit	6 fluid ounces	−5.5
Fruit Drink, Punch, Capri Sun	Fruit	6 fluid ounces	−5.5
Fruit Drink, Strawberry Smoothie, Nutripoint	Fruit	1 cup	13.0
Fruit Drink, Sunrise Cooler, Nutripoint	Fruit	½ cup	15.5
Fruit drink, w/sugar	Fruit	6 fluid ounces	−1.5
Fruit Drink, Tang	Sugar	6 fluid ounces	3.0
Fruit Drink Mix, Wild Grape, Sugar-Free, Wyler's	Miscellaneous	8 fluid ounces	1.0
Fruit leather	Fruit	1 ounce	2.0
Fruit Platter, Fresh, Nutripoint	Fruit	½ cup	17.0
Fruit leather, with sugar	Fruit	1 piece	−2.0
Fruit Salad Plate, Nutripoint	Fruit	½ cup	14.5
Fruit salad, fresh	Fruit	½ cup	13.0
Fruit Slices, Fresh, Nutripoint	Fruit	½ cup	23.5
Fruit, Rainbow Compote, Nutripoint	Fruit	1 cup	18.0
Fruitcake	Grain	1 piece	−1.0
Fudge, chocolate	Sugar	1 ounce	−5.5
Fudge, chocolate w/nuts	Sugar	1 piece	−3.5
Fudge, divinity	Sugar	1 piece	−3.5
Fudge, peanut butter	Sugar	1 piece	−2.5
Fudge, vanilla	Sugar	1 piece	−4.0
Fudge, vanilla, w/nuts	Sugar	1 piece	−3.5

Food Name	Nutrigroup	Serving Size	Nutripoints
Garlic powder	Condiment	1 teaspoon	0.5
Garlic, raw	Condiment	1 piece	0.5
Gatorade	Sugar	2 cups	−8.0
Gazpacho	Vegetable	1 cup	1.5
Gelatin, Cherry, Jell-O	Fruit	½ cup	−5.0
Gelatin, Cherry, Sugar-Free, Jell-O	Fruit	1 cup	1.0
Gelatin, Strawberry-Banana, Royal	Fruit	½ cup	−4.0
Gin	Alcohol	2 fluid ounces	−17.5
Gin and tonic	Alcohol	8 fluid ounces	−11.0
Gin rickey	Alcohol	6 fluid ounces	−15.5
Ginger	Condiment	1 teaspoon	0.5
Gingerbread	Grain	1 piece	0.0
Goat	Meat/Fish/Poultry	3 ounces	0.5
Gold Cadillac	Alcohol	2 fluid ounces	−9.5
Goose, meat and skin, baked	Meat/Fish/Poultry	3 ounces	0.0
Goulash	Vegetable	½ cup	1.5
Graham Crumbs, Keebler	Grain	¼ cup	−0.5
Granola	Grain	¼ cup	0.0
Granola bar	Grain	1 bar	−0.5
Granola Bar, Chewy Chocolate Chip, Quaker	Grain	1 bar	0.5
Granola Bar, Chewy Fruit, Quaker	Grain	1 bar	−1.5
Granola Bar, Chewy Honey and Oats, Quaker	Grain	1 bar	−1.0
Granola Bar, Chewy Fruit and Nut, Jack La Lanne	Grain	1 bar	4.0
Granola Bar, Oats 'n Honey, Nature Valley	Grain	1 bar	−2.0

Food Name	Nutrigroup	Serving Size	Nutripoints
Granola Bar, w/Roasted Almonds, Nature Valley	Grain	1 bar	−1.5
Granola, Heartland	Grain	¼ cup	1.0
Granola, Maple Nut, Arrowhead Mills	Grain	¼ cup	1.5
Granola, no sugar	Grain	¼ cup	1.5
Grapefruit, fresh	Fruit	½ piece	13.0
Grapes, raw	Fruit	20 grapes	4.5
Grasshopper	Alcohol	2 fluid ounces	−8.5
Gravy	Fat/Oil	¼ cup	−2.5
Gravy Mix, Brown, French's	Fat/Oil	¼ cup	−4.0
Gravy Mix, Chicken, McCormick's	Fat/Oil	¼ cup	−4.5
Gravy mix, chicken, prepared	Fat/Oil	¼ cup	0.0
Gravy mix, chicken, prepared w/milk and butter	Fat/Oil	¼ cup	−2.5
Gravy Mix, Mushroom, French's	Fat/Oil	¼ cup	−4.0
Gravy mix, mushroom, prepared	Fat/Oil	¼ cup	−0.5
Gravy mix, pork, prepared	Fat/Oil	¼ cup	−2.0
Gravy mix, turkey, prepared	Fat/Oil	¼ cup	−0.5
Gravy mix, turkey, prepared w/milk and butter	Fat/Oil	¼ cup	−2.5
Gravy, beef, canned	Fat/Oil	¼ cup	1.0
Gravy, chicken, canned	Fat/Oil	¼ cup	−1.5
Gravy, Chicken, Franco-American	Fat/Oil	¼ cup	−4.0
Gravy, dehydrated	Miscellaneous	1 tablespoon	−3.0

Food Name	Nutrigroup	Serving Size	Nutripoints
Gravy, mushroom, canned	Fat/Oil	1/4 cup	0.0
Gravy, Mushroom, Franco-American	Fat/Oil	1/4 cup	−3.5
Gravy, turkey, canned	Fat/Oil	1/4 cup	0.0
Green pepper, raw	Vegetable	2 whole	37.5
Green Pepper, Stuffed w/Beef and Tomato Sauce, frozen, Stouffer's	Meat/Fish/Poultry	1 piece	−0.5
Green pepper, stuffed w/meat	Meat/Fish/Poultry	1 piece	2.5
Grits, cooked	Grain	1 cup	3.0
Grouper, baked	Meat/Fish/Poultry	5 ounces	3.0
Guacamole	Fruit	1/4 cup	4.5
Guava	Fruit	1 piece	21.0
Gum	Sugar	10 pieces	−3.0
Gum, Bubble, Original, Hubba Bubba	Sugar	5 pieces	−6.0
Gum, Doublemint, Wrigley's	Sugar	10 pieces	−4.5
Haddock Fillet, Light, Mrs. Paul's	Meat/Fish/Poultry	1 piece	0.0
Haddock, baked	Meat/Fish/Poultry	4 ounces	2.5
Haddock, floured/breaded, fried	Meat/Fish/Poultry	3 ounces	−1.0
Haddock, smoked	Meat/Fish/Poultry	6 ounces	2.0
Halibut fillet, batter-fried	Meat/Fish/Poultry	3 ounces	3.5
Halibut, baked	Meat/Fish/Poultry	4 ounces	7.5
Halibut, smoked	Meat/Fish/Poultry	3 ounces	−1.5
Halibut, w/Yellow Bell Pepper Sauce, Nutripoint	Meat/Fish/Poultry	4 ounces	7.0
Halvah, plain	Sugar	1 ounce	−2.0
Ham and cheese loaf/roll	Meat/Fish/Poultry	2 pieces	0.0

Food Name	Nutrigroup	Serving Size	Nutripoints
Ham Dinner, frozen, Morton	Meat/Fish/Poultry	1 portion	5.0
Ham salad	Meat/Fish/Poultry	½ cup	1.0
Ham, Aparagus au Gratin, Slim, frozen, Budget Gourmet	Meat/Fish/Poultry	1 portion	0.0
Ham, baked, canned, 13-percent fat	Meat/Fish/Poultry	3 ounces	2.0
Ham, canned, Armour Golden Star	Meat/Fish/Poultry	4 ounces	1.0
Ham, chopped	Meat/Fish/Poultry	2 pieces	0.5
Ham, Deviled, Underwood	Meat/Fish/Poultry	2 ounces	−3.5
Ham, frozen dinner	Meat/Fish/Poultry	½ portion	2.5
Ham, Land O' Frost	Meat/Fish/Poultry	3 ounces	−3.5
Ham, lean, baked, canned, 4-percent fat	Meat/Fish/Poultry	4 ounces	5.0
Ham, minced	Meat/Fish/Poultry	2 ounces	0.0
Ham, Slices, Jubilee, Oscar Mayer	Meat/Fish/Poultry	4 pieces	5.5
Ham, Turkey, Mr. Turkey	Meat/Fish/Poultry	4 ounces	−2.0
Hamburger Helper, Prepared	Meat/Fish/Poultry	¼ cup	1.0
Hamburger patty, broiled	Meat/Fish/Poultry	3 ounces	0.0
Hamburger Patty, Grillers, frozen, Morningstar Farms	Legume/Nut/Seed	1 piece	3.5
Hamburger patty, lean, broiled	Meat/Fish/Poultry	3 ounces	3.0
Hamburger patty, lean, fried	Meat/Fish/Poultry	3 ounces	1.5
Hamburger w/bun, fast-food, small, plain	Meat/Fish/Poultry	½ piece	1.5

Food Name	Nutrigroup	Serving Size	Nutripoints
Hamburger w/bun/ lettuce/tomato, fast-food	Meat/Fish/Poultry	1/2 piece	3.0
Hamburger, Aerobics, Nutripoint	Meat/Fish/Poultry	1 burger	5.0
Hash	Meat/Fish/Poultry	1/2 cup	−0.5
Herring, canned	Meat/Fish/Poultry	1/2 cup	1.5
Herring, pickled	Meat/Fish/Poultry	2 pieces	0.5
Honey	Sugar	2 tablespoons	−5.5
Horseradish	Condiment	1 tablespoon	0.0
Hush puppies	Grain	2 pieces	−1.0
Ice Cream Bar, Chocolate Peanut Butter, Milk Chocolate, Häagen-Dazs	Milk/Dairy	1/2 piece	−3.0
Ice Cream Bar, Eskimo Pie	Milk/Dairy	1 piece	−3.5
Ice Cream Bar, Nondairy, Chocolate-Covered, Mocha Mix	Milk/Dairy	1/2 piece	−2.5
Ice Cream Bar, Vanilla, Milk Chocolate, Almonds, Häagen-Dazs	Milk/Dairy	1/2 piece	−4.0
Ice Cream Bar, Vanilla, Milk Chocolate, Häagen-Dazs	Milk/Dairy	1/2 piece	−4.0
Ice cream cone, vanilla	Milk/Dairy	1/2 piece	−1.5
Ice cream sandwich	Milk/Dairy	1 piece	−2.5
Ice Cream Sandwich, Good Humor	Milk/Dairy	1/2 piece	−2.5
Ice cream soda	Milk/Dairy	6 fluid ounces	−3.5
Ice cream sundae, caramel	Milk/Dairy	1/2 serving	−2.0

Food Name	Nutrigroup	Serving Size	Nutripoints
Ice cream sundae, hot fudge	Milk/Dairy	½ serving	−1.0
Ice cream sundae, strawberry	Milk/Dairy	½ serving	0.0
Ice Cream, Butter Pecan, Meadow Gold	Milk/Dairy	½ cup	−5.0
Ice Cream, Buttered Pecan, Borden	Milk/Dairy	½ cup	−4.0
Ice Cream, Chocolate/ Chocolate Chip, Häagen-Dazs	Milk/Dairy	¼ cup	−3.5
Ice Cream, Chocolate, Schrafft's	Milk/Dairy	¼ cup	−4.0
Ice Cream, Coffee, Häagen-Dazs	Milk/Dairy	¼ cup	−3.5
Ice Cream, Dutch Chocolate, Borden	Milk/Dairy	½ cup	−2.0
Ice Cream, Extra Light, Blue Bell	Milk/Dairy	1 cup	1.5
Ice Cream, French Vanilla, Meadow Gold	Milk/Dairy	½ cup	−4.0
Ice Cream, Nondairy, Vanilla, Mocha Mix	Milk/Dairy	½ cup	−2.5
Ice cream, regular fat, vanilla	Milk/Dairy	½ cup	−2.0
Ice Cream, Simple Pleasures, (w/Simplesse)	Milk/Dairy	4 fluid ounces	−0.5
Ice Cream, Sorbet and Cream, Key Lime, Häagen-Dazs	Milk/Dairy	½ cup	−3.5
Ice Cream, Strawberry, Borden	Milk/Dairy	½ cup	−3.5
Ice Cream, Vanilla Swiss Almond, Häagen-Dazs	Milk/Dairy	¼ cup	−4.0

Food Name	Nutrigroup	Serving Size	Nutripoints
Ice Cream, Vanilla, Häagen-Dazs	Milk/Dairy	¼ cup	−4.0
Ice Cream, Vanilla, Louis Sherry	Milk/Dairy	½ cup	−3.5
Ice Cream, Vanilla, Party Time, Knudsen	Milk/Dairy	½ cup	−4.0
Ice Cream, Vanilla, premium (rich)	Milk/Dairy	¼ cup	−2.0
Ice cream, Vanilla, Soft Serve	Milk/Dairy	½ cup	−3.5
Ice Milk, Chocolate, Borden	Milk/Dairy	½ cup	−2.0
Ice Milk, Strawberry, Borden	Milk/Dairy	½ cup	−2.0
Ice milk, vanilla	Milk/Dairy	½ cup	−1.0
Ice Milk, Vanilla, Borden	Milk/Dairy	½ cup	−2.0
Iced Tea Mix, Sugar and Lemon Flavor, Nestea	Sugar	8 fluid ounces	−6.5
Instant Breakfast, Chocolate, Carnation	Milk/Dairy	½ cup	6.0
Instant Breakfast, Vanilla, Carnation	Milk/Dairy	½ cup	6.0
Instant Breakfast, w/low-fat milk, no sugar, all flavors, Carnation	Milk/Dairy	1 cup	12.0
Jack in the Box Bacon Cheeseburger	Meat/Fish/Poultry	½ piece	−1.0
Jack in the Box Beef Fajita Pita	Meat/Fish/Poultry	½ serving	1.5
Jack in the Box Bleu Cheese Dressing	Fat/Oil	1 tablespoon	−3.0
Jack in the Box Breakfast Jack	Meat/Fish/Poultry	½ piece	−2.5

Food Name	Nutrigroup	Serving Size	Nutripoints
Jack in the Box Buttermilk House Dressing	Fat/Oil	1 tablespoon	−3.0
Jack in the Box Canadian Crescent Breakfast	Meat/Fish/Poultry	½ piece	−3.0
Jack in the Box Cheeseburger	Meat/Fish/Poultry	½ piece	0.0
Jack in the Box Cheesecake	Milk/Dairy	½ piece	−3.0
Jack in the Box Chef Salad	Vegetable	¼ cup	−2.5
Jack in the Box Chicken Fajita Pita	Meat/Fish/Poultry	½ serving	2.0
Jack in the Box Chicken Strips (4 pieces)	Meat/Fish/Poultry	½ serving	−1.0
Jack in the Box Chicken Strips (6 pieces)	Meat/Fish/Poultry	3 pieces	−1.0
Jack in the Box Chicken Supreme	Meat/Fish/Poultry	½ piece	−1.5
Jack in the Box Club Pita	Meat/Fish/Poultry	½ serving	2.5
Jack in the Box Double Cheeseburger	Meat/Fish/Poultry	½ piece	−1.0
Jack in the Box Egg Rolls (3 pieces)	Meat/Fish/Poultry	2 pieces	−1.0
Jack in the Box Egg Rolls (5 pieces)	Meat/Fish/Poultry	2 rolls	−0.5
Jack in the Box Fish Supreme	Meat/Fish/Poultry	½ piece	−1.0
Jack in the Box Grilled Chicken Fillet Sandwich	Meat/Fish/Poultry	½ piece	1.0
Jack in the Box Hamburger	Meat/Fish/Poultry	1 piece	0.0
Jack in the Box Hash Browns	Vegetable	1 serving	−2.0

Food Name	Nutrigroup	Serving Size	Nutripoints
Jack in the Box Hot Apple Turnover	Fruit	¼ piece	−2.5
Jack in the Box Hot Club Supreme	Meat/Fish/Poultry	½ piece	−0.5
Jack in the Box Jumbo Jack	Meat/Fish/Poultry	½ piece	0.0
Jack in the Box Jumbo Jack w/Cheese	Meat/Fish/Poultry	½ piece	−1.5
Jack in the Box Mexican Chicken Salad	Vegetable	¼ cup	−0.5
Jack in the Box Pancake Platter	Grain	½ serving	−0.5
Jack in the Box Reduced-Calorie French Dressing	Fat/Oil	2 tablespoons	−4.5
Jack in the Box Sausage Crescent Breakfast	Meat/Fish/Poultry	½ piece	−3.0
Jack in the Box Scrambled Egg Platter	Milk/Dairy	¼ serving	−3.5
Jack in the Box Shrimp (10 pieces)	Meat/Fish/Poultry	7 pieces	−2.5
Jack in the Box Side Salad	Vegetable	1 cup	−0.5
Jack in the Box Super Taco	Legume/Nut/Seed	½ serving	−2.0
Jack in the Box Supreme Crescent Breakfast	Meat/Fish/Poultry	½ piece	−2.5
Jack in the Box Swiss and Bacon Burger	Meat/Fish/Poultry	½ piece	−2.5
Jack in the Box Taco	Legume/Nut/Seed	1 serving	−1.5
Jack in the Box Taco Salad	Vegetable	¼ cup	−1.0
Jack in the Box Taquitos (7 pieces)	Meat/Fish/Poultry	½ piece	−0.5

Food Name	Nutrigroup	Serving Size	Nutripoints
Jack in the Box Thousand Island Dressing	Fat/Oil	1 tablespoon	−3.5
Jack in the Box Ultimate Cheeseburger	Meat/Fish/Poultry	¼ piece	−2.0
Jam, Grape, Welch's	Fruit	1 tablespoon	−5.5
Jam, low-cal.	Fruit	2 tablespoons	−0.5
Jam, preserves, all flavors	Fruit	1 tablespoon	−3.0
Jam, Strawberry, Smucker's	Fruit	1 tablespoon	−6.0
Jambalaya, Nutripoint	Grain	1 cup	7.5
Jelly beans	Sugar	15 pieces	−5.5
Jelly, all flavors	Sugar	2 tablespoons	−3.5
Jelly, Blackberry Spread, Smucker's	Fruit	2 tablespoons	−5.5
Jelly, cranberry	Fruit	2 tablespoons	−5.5
Jelly, fruit butters, all flavors	Fruit	1 tablespoon	0.0
Jelly, Grape, Concord, Smucker's	Fruit	1 tablespoon	−6.0
Jelly, Grape, Imitation, Smucker's	Fruit	2 tablespoons	0.5
Jelly, Grape, Welch's	Fruit	1 tablespoon	−5.5
Jelly, low-cal., all flavors	Sugar	4 tablespoons	−1.0
Juice, apple	Fruit	6 fluid ounces	2.5
Juice, Apple Sparkler, Sundance	Fruit	6 fluid ounces	2.5
Juice, Apple, from concentrate, frozen, Tree Top	Fruit	6 fluid ounces	1.0
Juice, Apple, from concentrate, Tree Top	Fruit	6 fluid ounces	1.5
Juice, Apple, frozen, Seneca	Fruit	6 fluid ounces	4.5

Food Name	Nutrigroup	Serving Size	Nutripoints
Juice, Apple, Lucky Leaf	Fruit	6 fluid ounces	1.0
Juice, Apple, Mott's	Fruit	6 fluid ounces	2.5
Juice, carrot	Vegetable	6 fluid ounces	15.0
Juice, Cranapple, Low-Cal., Ocean Spray	Fruit	8 fluid ounces	12.5
Juice, Cranapple, Ocean Spray	Fruit	6 fluid ounces	1.5
Juice, Cranberry Cocktail, frozen, Welch's	Fruit	6 fluid ounces	0.0
Juice, Cranberry Cocktail, Ocean Spray	Fruit	6 fluid ounces	7.0
Juice, Cranberry Sparkler, Sundance	Fruit	6 fluid ounces	2.0
Juice, cranberry, low-cal.	Fruit	1 cup	12.5
Juice, Cranberry, Low-Cal., Ocean Spray	Fruit	8 fluid ounces	10.5
Juice, cranberry, sweetened	Fruit	6 fluid ounces	3.5
Juice, Grape, Sweetened, frozen, Welch's	Fruit	6 fluid ounces	2.0
Juice, grape, unsweetened	Fruit	6 fluid ounces	5.5
Juice, Grape, Unsweetened, frozen, Welch's	Fruit	6 fluid ounces	5.5
Juice, Purple Grape, Welch's	Fruit	6 fluid ounces	3.5
Juice, Red Grape, Welch's	Fruit	6 fluid ounces	3.5
Juice, White Grape, Welch's	Fruit	6 fluid ounces	2.0
Juice, Grapefruit Sparkler, Sundance	Fruit	6 fluid ounces	7.0

Food Name	Nutrigroup	Serving Size	Nutripoints
Juice, Grapefruit, Ocean Spray	Fruit	6 fluid ounces	8.0
Juice, Grapefruit, Pink, Ocean Spray	Fruit	6 fluid ounces	6.0
Juice, grapefruit, sweetened	Fruit	6 fluid ounces	7.0
Juice, grapefruit, unsweetened	Fruit	6 fluid ounces	11.0
Juice, Kiwi Fruit, Sweetened, Kiwi Island	Fruit	6 fluid ounces	4.5
Juice, Kiwi-Lime Sparkler, Sundance	Fruit	6 fluid ounces	2.0
Juice, lemon	Condiment	1 tablespoon	1.0
Juice, Lemon, ReaLemon	Condiment	1 tablespoon	1.0
Juice, lime	Condiment	1 tablespoon	0.5
Juice, Orange Sparkler, Sundance	Fruit	6 fluid ounces	8.0
Juice, Orange, Calcium Fortified, Minute Maid	Fruit	6 fluid ounces	11.0
Juice, orange, fresh squeezed	Fruit	6 fluid ounces	11.5
Juice, Orange, frozen, Minute Maid	Fruit	6 fluid ounces	10.0
Juice, orange, frozen, reconstituted	Fruit	6 fluid ounces	11.0
Juice, Orange, Tropicana	Fruit	6 fluid ounces	11.0
Juice, Orange, w/Calcium, Citrus Hill	Fruit	6 fluid ounces	10.5
Juice, orange-grapefruit, unsweetened, canned	Fruit	6 fluid ounces	10.0
Juice, orange-pineapple	Fruit	6 fluid ounces	9.5
Juice, Pineapple, Dole	Fruit	6 fluid ounces	5.0

Food Name	Nutrigroup	Serving Size	Nutripoints
Juice, pineapple, unsweetened, canned	Fruit	6 fluid ounces	6.0
Juice, prune, canned	Fruit	4 fluid ounces	5.0
Juice, Prune, Sunsweet	Fruit	4 fluid ounces	4.0
Juice, Raspberry Sparkler, Sundance	Fruit	6 fluid ounces	2.0
Juice, tomato	Vegetable	6 fluid ounces	24.5
Juice, Tomato, Campbell's	Vegetable	¾ cup	12.0
Juice, tomato, low-sodium	Vegetable	6 fluid ounces	26.0
Juice, Vegetable, V-8	Vegetable	6 fluid ounces	24.5
Juice, Vegetable, No Salt Added, V-8	Vegetable	6 fluid ounces	28.5
Juice, Vegetable, Spicy, V-8	Vegetable	6 fluid ounces	26.0
Kale, chopped, cooked	Vegetable	1 cup	38.5
Kelp	Vegetable	½ cup	18.0
Kentucky Fried Chicken, Chicken Keel	Meat/Fish/Poultry	1 piece	−1.0
Kentucky Fried Chicken, Chicken Keel, Extra Crispy	Meat/Fish/Poultry	1 piece	−0.5
Kentucky Fried Chicken, Chicken Wing	Meat/Fish/Poultry	1 piece	−2.5
Kentucky Fried Chicken, Coleslaw	Vegetable	½ cup	1.5
Kentucky Fried Chicken, Corn	Vegetable	½ cup	2.5
Kentucky Fried Chicken, Drumstick	Meat/Fish/Poultry	1 piece	−1.5
Kentucky Fried Chicken, Drumstick, Extra Crispy	Meat/Fish/Poultry	1 piece	−1.5
Kentucky Fried Chicken, Gravy	Fat/Oil	¼ cup	−1.5

Food Name	Nutrigroup	Serving Size	Nutripoints
Kentucky Fried Chicken, Mashed Potatoes	Vegetable	½ cup	−2.5
Kentucky Fried Chicken, Roll	Grain	2 rolls	2.0
Kentucky Fried Chicken, Side Breast	Meat/Fish/Poultry	1 piece	−1.5
Kentucky Fried Chicken, Side Breast, Extra Crispy	Meat/Fish/Poultry	1 piece	−1.0
Kentucky Fried Chicken, Thigh	Meat/Fish/Poultry	1 piece	−2.5
Kentucky Fried Chicken, Thigh, Extra Crispy	Meat/Fish/Poultry	1 piece	−2.0
Kentucky Fried Chicken, Wing, Extra Crispy	Meat/Fish/Poultry	1 piece	−2.0
Kentucky Fried Chicken	Meat/Fish/Poultry	1 piece	−1.0
Ketchup, Heinz	Vegetable	2 tablespoons	−1.5
Ketchup, Low-Sodium, Heinz	Condiment	2 tablespoons	0.5
Kielbasa	Meat/Fish/Poultry	3 ounces	−1.5
Kiwi fruit	Fruit	1 piece	17.0
Knockwurst	Meat/Fish/Poultry	2 ounces	−2.0
Kohlrabi, raw	Vegetable	2 cups	24.5
Kumquat	Fruit	6 pieces	10.0
Lamb chop, loin, medium fat, baked	Meat/Fish/Poultry	2 ounces	−0.5
Lamb roast, leg, baked	Meat/Fish/Poultry	3 ounces	3.5
Lamb roast, leg, medium fat, baked	Meat/Fish/Poultry	3 ounces	0.5
Lamb shoulder, lean, baked	Meat/Fish/Poultry	3 ounces	3.0
Lamb shoulder, medium fat, baked	Meat/Fish/Poultry	3 ounces	−1.0

Food Name	Nutrigroup	Serving Size	Nutripoints
Lard	Fat/Oil	1 tablespoon	−5.0
Lasagna	Grain	½ cup	2.5
Lasagna, Italian Cheese, frozen, Weight Watchers	Grain	½ portion	1.0
Lasagna, Italian Sausage, frozen, Budget Gourmet	Grain	¼ portion	0.5
Lasagna, low-cal. frozen meal	Grain	½ portion	4.0
Lasagna, single serving, frozen, Stouffer's	Grain	½ portion	0.5
Lasagna, Spinach, Nutripoint	Grain	1 cup	9.0
Lasagna, Three-Cheese, frozen, Budget Gourmet	Grain	⅓ portion	1.5
Lasagna, Tuna, Spinach Noodles & Vegetables, frozen, Stouffer's	Meat/Fish/Poultry	1 portion	2.0
Lasagna, Vegetable, single serving, frozen, Stouffer's	Grain	½ portion	0.5
Lasagna, w/Bread, frozen, Morton	Grain	½ portion	1.5
Lasagna, w/Meat Sauce, Slim, frozen, Budget Gourmet	Grain	½ portion	0.5
Lasagna, w/Meat Sauce, frozen, Stouffer's	Grain	½ portion	0.5
Lasagna, w/Meat Sauce, frozen, Weight Watchers	Grain	½ portion	1.0

Food Name	Nutrigroup	Serving Size		Nutripoints
Lasagna, Zucchini, Lean Cuisine, Stouffer's	Grain	½	portion	2.0
Lasagne, frozen, Celentano	Grain	½	portion	1.5
Lasagne, Primavera, frozen, Celentano	Grain	½	portion	2.5
Leeks, cooked	Vegetable	1	cup	7.5
Leeks, raw	Vegetable	2	whole	16.0
Lemon	Condiment	¼	lemon	2.5
Lemonade Mix, Sugar-Free, Country Time	Miscellaneous	8	fluid ounces	1.0
Lemonade, Minute Maid	Fruit	6	fluid ounces	−5.0
Lentils and Wild Rice, Herbed, Nutripoint	Legume/Nut/Seed	1	cup	6.5
Lentils, cooked	Legume/Nut/Seed	1	cup	8.0
Lettuce and tomato	Vegetable	1	cup	18.5
Lettuce, butterhead/ Boston/Bibb, chopped	Vegetable	2	cups	34.0
Lettuce, iceberg	Vegetable	10	leaves	18.0
Lettuce, loose-leaf	Vegetable	10	leaves	30.5
Lettuce, romaine	Vegetable	2	cups	47.5
Lime	Condiment	¼	lime	1.0
Linguine, Buitoni (2 ounces dry = ¾ cup cooked)	Grain	2	ounces	3.0
Linguine, San Giorgio (2 ounces dry = ¾ cup cooked)	Grain	2	ounces	2.5
Linguine, Spinach, High-Protein, Buitoni	Grain	½	cup	3.5
Linguine, Thin, Ronzoni (2 ounces dry = ¾ cup cooked)	Grain	2	ounces	2.5

Food Name	Nutrigroup	Serving Size		Nutripoints
Linguini, Seafood, frozen, Weight Watchers	Grain	1	portion	2.0
Linguini, w/clam sauce, frozen, Stouffer's	Grain	½	portion	−0.5
Linguini, w/Scallops and Clams, Slim, frozen, Budget Gourmet	Grain	½	portion	−0.5
Linguini, w/Shrimp, frozen, Budget Gourmet	Grain	½	portion	0.5
Litchi, fresh	Fruit	6	pieces	16.0
Liverwurst	Meat/Fish/Poultry	2	ounces	4.5
Liverwurst, Original, Jones	Meat/Fish/Poultry	2	ounces	−3.0
Lobster Newburg, frozen dinner	Meat/Fish/Poultry	½	portion	1.0
Lobster, baked/broiled, w/butter	Meat/Fish/Poultry	4	ounces	−1.0
Lobster, floured/breaded, fried	Meat/Fish/Poultry	3	ounces	−0.5
Lobster, steamed/boiled	Meat/Fish/Poultry	6	ounces	2.5
Loquat, fresh	Fruit	5	pieces	10.0
Luncheon meat, beef	Meat/Fish/Poultry	2	ounces	−1.5
Luncheon meat, head cheese	Meat/Fish/Poultry	2	pieces	−1.5
Luncheon meat, honeyloaf	Meat/Fish/Poultry	3	pieces	3.5
Luncheon meat, olive loaf	Meat/Fish/Poultry	1	slice	−1.0
Luncheon Meat, Olive Loaf, Eckrich	Meat/Fish/Poultry	2	ounces	−2.5
Luncheon Meat, Olive Loaf, Oscar Mayer	Meat/Fish/Poultry	2	pieces	−2.0

Food Name	Nutrigroup	Serving Size		Nutripoints
Luncheon Meat, Oscar Mayer	Meat/Fish/Poultry	2	pieces	−3.5
Luncheon meat, pickle and pimiento loaf	Meat/Fish/Poultry	2	pieces	−1.0
Luncheon Meat, Picnic Loaf, Oscar Mayer	Meat/Fish/Poultry	2	pieces	−1.0
Luncheon meat, pimiento loaf	Meat/Fish/Poultry	2	ounces	−1.0
Luncheon meat, turkey ham	Meat/Fish/Poultry	4	ounces	2.0
Macadamia nuts, oil roasted, salted	Legume/Nut/Seed	8	pieces	0.5
Macaroni and cheese	Grain	1/4	cup	0.0
Macaroni and Cheese Dinner, Deluxe, Kraft	Grain	1/2	cup	0.0
Macaroni and Cheese, Casserole, frozen, Morton	Grain	1/2	portion	−1.5
Macaroni and Cheese, frozen, Budget Gourmet	Grain	1/2	portion	0.0
Macaroni and Cheese, frozen, Stouffer's	Grain	1/2	portion	−2.0
Macaroni and Spaghetti, Enriched, Prince	Grain	1/2	cup	4.0
Macaroni Ribbons, Spinach, Creamette, Borden	Grain	1/2	cup	3.0
Macaroni salad	Grain	1/2	cup	0.0
Macaroni, cooked, all shapes, Mueller's	Grain	1/2	cup	3.5
Macaroni, cooked, no salt (1 cup = 2 ounces dry)	Grain	1/2	cup	3.5
Macaroni, dry (2 ounces = 1 cup cooked)	Grain	1	ounce	3.5

Food Name	Nutrigroup	Serving Size	Nutripoints
Macaroni, Elbow, Creamette, Borden	Grain	1/2 cup	2.5
Macaroni, Superoni, Prince	Grain	1/2 cup	3.0
Mackerel, baked	Meat/Fish/Poultry	3 ounces	4.0
Mai tai	Alcohol	2 fluid ounces	−11.5
Malted milk powder	Milk/Dairy	1 tablespoon	1.0
Mandarin oranges, canned	Fruit	1/2 cup	5.0
Mandarin oranges, canned, unsweetened	Fruit	1/2 cup	15.5
Mango	Fruit	1/2 piece	17.5
Manhattan	Alcohol	3 fluid ounces	−13.5
Manicotti, 3-Cheese, Tomato Sauce, Le Menu	Milk/Dairy	1/2 portion	0.5
Manicotti, Cheese, frozen, Weight Watchers	Milk/Dairy	1/2 portion	0.0
Manicotti, Cheese, w/Meat Sauce, frozen, Budget Gourmet	Milk/Dairy	1/3 portion	0.5
Manicotti, frozen, Celentano	Milk/Dairy	1/2 portion	2.0
Margarine	Fat/Oil	1 tablespoon	−3.0
Margarine, Cookery, Parkay	Fat/Oil	1 tablespoon	−2.5
Margarine, corn oil	Fat/Oil	1 tablespoon	−2.5
Margarine, Corn Oil Spread, Light, Mazola	Fat/Oil	2 tablespoons	−2.5
Margarine, County Crock Spread, Shedd's	Fat/Oil	1 tablespoon	−3.0
Margarine, Diet Imitation, Mazola	Fat/Oil	2 tablespoons	−2.5
Margarine, Diet, Fleischmann's	Fat/Oil	2 tablespoons	−2.5

Food Name	Nutrigroup	Serving Size	Nutripoints
Margarine, Diet, Soft, Parkay	Fat/Oil	2 tablespoons	−2.5
Margarine, Extra Light, Promise	Fat/Oil	2 tablespoons	−2.5
Margarine, Family Spread, Mrs. Filbert's	Fat/Oil	1 tablespoon	−2.0
Margarine, hard, coconut, safflower and palm	Fat/Oil	1 tablespoon	−2.5
Margarine, Heart Beat	Fat/Oil	4 tablespoons	−3.0
Margarine, I Can't Believe It's Not Butter!	Fat/Oil	1 tablespoon	−2.5
Margarine, liquid, soybean and cottonseed	Fat/Oil	1 tablespoon	−3.0
Margarine, low-cal.	Fat/Oil	1 tablespoon	−1.0
Margarine, Mazola	Fat/Oil	1 tablespoon	−2.5
Margarine, Parkay	Fat/Oil	1 tablespoon	−2.5
Margarine, Promise	Fat/Oil	1 tablespoon	−2.0
Margarine, Reduced-Calorie Spread, Blue Bonnet	Fat/Oil	1 tablespoon	−2.5
Margarine, Reduced Calorie, Diet, Mazola	Fat/Oil	2 tablespoons	−2.5
Margarine, Reduced Calorie, Unsalted, Weight Watchers	Fat/Oil	2 tablespoons	−2.0
Margarine, Reduced Calorie, Weight Watchers	Fat/Oil	2 tablespoons	−2.5
Margarine, Safflower, Hain	Fat/Oil	1 tablespoon	−2.5
Margarine, Soft, Blue Bonnet	Fat/Oil	1 tablespoon	−3.0
Margarine, Soft, Chiffon	Fat/Oil	1 tablespoon	−3.0

Food Name	Nutrigroup	Serving Size	Nutripoints
Margarine, Soft, Corn Oil, Mrs. Filbert's	Fat/Oil	1 tablespoon	−2.5
Margarine, Soft, Imperial	Fat/Oil	1 tablespoon	−3.0
Margarine, Soft, Low-Salt, Country Morning Blend, Land O Lakes	Fat/Oil	1 tablespoon	−4.0
Margarine, Soft, Spread, Touch of Butter, Kraft	Fat/Oil	2 tablespoons	−2.5
Margarine, Squeeze, Parkay	Fat/Oil	1 tablespoon	−2.5
Margarine, Stick, Blue Bonnet	Fat/Oil	1 tablespoon	−3.0
Margarine, Stick, Fleischmann's	Fat/Oil	1 tablespoon	−3.0
Margarine, Stick, Imperial	Fat/Oil	1 tablespoon	−3.0
Margarine, Stick, Land O Lakes	Fat/Oil	1 tablespoon	−2.5
Margarine, Stick, Unsalted, Fleischmann's	Fat/Oil	1 tablespoon	−2.5
Margarine, Sweet Unsalted, Heart Beat	Fat/Oil	4 tablespoons	−2.0
Margarine, Unsalted, Mazola	Fat/Oil	1 tablespoon	−2.5
Margarine, Whipped Spread, Parkay	Fat/Oil	1 tablespoon	−2.5
Margarine, Whipped, Imperial	Fat/Oil	2 tablespoons	−2.5
Margarita	Alcohol	3 fluid ounces	−13.5
Marjoram	Condiment	1 teaspoon	0.5
Marmalade	Sugar	2 tablespoons	−5.0
Marmalade, Orange, Smucker's	Fruit	1 tablespoon	−6.0
Marshmallows, Jet-Puffed, Kraft	Sugar	4 pieces	−5.5

Food Name	Nutrigroup	Serving Size	Nutripoints
Martini	Alcohol	3 fluid ounces	−15.5
Mayo Mix, Lite, Nutripoint	Fat/Oil	¼ cup	1.5
Mayonnaise	Fat/Oil	1 tablespoon	−2.5
Mayonnaise, Blue Plate	Fat/Oil	1 tablespoon	−3.0
Mayonnaise, Cholesterol Free, Kraft	Fat/Oil	1 tablespoon	−2.5
Mayonnaise, Cholesterol Free, Miracle Whip	Fat/Oil	1 tablespoon	−2.5
Mayonnaise, imitation, milk cream	Fat/Oil	1 tablespoon	−3.5
Mayonnaise, imitation, soybean	Fat/Oil	1 tablespoon	−3.0
Mayonnaise, Light, Kraft	Fat/Oil	2 tablespoons	0.0
Mayonnaise, Light, Miracle Whip	Fat/Oil	2 tablespoons	−3.0
Mayonnaise, Light, Reduced Calorie, Hellman's	Fat/Oil	2 tablespoons	−3.0
Mayonnaise, Light, Reduced Calorie, Kraft	Fat/Oil	1 tablespoon	−2.5
Mayonnaise, low-cal.	Fat/Oil	2 tablespoons	−2.5
Mayonnaise, Real, Best Foods	Fat/Oil	1 tablespoon	−3.0
Mayonnaise, Real, Hellman's	Fat/Oil	1 tablespoon	−3.5
Mayonnaise, Real, Kraft	Fat/Oil	1 tablespoon	−3.5
Mayonnaise, Reduced Calorie, Light n'Lively	Condiment	1 teaspoon	0.5
McDonald's 1000 Island Dressing	Fat/Oil	2 tablespoons	−3.0
McDonald's Apple Danish	Grain	½ Danish	−1.5

Food Name	Nutrigroup	Serving Size	Nutripoints
McDonald's Apple Pie	Fruit	¼ piece	−2.0
McDonald's Bacon Bits	Meat/Fish/Poultry	1 tablespoon	−1.5
McDonald's Barbecue Sauce	Condiment	1 tablespoon	0.0
McDonald's Big Mac	Meat/Fish/Poultry	½ piece	−1.0
McDonald's Biscuit w/Bacon, Egg, and Cheese	Milk/Dairy	½ serving	−4.5
McDonald's Biscuit w/Biscuit Spread	Grain	½ serving	−0.5
McDonald's Biscuit w/Sausage	Meat/Fish/Poultry	½ piece	−1.5
McDonald's Biscuit w/Sausage and Egg	Meat/Fish/Poultry	½ serving	−4.5
McDonald's Bleu Cheese Dressing	Fat/Oil	1 tablespoon	−3.5
McDonald's Cheeseburger	Meat/Fish/Poultry	½ piece	0.0
McDonald's Chef Salad	Fruit	¼ serving	−0.5
McDonald's Chicken McNuggets	Meat/Fish/Poultry	1 serving	−1.5
McDonald's Chicken Salad Oriental	Meat/Fish/Poultry	1 serving	5.0
McDonald's Chocolate Milk Shake	Milk/Dairy	½ serving	−3.0
McDonald's Chocolaty Chip Cookies	Grain	1 cookie	−2.5
McDonald's Chow Mein Noodles	Grain	2 tablespoons	0.0
McDonald's Cinnamon Raisin Danish	Grain	½ Danish	−1.5
McDonald's Croutons	Grain	2 tablespoons	5.0
McDonald's Egg McMuffin	Milk/Dairy	½ serving	−4.0
McDonald's English Muffin w/Butter	Grain	1 whole	1.0

Food Name	Nutrigroup	Serving Size	Nutripoints
McDonald's			
Fillet-O-Fish	Meat/Fish/Poultry	1/2 piece	−1.0
McDonald's French			
Dressing	Fat/Oil	2 tablespoons	−2.5
McDonald's Garden			
Salad	Fruit	1/2 serving	0.5
McDonald's			
Hamburger	Meat/Fish/Poultry	1 piece	0.5
McDonald's			
Hashbrown			
Potatoes	Vegetable	1/2 serving	−2.0
McDonald's Hot			
Caramel Sundae	Milk/Dairy	1/2 serving	−1.5
McDonald's Hot			
Fudge Sundae	Milk/Dairy	1/2 serving	−1.5
McDonald's Hot			
Mustard Sauce	Condiment	1 tablespoon	−0.5
McDonald's Hotcakes			
w/Butter and			
Syrup	Grain	1/2 serving	−0.5
McDonald's Iced			
Cheese Danish	Grain	1/2 Danish	−2.0
McDonald's Lite			
Vinaigrette			
Dressing	Condiment	1 tablespoon	0.0
McDonald's			
McD.L.T.	Meat/Fish/Poultry	1/3 piece	−1.0
McDonald's			
McDonaldland			
Cookies	Grain	1 cookie	−2.0
McDonald's Oriental			
Dressing	Condiment	1 tablespoon	0.0
McDonald's Pork			
Sausage	Meat/Fish/Poultry	1 piece	−3.5
McDonald's Quarter			
Pounder	Meat/Fish/Poultry	1/2 piece	−0.5
McDonald's Quarter			
Pounder w/Cheese	Meat/Fish/Poultry	1/2 piece	−1.0
McDonald's Ranch			
Dressing	Fat/Oil	2 tablespoons	−3.0

Food Name	Nutrigroup	Serving Size	Nutripoints
McDonald's Raspberry Danish	Grain	½ Danish	−1.0
McDonald's Regular French Fries	Vegetable	¼ piece	−0.5
McDonald's Sausage McMuffin	Meat/Fish/Poultry	½ piece	−0.5
McDonald's Sausage McMuffin w/Egg	Meat/Fish/Poultry	½ serving	−4.0
McDonald's Scrambled Eggs	Milk/Dairy	1 serving	−19.5
McDonald's Shrimp Salad	Meat/Fish/Poultry	1 piece	−2.5
McDonald's Side Salad	Vegetable	1 piece	1.0
McDonald's Soft Serve Cone	Milk/Dairy	1 piece	−1.0
McDonald's Strawberry Milk Shake	Milk/Dairy	½ serving	−3.0
McDonald's Strawberry Sundae	Milk/Dairy	½ serving	−1.5
McDonald's Sweet and Sour Sauce	Condiment	1 tablespoon	0.0
McDonald's Vanilla Milk Shake	Milk/Dairy	½ serving	−3.0
Meatballs	Meat/Fish/Poultry	2 pieces	−0.5
Meatballs, Italian Style, w/Noodles and Peppers, frozen, Budget Gourmet	Meat/Fish/Poultry	½ portion	0.0
Meatballs, Swedish, w/Noodles, frozen, Budget Gourmet	Meat/Fish/Poultry	⅓ portion	−2.5
Meat loaf	Meat/Fish/Poultry	3 ounces	−0.5
Meat loaf, frozen dinner	Meat/Fish/Poultry	½ piece	1.5
Melon, cantaloupe	Fruit	¼ piece	29.0
Melon, casaba	Fruit	¼ piece	11.0

Food Name	Nutrigroup	Serving Size		Nutripoints
Melon, honeydew	Fruit	1/4	piece	14.0
Mexican Combination Dinner, frozen, Swanson	Legume/Nut/Seed	1/3	portion	−1.0
Mexican Dinner, frozen, Patio	Legume/Nut/Seed	1/4	portion	0.0
Mexican Style Combo Dinner, frozen, Patio	Legume/Nut/Seed	1/3	portion	0.0
Mexican Style Dinner, frozen, Morton	Legume/Nut/Seed	1/2	portion	4.5
Milk Drink Mix, Strawberry, Quik, Nestlé	Milk/Dairy	1/2	cup	−2.0
Milk Drink, Alba	Milk/Dairy	16	fluid ounces	3.5
Milk Drink, Diet, Lite, Sego	Milk/Dairy	10	fluid ounces	13.5
Milk Drink, Diet, Sego	Milk/Dairy	6	fluid ounces	7.5
Milk Drink, Nutrament	Milk/Dairy	6	fluid ounces	4.5
Milk Drink, Slim-Fast	Milk/Dairy	8	fluid ounces	13.0
Milk Drink, Ultra Slim-Fast	Milk/Dairy	8	fluid ounces	11.0
Milk, condensed, sweetened, canned	Milk/Dairy	2	ounces	−2.0
Milk, Condensed, Sweetened, Carnation	Milk/Dairy	1/4	cup	−2.0
Milk, canned, evaporated, unsweetened	Milk/Dairy	1/2	cup	1.0
Milk, canned, skim, evaporated	Milk/Dairy	1/2	cup	9.5
Milk, chocolate	Milk/Dairy	1/2	cup	−0.5
Milk, chocolate, low-fat (1-percent)	Milk/Dairy	1	cup	2.5
Milk, chocolate, low-fat (2-percent)	Milk/Dairy	6	fluid ounces	2.5
Milk shake, chocolate	Milk/Dairy	1/2	cup	−1.0
Milk shake, vanilla	Milk/Dairy	1/2	cup	−1.0

Food Name	Nutrigroup	Serving Size	Nutripoints
Milk, Condensed, Sweetened, Eagle Brand	Milk/Dairy	¼ cup	−3.0
Milk, Evaporated, Carnation	Milk/Dairy	½ cup	1.0
Milk, Evaporated, Skim, Carnation	Milk/Dairy	¾ cup	9.0
Milk, goat	Milk/Dairy	1 cup	1.5
Milk, Instant Natural Malted, Carnation	Milk/Dairy	½ cup	−0.5
Milk, Instant Nonfat Dry, Carnation	Milk/Dairy	2 cups	11.5
Milk, low-fat (1-percent)	Milk/Dairy	1 cup	8.0
Milk, Low-Fat (2-percent), Hi-Calcium, Borden	Milk/Dairy	1 cup	7.5
Milk, low-fat (2-percent), protein fortified	Milk/Dairy	1 cup	6.0
Milk, Nondairy, Soy, West Soy	Legume/Nut/Seed	1 cup	0.5
Milk, nonfat dry	Milk/Dairy	¼ cup	10.5
Milk, skim	Milk/Dairy	1 cup	9.5
Milk, Soy, Natural Creamy Original, Vitasoy	Legume/Nut/Seed	1 cup	1.0
Milk, Soy, Natural, Edensoy	Legume/Nut/Seed	1 cup	2.0
Milk, Soy, Solait, Miller Farms	Legume/Nut/Seed	8 fluid ounces	0.5
Milk, Soy, Soyamel, Worthington	Legume/Nut/Seed	8 fluid ounces	7.5
Milk, Soy, Soymoo, Health Valley	Legume/Nut/Seed	1 cup	0.0
Milk, whole (3.3-percent)	Milk/Dairy	1 cup	2.5
Milk, whole (3.7-percent)	Milk/Dairy	1 cup	2.0
Mint julep	Alcohol	2 fluid ounces	−15.0

Food Name	Nutrigroup	Serving Size	Nutripoints
Mixed Fruits, Dried, Sun-Maid	Fruit	2 ounces	3.5
Mixed nuts, dry roast, unsalted	Legume/Nut/Seed	1 ounce	1.0
Mixed nuts, oil roasted, salted	Legume/Nut/Seed	1 ounce	1.0
Mixed Vegetables, frozen, Veg-All	Vegetable	½ cup	21.0
Mixed Vegetables, Natural Pack, canned, Libby's	Vegetable	½ cup	18.5
Mixed Vegetables, w/Butter, frozen, Green Giant	Vegetable	½ cup	7.5
Molasses	Sugar	2 tablespoons	−3.0
Molasses, blackstrap	Sugar	2 tablespoons	3.5
Moose	Meat/Fish/Poultry	3 ounces	5.5
Mousse, Cheesecake, Sans Sucre de Paris	Milk/Dairy	½ cup	3.5
Mousse, chocolate	Sugar	½ cup	−5.5
Mousse, Chocolate, frozen, Weight Watchers	Milk/Dairy	1 piece	−1.5
Mousse, Chocolate, Light, Sara Lee	Grain	½ piece	−4.0
Mousse, Key Lime, Nutripoint	Milk/Dairy	½ cup	5.5
Mousse, Raspberry, frozen, Weight Watchers	Fruit	½ portion	−2.5
Muffin	Grain	1 muffin	0.5
Muffin Mix, Blueberry, Wild, Betty Crocker	Grain	1 muffin	−1.5
Muffin Mix, Blueberry, Wild, Duncan Hines	Grain	1 muffin	−1.5
Muffin Mix, Bran Date, "Jiffy"	Grain	1 muffin	−1.0

Food Name	Nutrigroup	Serving Size	Nutripoints
Muffin Mix, Bran, Original Wheat, Arrowhead Mills	Grain	1 muffin	2.0
Muffin Mix, Corn, Betty Crocker	Grain	1 muffin	−1.0
Muffin Mix, Corn, "Jiffy"	Grain	1 muffin	−1.0
Muffin Mix, Corn, Old-Fashioned, frozen, Pepperidge Farm	Grain	1 muffin	−1.0
Muffin Mix, Oat Bran, Wheat-Free, Arrowhead Mills	Grain	1 muffin	2.5
Muffin, blueberry	Grain	1 muffin	0.0
Muffin, bran	Grain	1 whole	3.0
Muffin, bran, w/raisins and nuts	Grain	1 whole	3.5
Muffin, cornbread	Grain	1 muffin	0.5
Muffin, English	Grain	1 whole	4.0
Muffin, English, cracked wheat	Grain	1 whole	3.5
Muffin, English, Health Nut, Oroweat	Grain	1 whole	3.0
Muffin, English, Honey Wheat, Thomas'	Grain	1 whole	2.0
Muffin, English, Pepperidge Farm	Grain	1 whole	4.0
Muffin, English, Regular, Thomas'	Grain	1 whole	2.5
Muffin, English, Roman Meal	Grain	1 whole	4.5
Muffin, English, w/raisins	Grain	1 whole	4.5
Muffin, English, whole wheat	Grain	1 whole	6.0
Muffin, Extra Crisp, Arnold	Grain	1 whole	3.5
Muffin, Nutripoint	Grain	1 whole	10.5

Food Name	Nutrigroup	Serving Size	Nutripoints
Muffin, Oat Bran, Nutripoint	Grain	1 whole	3.5
Muffin, oatmeal	Grain	1 whole	1.0
Muffin, Raisin Oat Bran, Health Valley	Grain	1 whole	5.0
Muffin, w/fruit and/or nuts	Grain	1 muffin	−0.5
Mushrooms, Canned, Green Giant	Vegetable	1 cup	13.0
Mushrooms, cooked	Vegetable	1 cup	19.0
Mushrooms, fresh	Vegetable	1 cup	32.5
Mushrooms, fried, w/breading	Vegetable	¼ cup	−1.0
Mussels, cooked	Meat/Fish/Poultry	6 ounces	2.0
Mustard	Condiment	1 teaspoon	0.0
Mustard greens, cooked	Vegetable	1 cup	62.0
Mustard greens, frozen, cooked	Vegetable	1 cup	48.0
Mustard, Bold 'n Spicy, French's	Condiment	1 tablespoon	−0.5
Mustard, dry	Condiment	1 teaspoon	0.5
Mustard, w/Horseradish, French's	Condiment	1 tablespoon	−0.5
Mustard, Yellow, Prepared, French's	Condiment	1 tablespoon	−0.5
Nachos, cheese/hot peppers	Grain	5 pieces	1.0
Nectarine, fresh	Fruit	1 piece	10.0
Noodles and Cheese Dinner, Deboles	Grain	¼ cup	1.0
Noodles, chow mein	Grain	¼ cup	1.0
Noodles, egg, cholesterol-free, no yolks	Grain	1 dry ounce	3.0
Noodles, Egg, Cooked, Mueller's	Grain	½ cup	2.0
Noodles, Egg, Ronzoni	Grain	½ cup	0.0

Food Name	Nutrigroup	Serving Size	Nutripoints
Noodles, Egg, Veggie, Hodgson Mill	Grain	1 ounce	2.5
Noodles, Egg, Whole Wheat, Hodgson Mill	Grain	1 ounce	2.0
Noodles, Spaghetti, Whole Wheat, Hodgson Mill	Grain	1 ounce	2.5
Noodles, spinach	Grain	½ cup	3.5
Noodles, Spinach, Whole Wheat, Hodgson Mill	Grain	1 ounce	2.0
Noodles, whole wheat	Grain	½ cup	4.0
Nut Meat, Nuteena, Loma Linda	Legume/Nut/Seed	2 ounces	2.0
Nutmeg	Condiment	1 teaspoon	0.0
Nuts, Mixed, w/Peanuts, Planters	Legume/Nut/Seed	1 ounce	−1.5
Ocean Perch Fillet, frozen, Gorton's	Meat/Fish/Poultry	4 ounces	2.5
Ocean Perch Fillet, Light, Mrs. Paul's	Meat/Fish/Poultry	1 piece	−1.0
Ocean perch, baked	Meat/Fish/Poultry	4 ounces	4.5
Octopus, fried	Meat/Fish/Poultry	3 ounces	2.0
Oil	Fat/Oil	1 tablespoon	−3.0
Oil, almond	Fat/Oil	1 tablespoon	−2.5
Oil, Canola, Puritan	Fat/Oil	1 tablespoon	−2.5
Oil, cocoa butter	Fat/Oil	1 tablespoon	−5.5
Oil, coconut	Fat/Oil	1 tablespoon	−7.0
Oil, Corn, Crisco	Fat/Oil	1 tablespoon	−3.0
Oil, Corn, Mazola	Fat/Oil	1 tablespoon	−3.0
Oil, cottonseed	Fat/Oil	1 tablespoon	−3.5
Oil, Crisco	Fat/Oil	1 tablespoon	−3.0
Oil, hazelnut	Fat/Oil	1 tablespoon	−2.5
Oil, linseed	Fat/Oil	1 tablespoon	−2.5
Oil, olive	Fat/Oil	1 tablespoon	−3.0
Oil, Olive, Bertolli	Fat/Oil	1 tablespoon	−3.0
Oil, palm	Fat/Oil	1 tablespoon	−5.0
Oil, palm kernel	Fat/Oil	1 tablespoon	−6.5

Food Name	Nutrigroup	Serving Size	Nutripoints
Oil, Pam Spray	Condiment	0.3 gm or 1 spray	−0.5
Oil, peanut	Fat/Oil	1 tablespoon	−3.0
Oil, Puritan	Fat/Oil	1 tablespoon	−2.5
Oil, safflower	Fat/Oil	1 tablespoon	−2.5
Oil, Safflower, Hollywood	Fat/Oil	1 tablespoon	−2.5
Oil, sesame	Fat/Oil	1 tablespoon	−3.0
Oil, soybean	Fat/Oil	1 tablespoon	−3.0
Oil, sunflower	Fat/Oil	1 tablespoon	−2.5
Oil, Sunlite	Fat/Oil	1 tablespoon	−2.5
Oil, Vegetable, Puritan	Fat/Oil	1 tablespoon	−2.5
Oil, walnut	Fat/Oil	1 tablespoon	−2.5
Oil, Wesson	Fat/Oil	1 tablespoon	−3.0
Oil, wheat germ	Fat/Oil	1 tablespoon	−3.0
Okra, cooked	Vegetable	½ cup	31.0
Okra, fried, w/breading	Vegetable	¼ cup	1.0
Okra, raw	Vegetable	1 cup	26.0
Old fashioned	Alcohol	2 fluid ounces	−15.5
Olives, black	Fruit	8 whole	−2.0
Olives, green	Fruit	8 whole	−4.0
Olives, Medium, Mammoth Queen, S&W	Fruit	8 whole	−3.0
Olives, Ripe, Lindsay	Fruit	4 whole	0.0
Onion powder	Condiment	1 teaspoon	0.5
Onion rings, fried	Vegetable	2 pieces	−0.5
Onion, green	Condiment	2 stalks	1.0
Onion, raw (1 tablespoon = 1 teaspoon dried onion flakes)	Vegetable	½ cup	8.5
Orange roughy, raw	Meat/Fish/Poultry	5 ounces	4.0
Orange, fresh	Fruit	1 piece	13.5
Oregano	Condiment	1 teaspoon	1.0
Oyster stew	Meat/Fish/Poultry	1 cup	3.0
Oysters, broiled, w/butter	Meat/Fish/Poultry	3 ounces	7.0
Oysters, eastern, raw	Meat/Fish/Poultry	12 oysters	13.0

Food Name	Nutrigroup	Serving Size	Nutripoints
Oysters, fried	Meat/Fish/Poultry	3 pieces	1.5
Oysters, Pacific, raw	Meat/Fish/Poultry	4 oysters	8.0
Pancake and Waffle Mix, Blue Corn	Grain	1 piece	−1.0
Pancake and Waffle Mix, Buttermilk, Hungry Jack	Grain	2 pancakes	−1.5
Pancake and Waffle Mix, Extra Light, Hungry Jack	Grain	2 pancakes	−1.0
Pancake Mix, Complete Buttermilk, Aunt Jemima	Grain	2 pancakes	3.5
Pancake Mix, Original Complete, Aunt Jemima	Grain	2 pancakes	2.5
Pancake, buckwheat	Grain	1 pancake	1.0
Pancake, cornmeal	Grain	1 pancake	1.0
Pancake, plain	Grain	1 pancake	0.5
Pancake, w/fruit	Grain	1 pancake	0.5
Pancake, Whole Grain, Nutripoint	Grain	4 pieces	5.5
Pancake, whole wheat	Grain	1 pancake	0.5
Pancakes, Lite, Buttermilk, Aunt Jemima	Grain	3 pancakes	7.0
Papaya	Fruit	1/2 piece	20.5
Papaya nectar, canned	Fruit	6 fluid ounces	4.0
Paprika	Condiment	1 teaspoon	2.5
Parsley, dried	Condiment	1 teaspoon	0.5
Parsley, fresh	Vegetable	1 cup	54.5
Parsnips, cooked	Vegetable	1/2 cup	8.5
Parsnips, raw	Vegetable	1/2 cup	11.5
Passion fruit, purple, fresh	Fruit	2 pieces	9.0

Food Name	Nutrigroup	Serving Size	Nutripoints
Pasta Accents, Cheddar Cheese, Green Giant	Grain	½ cup	4.0
Pasta Accents, Garlic Seasoning, Green Giant	Grain	½ cup	3.5
Pasta Alfredo, w/Broccoli, frozen, Budget Gourmet	Grain	½ portion	0.0
Pasta and Cheese, Baked, frozen, Celentano	Grain	½ portion	0.0
Pasta and Sauce, Marinara, Hain	Grain	¼ cup	1.0
Pasta and Sauce, Swiss, Creamy, Hain	Grain	¼ cup	− 1.5
Pasta Carbonara, frozen, Stouffer's	Grain	¼ portion	− 1.5
Pasta Casino, frozen, Stouffer's	Grain	½ portion	1.0
Pasta Mexicali, frozen, Stouffer's	Grain	½ portion	− 1.0
Pasta Oriental, frozen, Stouffer's	Grain	½ portion	1.0
Pasta Primavera, frozen, Weight Watchers	Grain	½ portion	2.5
Pasta Salad, Fresh, Nutripoint	Grain	½ cup	4.5
Pasta salad, home recipe	Grain	¼ cup	− 1.0
Pasta Salad, Italian, Cool Side, Lipton	Grain	½ cup	0.5
Pasta Shells and Beef, frozen, Budget Gourmet	Grain	½ piece	1.5
Pasta Shells, Cheese Stuffed, w/Meat Sauce, Stouffer's	Milk/Dairy	½ portion	− 0.5

Food Name	Nutrigroup	Serving Size	Nutripoints
Pasta, Angel Hair, w/Sunshine Sauce, Nutripoint	Grain	1½ cups	10.0
Pastrami, beef	Meat/Fish/Poultry	2 ounces	−2.5
Pastrami, Land O' Frost	Meat/Fish/Poultry	4 ounces	−2.0
Pastrami, turkey	Meat/Fish/Poultry	3 pieces	1.0
Pâté	Meat/Fish/Poultry	2 ounces	−3.5
Pâté, chicken liver, canned	Meat/Fish/Poultry	2 ounces	0.5
Pâté, de foie gras, canned (goose liver)	Meat/Fish/Poultry	1 ounce	−1.0
Peach nectar, canned	Fruit	6 fluid ounces	4.0
Peach, fresh	Fruit	1 piece	11.0
Peaches, canned in heavy syrup	Fruit	½ cup	0.0
Peaches, canned in juice	Fruit	1 piece	6.5
Peaches, canned, unsweetened	Fruit	½ cup	10.5
Peaches, dried, sulfured, uncooked	Fruit	2 pieces	5.0
Peaches, Dried, Sun-Maid	Fruit	4 pieces	5.0
Peaches, Light Yellow Cling, in Fruit Juice, canned, Libby's	Fruit	½ cup	6.5
Peaches, Yellow Cling, in Light Syrup, canned, Del Monte	Fruit	½ cup	4.0
Peanut butter	Legume/Nut/Seed	1 tablespoon	0.5
Peanut Butter, Chunky, Health Valley	Legume/Nut/Seed	2 tablespoons	1.5
Peanut Butter, Chunky, No Salt, Health Valley	Legume/Nut/Seed	2 tablespoons	1.5
Peanut Butter, Creamy, Jif	Legume/Nut/Seed	1 tablespoon	0.0

Food Name	Nutrigroup	Serving Size	Nutripoints
Peanut Butter, Creamy, Skippy	Legume/Nut/Seed	1 tablespoon	0.0
Peanut Butter, Crunchy, Peter Pan	Legume/Nut/Seed	1 tablespoon	0.0
Peanut butter, low-sodium	Legume/Nut/Seed	1 tablespoon	1.0
Peanut Butter, Natural, Smucker's	Legume/Nut/Seed	1 tablespoon	1.0
Peanut Butter, No Salt Added, Natural, Smucker's	Legume/Nut/Seed	1 tablespoon	1.0
Peanut Butter, Super Chunk, Skippy	Legume/Nut/Seed	1 tablespoon	0.0
Peanut butter, unsalted	Legume/Nut/Seed	1 tablespoon	1.0
Peanuts, chocolate-covered	Legume/Nut/Seed	1 ounce	−1.0
Peanuts, Cocktail, Planters	Legume/Nut/Seed	1 ounce	1.0
Peanuts, Dry Roasted, Salted, Frito-Lay	Legume/Nut/Seed	25 pieces	1.0
Peanuts, Dry Roasted, Salted, Planters	Legume/Nut/Seed	1 ounce	1.0
Peanuts, Dry Roasted, Unsalted, Planters	Legume/Nut/Seed	1 ounce	1.5
Peanuts, honey roasted	Legume/Nut/Seed	1 ounce	0.5
Peanuts, oil roasted, salted	Legume/Nut/Seed	25 pieces	1.0
Peanuts, oil roasted, unsalted	Legume/Nut/Seed	25 pieces	1.5
Peanuts, Spanish, Salted, Planters	Legume/Nut/Seed	1 ounce	1.0
Peanuts, yogurt-covered	Legume/Nut/Seed	1 ounce	−1.0
Pear nectar, canned	Fruit	6 fluid ounces	2.5
Pear, fresh	Fruit	1 whole	4.5
Pear, Poached, Nutripoint	Fruit	½ serving	4.0

Food Name	Nutrigroup	Serving Size	Nutripoints
Pears, Bartlett, in Light Syrup, canned, Del Monte	Fruit	1/2 cup	1.5
Pears, canned in heavy syrup	Fruit	1/2 cup	−1.0
Pears, canned, no sugar	Fruit	1/2 cup	3.5
Pears, dried	Fruit	2 pieces	3.0
Peas and carrots, canned	Vegetable	1/2 cup	25.0
Peas and carrots, frozen, cooked	Vegetable	1/2 cup	28.0
Peas, black-eyed, canned	Legume/Nut/Seed	1 cup	9.0
Peas, black-eyed, cooked	Legume/Nut/Seed	1 cup	8.5
Peas, canned	Legume/Nut/Seed	1 cup	7.5
Peas, Early June, canned, Le Sueur	Legume/Nut/Seed	1 cup	4.5
Peas, frozen, cooked	Legume/Nut/Seed	1 cup	14.0
Peas, Green, frozen, Birds Eye	Legume/Nut/Seed	1 cup	12.0
Peas, Green, No Salt Added, canned, Del Monte	Legume/Nut/Seed	1 cup	14.0
Peas, split	Legume/Nut/Seed	1/2 cup	8.0
Peas, Sweet, 50-Percent Less Salt, canned, Green Giant	Legume/Nut/Seed	1/2 cup	6.5
Peas, Sweet, canned, Green Giant	Legume/Nut/Seed	1/2 cup	6.5
Peas, Sweet, Early Garden, canned, Del Monte	Legume/Nut/Seed	1/2 cup	6.0
Pecans, oil roasted, salted	Legume/Nut/Seed	1 ounce	−0.5
Pecans, unsalted, raw	Legume/Nut/Seed	15 pieces	0.0

Food Name	Nutrigroup	Serving Size	Nutripoints
Pepper Steak, w/Rice, frozen, Budget Gourmet	Meat/Fish/Poultry	½ portion	0.0
Pepper, black	Condiment	1 teaspoon	0.5
Pepper, cayenne/red	Condiment	1 teaspoon	1.5
Pepper, jalapeño	Condiment	1 pepper	0.5
Pepperoni	Meat/Fish/Poultry	1 ounce	−5.0
Pepperoni, Gallo	Meat/Fish/Poultry	1 ounce	−6.0
Peppers, green, hot chili	Condiment	1 tablespoon	2.5
Peppers, sweet red, raw	Vegetable	2 whole	42.5
Peppers, Sweet, Stuffed, frozen, Celentano	Meat/Fish/Poultry	½ portion	2.0
Perch fillet, baked/broiled	Meat/Fish/Poultry	4 ounces	4.0
Perch, fried, w/breading	Meat/Fish/Poultry	3 ounces	1.0
Perrier Mineral Water	Miscellaneous	8 fluid ounces	0.0
Persimmon	Fruit	1 piece	7.5
Pheasant, w/o skin	Meat/Fish/Poultry	4 ounces	5.5
Pickle relish	Vegetable	2 tablespoons	−6.0
Pickles, Bread 'n Butter, Cucumber Slices, Heinz	Vegetable	8 pieces	−1.0
Pickles, dill	Vegetable	2 whole	−3.5
Pickles, Kosher Crunchy Dills, Half the Salt, Vlasic	Vegetable	2 whole	3.0
Pickles, Kosher Dill Spears, Vlasic	Vegetable	2 whole	0.5
Pickles, Kosher, Claussen	Vegetable	2 whole	−4.0
Pickles, sweet	Vegetable	1 whole	−5.0
Pickles, Sweet Butter Chips, Vlasic	Condiment	1 ounce	−1.0
Pickles, Sweet Gherkins, Heinz	Vegetable	1 whole	−2.5

Food Name	Nutrigroup	Serving Size	Nutripoints
Pickles, Sweet 'n Sour, Claussen	Vegetable	1 piece	2.5
Pie crust	Grain	1 piece	−3.0
Pie Crust Mix, Betty Crocker	Grain	1 piece	−2.5
Pie Crust, Pet Ritz	Grain	1 piece	−2.5
Pie Filling, Apple, Lite, Thank You	Fruit	½ cup	−1.5
Pie Filling, Apple, Thank You	Fruit	½ cup	−3.0
Pie Filling, Cherry, Thank You	Fruit	½ cup	−4.0
Pie, apple	Fruit	¼ piece	−2.0
Pie, Apple, frozen, Weight Watchers	Fruit	½ piece	−2.0
Pie, Apple, in Natural Juice, Mrs. Smith's	Fruit	¼ piece	−2.5
Pie, banana cream	Fruit	½ piece	−1.0
Pie, berry	Fruit	½ piece	−2.0
Pie, blackberry	Fruit	½ piece	−1.5
Pie, blueberry	Fruit	½ piece	−2.0
Pie, Blueberry, Hostess	Fruit	¼ piece	−2.0
Pie, Boston cream	Milk/Dairy	½ piece	−1.0
Pie, Boston Cream Classic, Betty Crocker	Milk/Dairy	½ piece	−2.5
Pie, Boston Cream, frozen, Weight Watchers	Milk/Dairy	1 piece	−2.5
Pie, cherry	Fruit	½ piece	−5.0
Pie, Cherry, Hostess	Fruit	¼ piece	−2.0
Pie, Cherry, in Natural Juice, Mrs. Smith's	Fruit	¼ piece	−2.0
Pie, cherry, w/cream cheese and sour cream	Fruit	¼ piece	−3.5
Pie, chiffon	Sugar	½ piece	−4.5
Pie, chocolate cream	Sugar	½ piece	−2.5

Food Name	Nutrigroup	Serving Size	Nutripoints
Pie, coconut cream	Fruit	½ piece	−3.5
Pie, custard	Milk/Dairy	½ piece	−3.5
Pie, fruit	Fruit	¼ piece	−2.0
Pie, Fruit Yogurt, Nutripoint	Milk/Dairy	1 piece	0.5
Pie, lemon meringue	Fruit	¼ piece	−4.0
Pie, mincemeat	Fruit	¼ piece	−1.0
Pie, peach	Fruit	½ piece	−2.0
Pie, Peach, Mrs. Smith's	Fruit	¼ piece	−2.5
Pie, pecan	Legume/Nut/Seed	½ piece	−3.5
Pie, Pumpkin Custard, Mrs. Smith's	Milk/Dairy	½ piece	−2.0
Pie, pumpkin, homemade	Fruit	½ piece	−3.0
Pie, raspberry	Fruit	½ piece	−1.0
Pie, rhubarb, homemade	Vegetable	¼ piece	−2.5
Pie, strawberry	Fruit	½ piece	−1.5
Pie, vanilla cream	Milk/Dairy	½ piece	−3.0
Pie, yogurt	Milk/Dairy	½ piece	−2.5
Pigeon peas, green, cooked	Legume/Nut/Seed	1 cup	11.0
Pike fillet, breaded, fried	Meat/Fish/Poultry	3 ounces	0.5
Pike, baked	Meat/Fish/Poultry	6 ounces	7.5
Pilaf, Breakfast, Seven Whole Grains and Sesame Seeds, Kashi	Grain	½ cup	3.5
Pilaf, Couscous, Casbah	Grain	½ cup	3.0
Pilaf, Vegetarian Amaranth, Health Valley	Grain	4 ounces	6.5
Piña colada	Alcohol	3 fluid ounces	−7.5
Pine Nuts, Pignolia	Legume/Nut/Seed	1 ounce	1.0
Pineapple, canned in heavy syrup	Fruit	½ cup	1.0

Food Name	Nutrigroup	Serving Size	Nutripoints
Pineapple, Chunks, in Juice, canned, Del Monte	Fruit	½ cup	4.0
Pineapple, fresh	Fruit	½ cup	8.0
Pineapple, Sliced, in Light Syrup, canned, Dole	Fruit	½ cup	2.0
Pineapple, Sliced, in Juice, canned, Del Monte	Fruit	½ cup	4.0
Pineapple, Sliced, in Juice, canned, Dole	Fruit	½ cup	4.0
Pistachios, dry roasted, salted	Legume/Nut/Seed	¼ cup	0.0
Pistachios, raw	Legume/Nut/Seed	1 ounce	1.0
Pizza Hut Cheese Pan Pizza	Grain	½ piece	2.5
Pizza Hut Cheese Thin 'n Crispy Pizza	Grain	1 piece	3.0
Pizza Hut Hand-Tossed Cheese Pizza	Grain	½ piece	2.0
Pizza Hut Pepperoni Hand-Tossed Pizza	Grain	½ piece	1.5
Pizza Hut Pepperoni Pan Pizza	Grain	½ piece	3.0
Pizza Hut Pepperoni Personal Pan Pizza	Grain	¼ piece	2.0
Pizza Hut Pepperoni Thin 'n Crispy Pizza	Grain	½ piece	1.5
Pizza Hut Super Supreme Hand-Tossed Pizza	Grain	½ piece	2.0
Pizza Hut Super Supreme Pan Pizza	Grain	½ piece	2.0
Pizza Hut Super Supreme Thin 'n Crispy Pizza	Grain	½ piece	2.0

Food Name	Nutrigroup	Serving Size	Nutripoints
Pizza Hut Supreme Hand-Tossed Pizza	Grain	½ piece	3.5
Pizza Hut Supreme Pan Pizza	Grain	½ piece	2.0
Pizza Hut Supreme Personal Pan Pizza	Grain	¼ piece	2.0
Pizza Hut Supreme Thin 'n Crispy Pizza	Grain	½ piece	2.0
Pizza, 9-Slice, frozen, Celentano	Grain	1 piece	0.5
Pizza, Cheese, Chef Boyardee	Grain	1 piece	0.5
Pizza, Cheese, Deluxe, frozen, Totino's	Grain	1 piece	1.0
Pizza, Cheese, French Bread, frozen, Weight Watchers	Grain	½ piece	0.5
Pizza, Cheese, French Bread, Lean Cuisine, Stouffer's	Grain	½ piece	2.0
Pizza, Cheese, frozen, Celeste	Grain	1 piece	0.0
Pizza, Cheese, frozen, Tree Tavern	Grain	½ piece	0.5
Pizza, Cheese, frozen, Weight Watchers	Grain	1 piece	1.5
Pizza, Cheese, Round Family Style, Ellio's	Grain	1 piece	0.0
Pizza, Combo, Deluxe, frozen, Weight Watchers	Grain	½ piece	1.5
Pizza, Combos	Grain	1 ounce	0.0
Pizza, French Bread Deluxe, frozen, Weight Watchers	Grain	½ piece	0.5
Pizza, French Bread Pepperoni, Stouffer's	Grain	½ piece	1.0

Food Name	Nutrigroup	Serving Size	Nutripoints
Pizza, French Bread, Cheese, frozen, Stouffer's	Grain	½ piece	0.5
Pizza, French Bread, Nutripoint	Grain	1 piece	6.0
Pizza, French Bread, Vegetable Deluxe, frozen, Stouffer's	Grain	½ piece	0.5
Pizza, French Bread, Pepperoni and Mushroom, frozen, Stouffer's	Grain	½ portion	0.0
Pizza, Party Cheese, frozen, Totino's	Grain	1 piece	0.5
Pizza, Pepperoni, Chef Boyardee	Grain	1 piece	−0.5
Pizza, Pepperoni, frozen, Ellio's	Grain	½ piece	0.0
Pizza, Pepperoni, frozen, Weight Watchers	Grain	½ piece	1.0
Pizza, Pepperoni, French Bread, frozen, Weight Watchers	Grain	½ portion	0.0
Pizza, Sausage, frozen, Weight Watchers	Grain	½ piece	1.0
Pizza, Thick Crust, frozen, Celentano	Grain	1 piece	0.5
Pizza, w/cheese	Grain	1 piece	1.0
Pizza, w/pepperoni	Grain	½ piece	−2.0
Pizza, w/sausage	Grain	½ piece	−1.0
Plantain, cooked	Fruit	½ cup	5.5
Plantain, fresh	Fruit	½ plantain	6.0
Plum, fresh	Fruit	2 whole	6.0
Plums, canned in heavy syrup	Fruit	½ cup	0.0

Food Name	Nutrigroup	Serving Size	Nutripoints
Plums, canned, unsweetened	Fruit	½ cup	14.0
Poi	Vegetable	½ cup	3.5
Pomegranate	Fruit	1 whole	3.5
Pompano, baked/broiled	Meat/Fish/Poultry	3 ounces	0.5
Pompano, floured/breaded, fried	Meat/Fish/Poultry	3 ounces	—0.5
Pop-Tarts, Blueberry, Kellogg's	Grain	1 tart	0.5
Pop-Tarts, Frosted Cherry w/Smucker's Fruit, Kellogg's	Grain	1 tart	0.5
Pop-Tarts, Frosted Strawberry, Kellogg's	Grain	1 tart	1.0
Popcorn, air-popped	Grain	2 cups	2.0
Popcorn, caramel	Grain	1 cup	0.0
Popcorn, cooked w/oil	Grain	2 cups	0.0
Popcorn, Gourmet, Microwave, Orville Redenbacher	Vegetable	2 cups	—0.5
Popcorn, Gourmet, Orville Redenbacher	Vegetable	2 cups	2.5
Popcorn, Light, Orville Redenbacher's	Vegetable	3 cups	3.0
Popcorn, Natural Salt Free, Orville Redenbacher's	Vegetable	2 cups	0.5
Popover	Grain	1 popover	—2.5
Poppy seed	Condiment	1 teaspoon	0.5
Pork chop, broiled	Meat/Fish/Poultry	2 ounces	—0.5
Pork chop, loin, lean, baked	Meat/Fish/Poultry	3 ounces	3.0
Pork chop, pan-fried	Meat/Fish/Poultry	1 piece	—1.0
Pork feet, pickled	Meat/Fish/Poultry	3 ounces	—1.0
Pork roast, baked	Meat/Fish/Poultry	2 ounces	0.0

Food Name	Nutrigroup	Serving Size	Nutripoints
Pork skins	Meat/Fish/Poultry	1 ounce	0.0
Pork spareribs	Meat/Fish/Poultry	3 pieces	−1.5
Pork, frozen dinner	Meat/Fish/Poultry	½ portion	2.0
Pork, sweet and sour	Meat/Fish/Poultry	¾ cup	0.0
Pork, Sweet and Sour, frozen, Chun King	Meat/Fish/Poultry	½ portion	2.0
Postum	Miscellaneous	6 fluid ounces	5.5
Potato chips	Vegetable	5 pieces	0.0
Potato Chips, Lay's	Vegetable	8 pieces	0.0
Potato Chips, Light, Pringle's	Vegetable	½ cup	−1.0
Potato Chips, Light, Ruffles	Vegetable	9 pieces	1.0
Potato Chips, Pringle's	Vegetable	½ cup	−2.0
Potato Chips, Ruffles	Vegetable	9 pieces	0.0
Potato Chips, Sour Cream 'n Onion, Pringle's	Vegetable	½ cup	−1.5
Potato Chips, Unsalted, Lay's	Vegetable	8 pieces	0.0
Potato Chips, Wise	Vegetable	5 pieces	−1.0
Potato salad, home recipe	Vegetable	¼ cup	−1.0
Potato Salad, Nutripoint	Vegetable	½ cup	9.0
Potato sticks, shoestring	Vegetable	¼ cup	0.0
Potato, baked	Vegetable	½ potato	8.5
Potato, Baked, Chicken Divan, frozen, Weight Watchers	Vegetable	¼ piece	1.5
Potato, Baked, w/Broccoli and Cheese, frozen, Weight Watchers	Vegetable	¼ piece	1.5
Potatoes au gratin	Vegetable	¼ cup	2.5
Potatoes au Gratin, Betty Crocker	Vegetable	½ cup	−0.5

Food Name	Nutrigroup	Serving Size	Nutripoints
Potatoes au Gratin, frozen, Stouffer's	Vegetable	½ piece	−0.5
Potatoes, Cheddared, w/Broccoli, frozen, Budget Gourmet	Vegetable	½ piece	1.5
Potatoes, Golden Crinkles, Ore-Ida	Vegetable	½ cup	0.5
Potatoes, hash-browned	Vegetable	¼ cup	0.5
Potatoes, Homestyle, Nutripoint	Vegetable	½ cup	5.5
Potatoes, Instant Mashed, Betty Crocker	Vegetable	½ cup	−0.5
Potatoes, Instant Mashed, Hungry Jack	Vegetable	¼ cup	0.0
Potatoes, mashed, from flakes	Vegetable	¼ cup	2.0
Potatoes, mashed, home recipe	Vegetable	¼ cup	1.0
Potatoes, scalloped	Vegetable	¼ cup	2.0
Potatoes, Scalloped, frozen, Stouffer's	Vegetable	½ portion	0.5
Potatoes, Tater Tots, Ore-Ida	Vegetable	¼ cup	−0.5
Preserves, all varieties, Kraft	Fruit	1 tablespoon	−5.0
Preserves, Raspberry, Smucker's	Fruit	1 tablespoon	−6.0
Preserves, Strawberry, Welch's	Fruit	1 tablespoon	−5.5
Pretzels, 3-ring	Grain	10 pieces	0.5
Pretzels, Keebler	Grain	½ cup	1.5
Pretzels, sticks	Grain	50 pieces	0.5
Pretzels, Twists, Rold Gold	Grain	1 ounce	1.0
Prickly pear	Fruit	1 piece	10.0
Protein powder	Miscellaneous	1 tablespoon	2.0

Food Name	Nutrigroup	Serving Size	Nutripoints
Prunes, canned in heavy syrup	Fruit	¼ cup	4.5
Prunes, cooked, unsweetened	Fruit	½ cup	6.5
Prunes, cooked, w/sugar	Fruit	¼ cup	4.0
Prunes, dried	Fruit	4 pieces	6.0
Prunes, Pitted, Bite-Size, Sunsweet	Fruit	1 ounce	5.0
Prunes, Whole, Sunsweet	Fruit	3 pieces	6.0
Pudding Mix, Americana Tapioca, Jell-O	Milk/Dairy	1 cup	−2.0
Pudding Mix, Vanilla, Jell-O	Milk/Dairy	1 cup	−2.5
Pudding Mix, Vanilla, Sugar-Free, Instant, Jell-O	Milk/Dairy	1 cup	2.0
Pudding, banana	Milk/Dairy	¼ cup	1.0
Pudding, bread	Grain	½ cup	−2.0
Pudding, Chocolate Pudding Snacks, Jell-O	Milk/Dairy	4 ounces	−3.5
Pudding, chocolate	Milk/Dairy	½ cup	−3.5
Pudding, Chocolate, Snack Pack, Hunt's	Milk/Dairy	4 ounces	−4.0
Pudding, low-cal.	Milk/Dairy	1 cup	3.0
Pudding, rice	Grain	¼ cup	−1.0
Pudding, Sustacal	Milk/Dairy	½ cup	2.0
Pudding, tapioca	Milk/Dairy	½ cup	−0.5
Pudding, vanilla	Milk/Dairy	½ cup	−1.5
Pudding, Vanilla, Snack Pack, Hunt's	Milk/Dairy	4 ounces	−4.0
Pumpkin, canned	Vegetable	½ cup	25.5
Pumpkin, cooked	Vegetable	½ cup	17.5
Quail, w/o skin	Meat/Fish/Poultry	4 ounces	6.0
Quiche, cheese	Milk/Dairy	½ piece	−6.0
Quiche, cheese/bacon	Milk/Dairy	¼ piece	−4.5

Food Name	Nutrigroup	Serving Size	Nutripoints
Quince	Fruit	1 whole	6.0
Quinine water	Sugar	8 fluid ounces	−5.5
Quinoa, Dry, Arrowhead Mills	Grain	1 ounce	5.5
Rabbit, domestic, breaded, fried	Meat/Fish/Poultry	3 ounces	3.0
Rabbit, stewed	Meat/Fish/Poultry	3 ounces	2.0
Rabbit, wild	Meat/Fish/Poultry	3 ounces	3.0
Radishes, raw	Vegetable	1 cup	29.0
Raisins	Fruit	¼ cup	4.0
Raisins, California Golden, Sun-Maid	Fruit	2 tablespoons	3.0
Raisins, carob-covered	Fruit	1 ounce	−1.0
Raisins, chocolate-covered	Fruit	1 ounce	−1.5
Raisins, Thompson Seedless, Natural, Sun-Maid	Fruit	2 tablespoons	3.0
Ramen, Natural Mushroom, Westbrae	Grain	½ cup	2.0
Ramen, Natural Spinach, Westbrae	Grain	1 ounce	2.0
Ramen, Natural Whole Wheat, Westbrae	Grain	1 ounce	2.0
Raspberries, fresh	Fruit	½ cup	12.5
Raspberries, frozen, sweetened	Fruit	¼ cup	4.5
Ratatouille, frozen dinner	Vegetable	1 piece	1.5
Ravioli	Grain	½ cup	4.5
Ravioli, Cheese, Slim, frozen, Budget Gourmet	Milk/Dairy	½ portion	0.5
Ravioli, frozen, Celentano	Grain	½ piece	0.0
Ravioli, Mini, frozen, Celentano	Grain	½ portion	2.0

Food Name	Nutrigroup	Serving Size	Nutripoints
Ravioli, w/Cheese, frozen, Weight Watchers	Milk/Dairy	½ portion	1.0
Red Snapper Veracruz, Nutripoint	Meat/Fish/Poultry	3 ounces	13.5
Red snapper, baked	Meat/Fish/Poultry	6 ounces	7.0
Relish, Hot Dog, Vlasic	Vegetable	2 tablespoons	−2.5
Relish, Sweet, Heinz	Vegetable	2 tablespoons	−3.5
Rhubarb, cooked, w/sugar	Vegetable	¼ cup	−2.5
Rice, Brown Pilaf, w/Vegetables and Herbs, Pritikin	Grain	½ cup	3.0
Rice, brown, cooked, w/o salt	Grain	½ cup	4.0
Rice, Brown, Instant, Minute	Grain	½ cup	3.5
Rice, Brown, Natural Long Grain, Mahatma	Grain	½ cup	3.5
Rice, Brown, Quick, w/Vegetables and Herbs, Arrowhead Mills	Grain	½ cup	2.5
Rice, Chicken Rice-A-Roni	Grain	½ cup	0.5
Rice, Converted, Uncle Ben's	Grain	½ cup	2.5
Rice, Extra Long Grain Enriched, Carolina	Grain	½ cup	2.0
Rice, Fried, w/Chicken, frozen, Chun King	Grain	½ portion	1.5
Rice, Fried, w/Pork, frozen, Chun King	Grain	½ portion	1.0
Rice, Long Grain Enriched, Mahatma	Grain	½ cup	2.0

Food Name	Nutrigroup	Serving Size	Nutripoints
Rice, Minute Rice	Grain	½ cup	2.5
Rice, Oriental, w/Vegetables, frozen, Budget Gourmet	Grain	½ portion	0.0
Rice, pilaf	Grain	½ cup	2.0
Rice, Rice-A-Roni	Grain	½ cup	0.0
Rice, Rice-A-Roni, Spanish	Grain	½ cup	1.5
Rice, Spanish	Grain	½ cup	4.0
Rice, white, instant, cooked	Grain	⅔ cup	3.0
Rice, white, regular, cooked, w/o salt	Grain	½ cup	3.0
Rice, white, regular, w/salt	Grain	½ cup	3.0
Rice, Whole Grain Brown, Uncle Ben's	Grain	⅗ cup	4.5
Rice, wild, cooked, w/o salt	Grain	½ cup	5.5
Rice, Wild, Sherry, frozen, Green Giant	Grain	½ cup	4.5
Rigatoni, w/Meat Sauce and Cheese, frozen, Stouffer's	Grain	½ portion	0.5
Roll, cracked wheat	Grain	1 whole	3.0
Roll, diet	Grain	1 whole	2.5
Roll, Dinner, Wheat Loaf, Pipin' Hot	Grain	2 rolls	1.5
Roll, Dinner, White Loaf, Pipin' Hot	Grain	2 rolls	1.5
Roll, Frankfurter, Side-Sliced, Pepperidge Farm	Grain	1 whole	1.5
Roll, Frankfurter, Wonder	Grain	1 whole	2.0
Roll, French or Vienna	Grain	1 whole	2.5

Food Name	Nutrigroup	Serving Size	Nutripoints
Roll, French, Brown 'n Serve, Pepperidge Farm	Grain	½ roll	2.5
Roll, hard	Grain	1 whole	2.0
Roll, rye	Grain	1 whole	3.5
Roll, sourdough	Grain	1 whole	2.5
Roll, Sourdough, French Extra, Earth Grains	Grain	2 whole	2.5
Roll, sweet	Grain	½ roll	−2.5
Roll, Sweet, Apple, frozen, Weight Watchers	Grain	1 roll	−1.5
Roll, sweet, cinnamon bun, frosted	Grain	1 roll	−1.0
Roll, Sweet, Cinnamon, w/Icing, Pillsbury	Grain	1 roll	−2.5
Roll, sweet, w/fruit	Grain	1 roll	1.5
Roll, sweet, w/fruit and nuts, frosted	Grain	1 roll	0.0
Roll, sweet, w/fruit, frosted	Grain	1 roll	0.0
Roll, white	Grain	1 whole	2.0
Roll, whole wheat	Grain	1 whole	4.5
Rosemary	Condiment	1 teaspoon	0.5
Rotini, w/Cheddar Cheese, Garden Gourmet, Green Giant	Grain	½ cup	4.0
Rotini, Rainbow, Creamette	Grain	1 ounce	3.0
Roy Rogers Apple Danish	Grain	½ Danish	−2.0
Roy Rogers Bacon Cheeseburger	Meat/Fish/Poultry	½ piece	−1.5
Roy Rogers Bar Burger	Meat/Fish/Poultry	½ piece	−1.5
Roy Rogers Biscuit	Grain	½ biscuit	−1.0

Food Name	Nutrigroup	Serving Size	Nutripoints
Roy Rogers Breakfast Crescent Sandwich	Grain	¼ serving	−3.5
Roy Rogers Breakfast Crescent Sandwich w/Bacon	Grain	¼ serving	−3.5
Roy Rogers Breakfast Crescent Sandwich w/Ham	Grain	¼ serving	−3.5
Roy Rogers Breakfast Crescent Sandwich w/Sausage	Grain	¼ serving	−3.0
Roy Rogers Brownie	Grain	½ piece	−2.0
Roy Rogers Caramel Sundae	Milk/Dairy	½ serving	−2.0
Roy Rogers Cheese Danish	Grain	½ Danish	−1.5
Roy Rogers Cheeseburger	Meat/Fish/Poultry	½ piece	−2.0
Roy Rogers Cherry Danish	Grain	½ Danish	−2.0
Roy Rogers Chicken Breast	Meat/Fish/Poultry	½ piece	−1.0
Roy Rogers Chicken Breast and Wing	Meat/Fish/Poultry	½ piece	−1.5
Roy Rogers Chicken Drumstick/Leg	Meat/Fish/Poultry	1 piece	−1.0
Roy Rogers Chicken Thigh	Meat/Fish/Poultry	½ piece	−2.0
Roy Rogers Chicken Thigh and Leg	Meat/Fish/Poultry	½ piece	−1.5
Roy Rogers Chicken Wing	Meat/Fish/Poultry	1 piece	−2.0
Roy Rogers Chocolate Shake	Milk/Dairy	½ serving	−2.0
Roy Rogers Coleslaw	Vegetable	½ serving	6.0
Roy Rogers Crescent Roll	Grain	¼ roll	−1.5
Roy Rogers Egg and Biscuit Platter	Milk/Dairy	¼ serving	−5.5

Food Name	Nutrigroup	Serving Size	Nutripoints
Roy Rogers Egg and Biscuit Platter w/Bacon	Milk/Dairy	¼ serving	−5.5
Roy Rogers Egg and Biscuit Platter w/Ham	Milk/Dairy	¼ serving	−5.0
Roy Rogers Egg and Biscuit Platter w/Sausage	Milk/Dairy	¼ serving	−5.5
Roy Rogers French Fries	Vegetable	¼ serving	−1.5
Roy Rogers Hamburger	Meat/Fish/Poultry	½ piece	−1.5
Roy Rogers Hot Fudge Sundae	Milk/Dairy	½ serving	−2.5
Roy Rogers Hot Topped Potato w/Bacon and Cheese	Vegetable	¼ serving	−0.5
Roy Rogers Hot Topped Potato w/Broccoli and Cheese	Vegetable	¼ piece	0.5
Roy Rogers Hot Topped Potato, w/margarine	Vegetable	¼ serving	2.5
Roy Rogers Hot Topped Potato w/Sour Cream and Chives	Vegetable	¼ serving	0.0
Roy Rogers Hot Topped Potato w/Taco Beef and Cheese	Vegetable	¼ serving	0.0
Roy Rogers Hot Topped Potato, plain	Vegetable	½ serving	4.0
Roy Rogers Large Roast Beef Sandwich	Meat/Fish/Poultry	½ piece	0.5

Food Name	Nutrigroup	Serving Size	Nutripoints
Roy Rogers Large Roast Beef Sandwich w/Cheese	Meat/Fish/Poultry	½ piece	−0.5
Roy Rogers Macaroni	Grain	½ cup	−2.0
Roy Rogers Pancake Platter w/Syrup and Butter	Grain	¼ serving	−0.5
Roy Rogers Pancake Platter w/Syrup/ Butter/Bacon	Grain	¼ serving	−1.0
Roy Rogers Pancake Platter w/Syrup/ Butter/Ham	Grain	¼ serving	−0.5
Roy Rogers Pancake Platter w/Syrup/ Butter/Sausage	Grain	¼ serving	−1.5
Roy Rogers Potato Salad	Vegetable	¼ cup	−1.0
Roy Rogers Roast Beef Sandwich	Meat/Fish/Poultry	½ piece	1.0
Roy Rogers Roast Beef Sandwich w/Cheese	Meat/Fish/Poultry	½ piece	−0.5
Roy Rogers Strawberry Shake	Milk/Dairy	½ serving	−2.0
Roy Rogers Strawberry Shortcake	Grain	¼ piece	−1.5
Roy Rogers Strawberry Sundae	Milk/Dairy	½ serving	−1.5
Roy Rogers Vanilla Shake	Milk/Dairy	½ serving	−2.0
Rum	Alcohol	2 fluid ounces	−16.5
Rum and carbonated beverage	Alcohol	6 fluid ounces	−10.5
Rum, hot buttered	Alcohol	3 fluid ounces	−12.5
Rutabagas, cooked	Vegetable	½ cup	18.0
Sage	Condiment	1 teaspoon	0.5

Food Name	Nutrigroup	Serving Size	Nutripoints
Salad Greens, w/ Balsamic Vinegar, Nutripoint	Vegetable	1 cup	42.0
Salad, chef, w/ham and cheese, w/o dressing	Vegetable	½ cup	−1.5
Salad, Mixed Vegetable, Nutripoint	Vegetable	½ cup	17.0
Salad, Spinach, Nutripoint	Vegetable	2 cups	65.0
Salad, spinach, w/egg/bacon/tom-ato	Vegetable	½ cup	4.0
Salad, three-bean	Legume/Nut/Seed	1 cup	1.5
Salad, tossed, no dressing	Vegetable	1 cup	33.0
Salad, Tossed, Nutripoint	Vegetable	2 cups	51.5
Salad, tossed, w/tomato	Vegetable	1 cup	21.5
Salad, Waldorf	Fruit	½ cup	−2.0
Salami, beef	Meat/Fish/Poultry	2 ounces	0.0
Salami, Cooked, Armour	Meat/Fish/Poultry	2 ounces	−4.0
Salami, Cotto Beef, Eckrich	Meat/Fish/Poultry	1 ounce	−4.0
Salami, Cotto, Oscar Mayer	Meat/Fish/Poultry	2 pieces	−2.0
Salami, Hard (Genoa), Oscar Mayer	Meat/Fish/Poultry	4 pieces	−2.5
Salami, pork	Meat/Fish/Poultry	4 pieces	1.0
Salami, Slices, frozen, Loma Linda	Legume/Nut/Seed	2 ounces	5.5
Salami, Turkey Cotto, Louis Rich	Meat/Fish/Poultry	3 pieces	−2.0
Salmon patty, fried	Meat/Fish/Poultry	3 ounces	1.0
Salmon, baked, w/butter	Meat/Fish/Poultry	3 ounces	2.0
Salmon, baked/broiled	Meat/Fish/Poultry	3 ounces	5.5

Food Name	Nutrigroup	Serving Size	Nutripoints
Salmon, canned in water	Meat/Fish/Poultry	½ cup	6.5
Salmon, Lettuce-Wrapped, w/Herb Sauce, Nutripoint	Meat/Fish/Poultry	4 ounces	10.5
Salmon, Pink, Bumble Bee	Meat/Fish/Poultry	½ cup	4.0
Salmon, Pink, Chunk, Skinless and Boneless, in Water, Chicken of the Sea	Meat/Fish/Poultry	¾ cup	4.5
Salmon, Red Sockeye, Bumble Bee	Meat/Fish/Poultry	½ cup	3.0
Salmon, Red, Chunk, Skinless and Boneless, Chicken of the Sea	Meat/Fish/Poultry	½ cup	3.5
Salmon, smoked	Meat/Fish/Poultry	3 ounces	3.0
Salmon, steamed/poached	Meat/Fish/Poultry	3 ounces	7.5
Salt	Condiment	1 teaspoon	0.0
Salt pork, raw	Meat/Fish/Poultry	1 ounce	−4.0
Salt, Iodized, Morton	Condiment	1 teaspoon	0.0
Salt, Lite, Morton	Condiment	1 teaspoon	0.0
Sandwich, BLT, white bread	Meat/Fish/Poultry	½ piece	1.0
Sandwich, BLT, whole wheat bread	Meat/Fish/Poultry	½ piece	2.0
Sandwich, chicken salad, white bread	Meat/Fish/Poultry	½ piece	3.5
Sandwich, chicken salad, whole wheat bread	Meat/Fish/Poultry	½ piece	4.0
Sandwich, chicken, white bread	Meat/Fish/Poultry	½ piece	2.0
Sandwich, chicken, whole wheat bread	Meat/Fish/Poultry	½ piece	2.0
Sandwich, corned beef, rye bread	Meat/Fish/Poultry	½ piece	1.5

Food Name	Nutrigroup	Serving Size	Nutripoints
Sandwich, egg salad, white bread	Milk/Dairy	½ piece	−3.5
Sandwich, egg salad, whole wheat bread	Milk/Dairy	½ piece	−3.0
Sandwich, grilled cheese, white	Milk/Dairy	½ piece	0.0
Sandwich, ham salad, white	Meat/Fish/Poultry	½ piece	−0.5
Sandwich, ham salad, whole wheat	Meat/Fish/Poultry	½ piece	0.0
Sandwich, ham/cheese, rye bread	Meat/Fish/Poultry	½ piece	0.5
Sandwich, ham/cheese, white bread	Meat/Fish/Poultry	½ piece	0.0
Sandwich, ham/cheese, whole wheat bread	Meat/Fish/Poultry	½ piece	0.5
Sandwich, Manwich, Original, Hunt's	Condiment	2 tablespoons	0.0
Sandwich, Open-Face Pita, Nutripoint	Grain	½ serving	5.0
Sandwich, peanut butter, white bread	Legume/Nut/Seed	½ piece	1.5
Sandwich, peanut butter, whole wheat bread	Legume/Nut/Seed	½ piece	2.0
Sandwich, peanut butter/jelly, white bread	Legume/Nut/Seed	½ piece	0.5
Sandwich, peanut butter/jelly, whole wheat	Legume/Nut/Seed	½ piece	0.5
Sandwich, roast beef, hot	Meat/Fish/Poultry	½ piece	1.0
Sandwich, sloppy joe, w/bun	Meat/Fish/Poultry	½ piece	1.0
Sandwich, Steak, frozen, Steak-Umm	Meat/Fish/Poultry	2 ounces	−3.0

Food Name	Nutrigroup	Serving Size	Nutripoints
Sandwich, submarine	Meat/Fish/Poultry	¼ piece	0.0
Sandwich, tuna salad, white bread	Meat/Fish/Poultry	½ piece	3.0
Sandwich, tuna salad, whole wheat bread	Meat/Fish/Poultry	½ piece	3.5
Sandwich, Turkey, Nutripoint	Meat/Fish/Poultry	1 whole	4.0
Sandwich, turkey, white bread	Meat/Fish/Poultry	½ piece	− 1.5
Sandwich, turkey, whole wheat bread	Meat/Fish/Poultry	½ piece	2.5
Sardines, canned in oil	Meat/Fish/Poultry	3 pieces	4.5
Sardines, canned in mustard sauce	Meat/Fish/Poultry	6 pieces	1.5
Sardines, canned in tomato sauce	Meat/Fish/Poultry	6 pieces	3.5
Sauce mix, Béarnaise, w/milk-butter	Fat/Oil	¼ cup	−5.5
Sauce mix, curry, w/milk	Fat/Oil	¼ cup	0.0
Sauce mix, mushroom, prepared w/milk	Fat/Oil	¼ cup	1.0
Sauce mix, Stroganoff, prepared w/milk and water	Fat/Oil	¼ cup	1.5
Sauce mix, sweet and sour, prepared	Fat/Oil	¼ cup	0.0
Sauce mix, teriyaki, prepared	Fat/Oil	¼ cup	−2.5
Sauce, Banana Mint, Nutripoint	Milk/Dairy	¼ cup	6.5
Sauce, barbecue	Condiment	1 tablespoon	0.0
Sauce, Barbecue, All-Natural Hot and Zesty, Hunt's	Condiment	1 tablespoon	− 1.5
Sauce, Barbecue, All-Natural Original Flavor, Hunt's	Condiment	1 tablespoon	−0.5

Food Name	Nutrigroup	Serving Size	Nutripoints
Sauce, Barbecue, Hickory Smoke Flavor, Open Pit	Condiment	1 tablespoon	−1.0
Sauce, Barbecue, Kraft	Condiment	1 tablespoon	−2.5
Sauce, Barbecue, Original Flavor, Open Pit	Condiment	1 tablespoon	−1.5
Sauce, Barbecue, w/Onion Bits, Kraft	Condiment	1 tablespoon	−1.5
Sauce, butterscotch	Sugar	2 tablespoons	−4.5
Sauce, Butterscotch, Smucker's	Sugar	2 tablespoons	−5.0
Sauce, cheese	Milk/Dairy	1/4 cup	−5.5
Sauce, chili	Condiment	1 tablespoon	1.0
Sauce, chocolate	Sugar	2 tablespoons	−5.0
Sauce, chocolate fudge	Sugar	2 tablespoons	−3.5
Sauce, cranberry, canned, sweetened	Fruit	2 tablespoons	−3.0
Sauce, Cranberry, Whole Berry, Ocean Spray	Fruit	1/4 cup	−4.5
Sauce, custard	Milk/Dairy	1/4 cup	−4.0
Sauce, Heinz 57	Condiment	1 tablespoon	−1.0
Sauce, Hollandaise	Fat/Oil	1/4 cup	−5.0
Sauce, Juniper Berry, Nutripoint	Condiment	2 tablespoons	0.0
Sauce, picante	Condiment	1/4 cup	4.0
Sauce, soy	Condiment	1 teaspoon	0.0
Sauce, Soy, Kikkoman	Condiment	1 teaspoon	−0.5
Sauce, Spaghetti, Extra Chunky Mushroom and Onion, Prego	Vegetable	1/4 cup	−0.5
Sauce, Spaghetti, Extra Thick and Zesty, Flavored w/Meat, Ragú	Vegetable	1/2 cup	−0.5

Food Name	Nutrigroup	Serving Size	Nutripoints
Sauce, Spaghetti, Flavored w/Meat, Ragú	Vegetable	1/2 cup	0.0
Sauce, Spaghetti, Garden Tomato w/Mushrooms, Prego	Vegetable	1/4 cup	−0.5
Sauce, Spaghetti, Meat Flavor, Prego	Vegetable	1/4 cup	−1.0
Sauce, Spaghetti, Meatless, Aunt Millie's	Vegetable	1/2 cup	4.0
Sauce, Spaghetti, No Salt Added, Prego	Vegetable	1/2 cup	4.0
Sauce, Spaghetti, plain, Extra Thick and Zesty, Ragú	Vegetable	1/2 cup	0.0
Sauce, Spaghetti, plain, Ragú	Vegetable	1/2 cup	0.0
Sauce, Spaghetti, Prego	Vegetable	1/2 cup	0.5
Sauce, Spaghetti, Pritikin	Vegetable	1/2 cup	9.5
Sauce, Spaghetti, w/Mushrooms, Homestyle, Ragú	Vegetable	1/2 cup	3.0
Sauce, Spaghetti, w/Mushrooms, Prego	Vegetable	1/2 cup	0.5
Sauce, Spaghetti, w/Peppers and Sausage, Aunt Millie's	Vegetable	1/2 cup	3.5
Sauce, steak	Condiment	1 tablespoon	1.5
Sauce, sweet and sour	Condiment	1 tablespoon	−1.5
Sauce, tartar	Fat/Oil	2 tablespoons	−3.5
Sauce, Tartar, Sauce Works, Kraft	Fat/Oil	1 tablespoon	−0.5

Food Name	Nutrigroup	Serving Size	Nutripoints
Sauce, teriyaki	Condiment	1 tablespoon	−0.5
Sauce, tomato, canned	Vegetable	1/2 cup	17.5
Sauce, Tomato, Del Monte	Vegetable	1/2 cup	10.5
Sauce, Tomato, Hunt's	Vegetable	1/2 cup	9.0
Sauce, Tomato, Nutripoint	Vegetable	1/2 cup	19.0
Sauce, Tomato, Thick and Zesty, Contadina	Vegetable	1/2 cup	15.5
Sauce, Traditional Pizza Quick, Ragú	Vegetable	3 tablespoons	−0.5
Sauce, white	Fat/Oil	1/4 cup	−1.0
Sauce, Worcestershire	Condiment	1 teaspoon	1.0
Sauerkraut, canned	Vegetable	1 cup	17.0
Sausage, link, pork	Meat/Fish/Poultry	2 pieces	−2.5
Sausage patty	Meat/Fish/Poultry	1 piece	3.0
Sausage Patty, Breakfast, frozen, Morningstar Farms	Legume/Nut/Seed	2 pieces	3.5
Sausage, Breakfast Links, frozen, Morningstar Farms	Legume/Nut/Seed	3 pieces	3.5
Sausage, Italian	Meat/Fish/Poultry	2 ounces	−0.5
Sausage, Italian, 1 link	Meat/Fish/Poultry	3 ounces	−1.5
Sausage, Little, Jones	Meat/Fish/Poultry	2 ounces	−3.0
Sausage, Polish	Meat/Fish/Poultry	2 ounces	0.0
Sausage, Pork, Jimmy Dean	Meat/Fish/Poultry	2 ounces	−3.5
Sausage, summer	Meat/Fish/Poultry	2 pieces	−1.0
Sausage, Vienna	Meat/Fish/Poultry	3 pieces	−3.5
Scallions	Vegetable	10 stalks	24.0
Scallop Kabob, Nutripoint	Meat/Fish/Poultry	2 kabobs	16.0
Scallops and Shrimp Mariner, frozen, Budget Gourmet	Meat/Fish/Poultry	1/2 portion	0.5

Food Name	Nutrigroup	Serving Size	Nutripoints
Scallops, baked/broiled	Meat/Fish/Poultry	6 ounces	4.0
Scallops, fried	Meat/Fish/Poultry	3 ounces	1.0
Screwdriver	Alcohol	8 fluid ounces	−9.0
Scrod, Baked, Stuffed, frozen, Gorton's	Meat/Fish/Poultry	4 ounces	−2.5
Seafood Newburg, frozen, Budget Gourmet	Meat/Fish/Poultry	½ portion	−0.5
Seasoning, poultry	Condiment	1 teaspoon	0.5
Seasoning, Shake 'n Bake for Pork	Condiment	1 tablespoon	−1.0
Seasoning, Shake 'n Bake Original Chicken	Condiment	1 tablespoon	0.0
Seeds, pumpkin and squash	Legume/Nut/Seed	¼ cup	2.0
Seeds, pumpkin and squash, roasted, salted	Legume/Nut/Seed	1 ounce	2.5
Seeds, pumpkin and squash, roasted, unsalted	Legume/Nut/Seed	1 ounce	2.5
Seeds, sesame	Legume/Nut/Seed	¼ cup	0.0
Seeds, Sunflower, Hulled, Arrowhead Mills	Legume/Nut/Seed	2 tablespoons	2.0
Seeds, sunflower, unsalted	Legume/Nut/Seed	¼ cup	4.5
Sesame butter (tahini)	Legume/Nut/Seed	1 ounce	1.5
Shallots, raw	Vegetable	¼ cup	8.5
Shark, mixed species, batter-dipped and fried	Meat/Fish/Poultry	3 ounces	0.0
Shark, mixed species, raw	Meat/Fish/Poultry	4 ounces	4.0
Shells and Cheese Dinner, Velveeta	Grain	½ cup	0.0
Shells, frozen, Broccoli Stuffed, Celentano	Milk/Dairy	¼ piece	1.5

Food Name	Nutrigroup	Serving Size	Nutripoints
Shells, Stuffed, 3-Cheese, frozen, Le Menu	Milk/Dairy	½ portion	1.0
Shells, Stuffed, frozen, Celentano	Milk/Dairy	½ portion	2.0
Sherbet, orange	Fruit	½ cup	−2.5
Sherbet, Orange, Borden	Milk/Dairy	½ cup	−4.0
Shortbread, Lorna Doone	Grain	3 pieces	−2.5
Shortcake, sponge type w/fruit	Grain	½ piece	−1.0
Shortcake, Strawberry, frozen, Weight Watchers	Grain	1 piece	−2.0
Shortening, Crisco	Fat/Oil	1 tablespoon	−3.5
Shortening, lard and vegetable oil	Fat/Oil	1 tablespoon	−4.5
Shortening, soybean and cottonseed	Fat/Oil	1 tablespoon	−3.5
Shortening, soybean and palm	Fat/Oil	1 tablespoon	−4.0
Shrimp Creole, frozen, Healthy Choice	Meat/Fish/Poultry	1 piece	0.5
Shrimp étouffée (1 serving = 1½ cup)	Meat/Fish/Poultry	1 serving	2.0
Shrimp Primavera, frozen, Stouffer's Right Course	Meat/Fish/Poultry	1 portion	1.0
Shrimp, fried	Meat/Fish/Poultry	3 pieces	−1.0
Shrimp, Fried, frozen, Mrs. Paul's	Meat/Fish/Poultry	3 ounces	−4.0
Shrimp, steamed	Meat/Fish/Poultry	15 pieces	0.5
Singapore sling	Alcohol	6 fluid ounces	−13.5
Sloe gin fizz	Alcohol	8 fluid ounces	−14.5
Smelt, rainbow, baked	Meat/Fish/Poultry	4 ounces	4.5
Snack Cake, Apple Delight, Little Debbie	Grain	2 pieces	−5.5

Food Name	Nutrigroup	Serving Size	Nutripoints
Snack Cake, Desert Light, Apple 'n' Spice, Pepperidge Farm	Grain	1 piece	−2.0
Snack Cake, Ding Dong, Hostess	Grain	1 piece	−2.0
Snack Cake, Drake's Devil Dogs	Grain	1 piece	−2.5
Snack Cake, Drake's Ring Ding Jr.	Grain	1 piece	−3.0
Snack Cake, Lights Hostess	Grain	1 piece	−1.0
Snack Cake, Oatmeal Creme Pie, Little Debbie	Grain	2 pieces	−6.5
Snack Cake, Peanut Butter Bar, Little Debbie	Grain	2 pieces	−7.0
Snack Cake, Star Crunch, Little Debbie	Grain	2 pieces	−8.5
Snack Cake, Suzy Q's	Grain	½ piece	−3.5
Snails	Meat/Fish/Poultry	4 ounces	4.0
Soft Drink, 7-Up	Sugar	12 fluid ounces	−5.5
Soft drink, Coke w/caffeine	Sugar	12 fluid ounces	−6.0
Soft drink, cream soda	Sugar	12 fluid ounces	−5.5
Soft drink, diet, w/caffeine	Miscellaneous	12 fluid ounces	−2.5
Soft drink, diet, w/o caffeine	Miscellaneous	12 fluid ounces	0.0
Soft drink, Dr Pepper	Sugar	12 fluid ounces	−5.5
Soft drink, ginger ale	Sugar	12 fluid ounces	−5.0
Soft drink, lemon-lime, w/o caffeine	Sugar	12 fluid ounces	−5.5
Soft drink, Mountain Dew	Sugar	12 fluid ounces	−6.5
Soft drink, w/caffeine	Sugar	12 fluid ounces	−7.0
Soft drink, w/o caffeine	Sugar	12 fluid ounces	−5.0

Food Name	Nutrigroup	Serving Size	Nutripoints
Sole au Gratin, frozen, Healthy Choice	Meat/Fish/Poultry	1 portion	1.5
Sole Fillet, Fishmarket Fresh, frozen, Gorton's	Meat/Fish/Poultry	4 ounces	−2.0
Sole Fillet, Light, Mrs. Paul's	Meat/Fish/Poultry	1 piece	−1.0
Sole, baked	Meat/Fish/Poultry	6 ounces	6.0
Sole, Stuffed, w/Newburg Sauce, frozen, Weight Watchers	Meat/Fish/Poultry	½ portion	1.5
Sopaipilla	Grain	1 piece	−3.0
Soufflé, cheese	Milk/Dairy	½ cup	−3.0
Soufflé, Corn, frozen, Stouffer's	Vegetable	½ piece	0.5
Soufflé, spinach	Vegetable	½ cup	−3.0
Soup mix, chicken noodle, dehydrated	Miscellaneous	1 serving	−1.5
Soup Mix, Chicken Noodle, w/Meat, Lipton	Meat/Fish/Poultry	1 cup	−2.5
Soup Mix, Chicken Rice, Lipton	Meat/Fish/Poultry	1 cup	−2.5
Soup Mix, Country Vegetable, Lipton	Vegetable	1 cup	2.0
Soup Mix, Cream of Mushroom, Cup-A-Soup, Lipton	Vegetable	1 cup	−2.5
Soup Mix, Green Pea, Cup-A-Soup, Lipton	Vegetable	½ cup	0.5
Soup mix, onion, dehydrated	Miscellaneous	2 tablespoons	−1.5
Soup Mix, Onion, Lipton	Vegetable	1 cup	−5.5
Soup Mix, Tomato, Cup-A-Soup, Lipton	Vegetable	1 cup	−2.5
Soup, bean	Legume/Nut/Seed	1 cup	3.5
Soup, black bean	Legume/Nut/Seed	1 cup	5.0

Food Name	Nutrigroup	Serving Size	Nutripoints
Soup, Black Bean, Health Valley	Legume/Nut/Seed	1 cup	7.5
Soup, beef	Meat/Fish/Poultry	1 cup	4.0
Soup, beef noodle	Meat/Fish/Poultry	1 cup	1.0
Soup, Beef, Campbell's	Meat/Fish/Poultry	1 cup	0.5
Soup, Blueberry, Chilled, Nutripoint	Fruit	3/4 cup	6.0
Soup, cheese	Milk/Dairy	1/2 cup	—1.0
Soup, chicken	Meat/Fish/Poultry	1 cup	1.5
Soup, Chicken Broth, Low-Sodium, Campbell's	Condiment	1 cup	3.5
Soup, chicken gumbo	Meat/Fish/Poultry	3/4 cup	5.5
Soup, chicken noodle	Meat/Fish/Poultry	1 cup	0.5
Soup, Chicken Noodle, Campbell's	Meat/Fish/Poultry	1 cup	—1.5
Soup, chicken rice	Meat/Fish/Poultry	1 cup	—1.5
Soup, Chicken Vegetable, Campbell's	Meat/Fish/Poultry	1 cup	2.0
Soup, Chicken Vegetable, Couscous, Nile Spice Foods	Meat/Fish/Poultry	1 cup	2.0
Soup, Chicken w/Noodles, Low-sodium, Campbell's	Meat/Fish/Poultry	1 cup	1.5
Soup, Chicken, Home Style, Progresso	Meat/Fish/Poultry	1 1/2 cups	5.5
Soup, Chicken, w/Ribbon Pasta, Pritikin	Meat/Fish/Poultry	1 cup	4.5
Soup, chowder, fish	Meat/Fish/Poultry	1 cup	1.0
Soup, Chunky Beef, Campbell's	Meat/Fish/Poultry	1 cup	4.0
Soup, Chunky Chicken Noodle, Campbell's	Meat/Fish/Poultry	1 cup	0.5

Food Name	Nutrigroup	Serving Size	Nutripoints
Soup, Chunky Five-Bean Vegetable, Health Valley	Vegetable	1 cup	11.0
Soup, Chunky Minestrone, Campbell's	Vegetable	1 cup	3.5
Soup, Chunky Old-Fashioned Bean 'n Ham, Campbell's	Legume/Nut/Seed	½ cup	2.0
Soup, Chunky Steak 'n Potato, Campbell's	Meat/Fish/Poultry	1 cup	0.5
Soup, Chunky Vegetable, Campbell's	Vegetable	1 cup	5.0
Soup, clam chowder, Manhattan tomato base	Meat/Fish/Poultry	2 cups	0.0
Soup, clam chowder, New England milk base	Meat/Fish/Poultry	1 cup	4.5
Soup, cream	Milk/Dairy	1 cup	1.5
Soup, cream of asparagus	Vegetable	½ cup	1.0
Soup, cream of celery	Vegetable	½ cup	−0.5
Soup, Cream of Celery, Campbell's	Vegetable	1 cup	−3.0
Soup, cream of chicken	Meat/Fish/Poultry	1 cup	0.0
Soup, Cream of Chicken, Campbell's	Meat/Fish/Poultry	1 cup	−2.0
Soup, Cream of Chicken, ⅓ Less Salt, Campbell's	Meat/Fish/Poultry	1 cup	−1.5
Soup, cream of mushroom	Vegetable	¼ cup	−1.0

Food Name	Nutrigroup	Serving Size	Nutripoints
Soup, Cream of Mushroom, Campbell's	Vegetable	1 cup	−4.5
Soup, Cream of Mushroom, 1/3 Less Salt, Campbell's	Vegetable	1 cup	−2.0
Soup, Creamy Natural Broccoli, Campbell's	Vegetable	1 cup	−1.0
Soup, Creamy Natural Broccoli, w/Milk, Campbell's	Vegetable	1/2 cup	−1.0
Soup, Creamy Natural Potato, Campbell's	Vegetable	1/2 cup	−4.0
Soup, Creamy Natural Potato, w/milk, Campbell's	Vegetable	1/2 cup	−2.5
Soup, French Market, Nutripoint	Legume/Nut/Seed	1 1/2 cups	17.0
Soup, French Onion, Campbell's	Vegetable	1 cup	−3.5
Soup, Green Pea, Campbell's	Legume/Nut/Seed	8 ounces	2.5
Soup, Hot and Sour, Nutripoint	Legume/Nut/Seed	1 cup	4.0
Soup, lentil	Legume/Nut/Seed	1 cup	5.5
Soup, Lentil Curry, Couscous, Nile Spice Foods	Legume/Nut/Seed	1 cup	6.5
Soup, Lentil, Health Valley	Legume/Nut/Seed	1/2 cup	8.0
Soup, Lentil, Nutripoint	Legume/Nut/Seed	1 cup	13.5
Soup, lentil, w/ham	Legume/Nut/Seed	1 cup	4.5
Soup, minestrone	Vegetable	1 cup	5.0
Soup, Minestrone, Campbell's	Vegetable	1 cup	3.5
Soup, Minestrone, Health Valley	Legume/Nut/Seed	1 1/2 cups	14.0

Food Name	Nutrigroup	Serving Size	Nutripoints
Soup, Minestrone, Progresso	Legume/Nut/Seed	1 cup	4.0
Soup, Mushroom, Beefy, Campbell's	Meat/Fish/Poultry	1 cup	−3.5
Soup, Mushroom, Cream of, Campbell's	Vegetable	¼ cup	−1.0
Soup, New England Clam Chowder, w/Milk, Campbell's	Meat/Fish/Poultry	1 cup	−0.5
Soup, onion	Vegetable	1 cup	−1.5
Soup, Oyster Stew, w/milk, Campbell's	Meat/Fish/Poultry	8 ounces	−1.5
Soup, pea	Legume/Nut/Seed	1 cup	4.0
Soup, Pea, Split, Green, Health Valley	Legume/Nut/Seed	½ cup	10.0
Soup, Pea, Split, Green, Progresso	Legume/Nut/Seed	½ cup	2.5
Soup, Pea, Split, Natural, Hain	Legume/Nut/Seed	1 cup	4.0
Soup, potato	Vegetable	½ cup	0.5
Soup, seafood gumbo	Meat/Fish/Poultry	1 cup	3.5
Soup, Spinach, Clear, Nutripoint	Vegetable	1 cup	23.5
Soup, tomato	Vegetable	1 cup	2.5
Soup, Tomato Minestrone, Couscous, Nile Spice Foods	Vegetable	½ cup	2.5
Soup, Tomato Rice, Old-Fashioned, Campbell's	Vegetable	1 cup	−1.5
Soup, Tomato w/Vegetables, Progresso	Vegetable	1 cup	6.5
Soup, Tomato, ⅓ Less Salt, Campbell's	Vegetable	1 cup	0.5

Food Name	Nutrigroup	Serving Size	Nutripoints
Soup, Tomato, Campbell's	Vegetable	1 cup	0.5
Soup, Tomato, Health Valley	Vegetable	½ cup	11.5
Soup, Tomato, Low Sodium, w/Tomato Pieces, Campbell's	Vegetable	½ cup	1.0
Soup, Tomato, No Salt, Health Valley	Vegetable	½ cup	12.0
Soup, Tomato, w/Milk, Campbell's	Vegetable	½ cup	−1.0
Soup, Tomato, w/Milk, ⅓ Less Salt, Campbell's	Vegetable	½ cup	0.0
Soup, Turkey Vegetable, Campbell's	Meat/Fish/Poultry	1 cup	2.5
Soup, vegetable	Vegetable	1 cup	12.0
Soup, vegetable beef	Vegetable	1 cup	4.5
Soup, Vegetable Parmesan, Couscous, Nile Spice Foods	Vegetable	½ cup	2.5
Soup, Vegetable, ⅓ Less Salt, Campbell's	Vegetable	1 cup	3.0
Soup, Vegetable, Campbell's	Vegetable	1 cup	2.0
Soup, Vegetable, Health Valley	Vegetable	1 cup	12.5
Soup, Vegetable, No Salt, Health Valley	Vegetable	1 cup	13.0
Soup, Vegetable, Pritikin	Vegetable	1 cup	6.5
Soup, Vegetarian Vegetable, Campbell's	Vegetable	8 ounces	4.5
Soup, Wild Rice, Nutripoint	Grain	1 cup	10.5

Food Name	Nutrigroup	Serving Size	Nutripoints
Soup, wonton	Miscellaneous	1 cup	−1.0
Soybean nuts, roasted, salted	Legume/Nut/Seed	1 ounce	5.0
Soybeans, cooked	Legume/Nut/Seed	¾ cup	7.0
Soybeans, Dry, Arrowhead Mills	Legume/Nut/Seed	1 ounce	7.5
Soybeans, roasted, unsalted	Legume/Nut/Seed	1 ounce	3.5
Soyburger patty	Legume/Nut/Seed	3 ounces	4.0
Soyburger, w/bun	Legume/Nut/Seed	½ piece	3.0
Spaghetti Substitute, Spinach, Deboles	Grain	1 ounce	2.5
Spaghetti, cooked (1 cup = 2 ounces dry)	Grain	½ cup	3.0
Spaghetti, Creamette, Borden	Grain	½ cup	2.5
Spaghetti, high-protein	Grain	½ cup	4.0
Spaghetti, low-cal., frozen dinner	Grain	½ portion	2.5
Spaghetti, Ronzoni	Grain	½ cup	3.0
Spaghetti, San Giorgio	Grain	½ cup	3.0
Spaghetti, w/Beef and Mushroom Sauce, frozen, Stouffer's	Grain	½ portion	0.5
Spaghetti, w/meat sauce	Grain	½ cup	2.0
Spaghetti, w/Meat Sauce, frozen, Weight Watchers	Grain	½ portion	2.5
Spaghetti, w/Meat Sauce, frozen, Stouffer's	Grain	½ portion	0.0
Spaghetti, w/Meatball Dinner, frozen, Morton	Grain	1 dinner	3.5
Spaghetti, w/meatballs	Grain	½ cup	1.5

Food Name	Nutrigroup	Serving Size	Nutripoints
Spaghetti, w/Meatballs in Tomato Sauce, Chef Boyardee	Grain	1 cup	−1.0
Spaghetti, w/sauce	Grain	½ cup	2.0
Spam	Meat/Fish/Poultry	2 ounces	−1.5
Spinach au Gratin, frozen, Budget Gourmet	Vegetable	½ portion	3.0
Spinach, Cut Leaf, in Butter, frozen, Green Giant	Vegetable	½ cup	20.0
Spinach, Early Garden, canned, Del Monte	Vegetable	¾ cup	35.5
Spinach, fresh, cooked	Vegetable	1 cup	53.5
Spinach, frozen, cooked	Vegetable	¾ cup	42.5
Spinach, Leaf, No Salt Added, canned, Del Monte	Vegetable	1 cup	29.5
Spinach, raw, chopped	Vegetable	2 cups	75.0
Spinach, Whole Leaf, frozen, Birds Eye	Vegetable	1 cup	57.0
Squash, acorn, baked	Vegetable	½ cup	11.5
Squash, butternut, baked	Vegetable	½ cup	26.5
Squash, fried, w/breading	Vegetable	¼ cup	−1.0
Squash, summer, cooked	Vegetable	1 cup	24.5
Squash, winter, baked	Vegetable	½ cup	16.0
Squash, Winter, Cooked, frozen, Birds Eye	Vegetable	½ cup	23.0
Squid, boiled	Meat/Fish/Poultry	6 ounces	−1.5
Squid, fried	Meat/Fish/Poultry	3 ounces	0.0
Squid, raw	Meat/Fish/Poultry	6 ounces	2.0

Food Name	Nutrigroup	Serving Size	Nutripoints
Squirrel	Meat/Fish/Poultry	3 ounces	3.0
Stinger	Alcohol	2 fluid ounces	−12.5
Strawberries, fresh	Fruit	1 cup	19.0
Strawberries, frozen, in Heavy Syrup, Birds Eye	Fruit	¼ cup	5.0
Strawberries, frozen, sweetened	Fruit	½ cup	6.5
Strawberries, frozen, unsweetened	Fruit	1 cup	17.0
Strawberries, Halved, frozen, in Light Syrup, Birds Eye	Fruit	½ cup	8.5
Stuffing	Grain	½ cup	−1.5
Stuffing Mix, American New England, Stove Top	Grain	½ cup	−0.5
Stuffing Mix, Cornbread, w/Butter, Stove Top	Grain	½ cup	−1.5
Stuffing Mix, Herb Seasoned, Pepperidge Farm	Grain	½ cup	1.0
Sturgeon, steamed	Meat/Fish/Poultry	4 ounces	5.5
Succotash, cooked	Vegetable	½ cup	7.5
Succotash, frozen, cooked	Vegetable	½ cup	7.0
Sugar, brown	Sugar	2 tablespoons	−5.0
Sugar, cinnamon	Sugar	2 tablespoons	−5.5
Sugar, maple	Sugar	3 tablespoons	−5.5
Sugar, powdered	Sugar	3 tablespoons	−4.5
Sugar, raw	Sugar	2 tablespoons	−5.0
Sugar, white	Sugar	2 tablespoons	−6.0
Sugar, white confectioner's	Sugar	4 tablespoons	−5.5
Sushi/raw fish	Meat/Fish/Poultry	6 ounces	2.5
Sustacal	Milk/Dairy	4 fluid ounces	8.0
Sweet potato/yam, baked	Vegetable	½ potato/yam	12.0

Food Name	Nutrigroup	Serving Size	Nutripoints
Sweet potato/yam, canned	Vegetable	½ potato/yam	8.0
Sweet potatoes, candied	Vegetable	½ potato	4.0
Sweetbreads	Meat/Fish/Poultry	3 ounces	−52.0
Swiss chard, cooked	Vegetable	1 cup	42.0
Swordfish fillet, breaded, fried	Meat/Fish/Poultry	3 ounces	1.0
Swordfish, baked	Meat/Fish/Poultry	3 ounces	6.5
Syrup, butter blends	Sugar	2 teaspoons	−6.0
Syrup, cane	Sugar	2 teaspoons	−5.0
Syrup, corn	Sugar	2 teaspoons	−5.0
Syrup, maple	Sugar	2 tablespoons	−5.0
Syrup, maple, low-cal.	Sugar	2 tablespoons	−4.0
Syrup, sorghum	Sugar	2 teaspoons	−3.5
Taco Bell Bean Burrito w/Green Sauce	Legume/Nut/Seed	½ serving	4.0
Taco Bell Bean Burrito w/Red Sauce	Legume/Nut/Seed	½ serving	4.0
Taco Bell Beef Burrito w/Green Sauce	Legume/Nut/Seed	½ serving	1.5
Taco Bell Beef Burrito w/Red Sauce	Legume/Nut/Seed	½ piece	1.0
Taco Bell Beef Enchirito w/Green Sauce	Meat/Fish/Poultry	½ piece	0.0
Taco Bell Beef Enchirito w/Red Sauce	Meat/Fish/Poultry	½ piece	0.0
Taco Bell Burrito Supreme w/Green Sauce	Legume/Nut/Seed	½ serving	2.0
Taco Bell Burrito Supreme w/Red Sauce	Legume/Nut/Seed	½ serving	2.0
Taco Bell Chicken Fajita	Meat/Fish/Poultry	1 piece	0.5
Taco Bell Cinnamon Crispas	Grain	½ serving	−2.0

Food Name	Nutrigroup	Serving Size	Nutripoints
Taco Bell Double Beef Burrito Supreme w/Green Sauce	Meat/Fish/Poultry	½ piece	1.0
Taco Bell Double Beef Burrito Supreme w/Red Sauce	Meat/Fish/Poultry	½ piece	1.0
Taco Bell Guacamole	Fruit	1 tablespoon	1.0
Taco Bell Jalapeño Peppers	Condiment	2 tablespoons	-1.5
Taco Bell Mexican Pizza	Grain	¼ piece	-0.5
Taco Bell Meximelt	Grain	½ serving	-1.0
Taco Bell Nachos	Grain	½ serving	-0.5
Taco Bell Nachos Bellgrande	Grain	¼ serving	0.0
Taco Bell Pico De Gallo	Condiment	2 tablespoons	1.0
Taco Bell Pintos and Cheese, w/Green Sauce	Legume/Nut/Seed	1 serving	2.5
Taco Bell Pintos and Cheese, w/Red Sauce	Legume/Nut/Seed	1 serving	2.5
Taco Bell Ranch Dressing	Fat/Oil	1 tablespoon	-4.0
Taco Bell Salsa	Condiment	1 teaspoon	2.0
Taco Bell Soft Taco	Meat/Fish/Poultry	1 piece	0.0
Taco Bell Sour Cream	Fat/Oil	2 tablespoons	-3.5
Taco Bell Steak Fajita	Meat/Fish/Poultry	1 piece	1.0
Taco Bell Super Combo Taco	Meat/Fish/Poultry	1 piece	-0.5
Taco Bell Supreme Soft Taco	Meat/Fish/Poultry	1 piece	-0.5
Taco Bell Taco	Meat/Fish/Poultry	1 piece	-1.0
Taco Bell Taco Bellgrande	Meat/Fish/Poultry	½ piece	-1.5
Taco Bell Taco Hot Sauce	Condiment	1 teaspoon	0.0
Taco Bell Taco Light	Meat/Fish/Poultry	½ piece	-1.5

Food Name	Nutrigroup	Serving Size	Nutripoints
Taco Bell Taco Salad, w/o shell	Vegetable	¼ serving	0.0
Taco Bell Taco Salad, w/Salsa, w/o shell	Vegetable	¼ serving	0.5
Taco Bell Taco Salad, w/Salsa, w/shell	Vegetable	⅛ serving	0.0
Taco Bell Taco Sauce	Condiment	1 teaspoon	0.0
Taco Bell Tostada Green Sauce	Vegetable	¼ piece	1.5
Taco Bell Tostada Red Sauce	Vegetable	¼ piece	1.5
Taco salad	Vegetable	½ cup	1.5
Taco, bean/cheese	Legume/Nut/Seed	½ piece	0.5
Taco, beef/cheese	Meat/Fish/Poultry	1 piece	2.5
Taco, chicken	Meat/Fish/Poultry	½ piece	2.0
Tamale	Grain	½ tamale	−1.5
Tamales, in Chili Sauce, Old El Paso	Grain	1 whole	−0.5
Tangerine	Fruit	1 piece	13.0
Tarragon	Condiment	1 teaspoon	0.5
Tea Mix, Iced, Lemon, Sugar-Free, Lipton	Miscellaneous	8 fluid ounces	−2.5
Tea Mix, Iced, Lipton	Sugar	8 fluid ounces	−7.5
Tea, American black	Miscellaneous	1 cup	−3.0
Tea, decaffeinated	Miscellaneous	1 cup	0.0
Tea, herb	Miscellaneous	6 fluid ounces	0.5
Tequila sunrise	Alcohol	6 fluid ounces	−10.0
Thyme	Condiment	1 teaspoon	0.5
Tofu	Legume/Nut/Seed	½ cup	5.0
Tofu Burger, frozen, Island Spring Oriental	Legume/Nut/Seed	1 piece	0.0
Tom Collins	Alcohol	8 fluid ounces	−14.0
Tomato paste, canned	Vegetable	¼ cup	20.0
Tomato Paste, Contadina	Vegetable	¼ cup	12.5
Tomato, fresh	Vegetable	1 piece	30.0
Tomatoes, canned	Vegetable	½ cup	23.0
Tomatoes, Peeled, Del Monte	Vegetable	1 cup	14.0

Food Name	Nutrigroup	Serving Size	Nutripoints
Tomatoes, Stewed, Hunt's	Vegetable	½ cup	7.0
Tonic water, sweetened	Sugar	12 fluid ounces	−5.5
Topping, Blueberry, Hot, Nutripoint	Fruit	½ cup	2.5
Topping, Extra Creamy, Cool Whip, Birds Eye	Milk/Dairy	¼ cup	−6.0
Topping, Lite, Cool Whip	Milk/Dairy	½ cup	−3.0
Topping, marshmallow cream	Sugar	2 tablespoons	−5.5
Topping, Nondairy, Cool Whip, Birds Eye	Milk/Dairy	¼ cup	−4.5
Topping, Peach, Hot, Nutripoint	Fruit	½ cup	7.0
Topping, Red Raspberry, Hot, Nutripoint	Fruit	½ cup	9.0
Topping, Strawberry, Smucker's	Fruit	1 tablespoon	−4.0
Topping, Whipped, La Creme	Milk/Dairy	¼ cup	−5.5
Tortellini, Cheese, w/Tomato Sauce, frozen, Stouffer's	Milk/Dairy	½ portion	0.0
Tortellini, Veal, Alfredo, frozen, Stouffer's	Meat/Fish/Poultry	½ piece	−1.0
Tortellini, Veal, w/Tomato Sauce, frozen, Stouffer's	Meat/Fish/Poultry	½ portion	1.5
Tortilla chips	Grain	15 pieces	0.5
Tortilla Chips, Doritos	Grain	18 pieces	−0.5
Tortilla Chips, Light Nacho Cheese, Doritos	Grain	15 pieces	1.0

Food Name	Nutrigroup	Serving Size	Nutripoints
Tortilla Chips, Nacho Cheese, Doritos	Grain	15 pieces	−0.5
Tortilla, corn	Grain	2 whole	4.0
Tortilla, flour	Grain	1 whole	2.0
Tortilla, whole wheat	Grain	1 whole	4.5
Tostada	Vegetable	1/4 piece	1.0
Trail mix	Legume/Nut/Seed	1/4 cup	2.0
Treet	Meat/Fish/Poultry	2 ounces	−4.5
Trout, baked	Meat/Fish/Poultry	3 ounces	5.0
Tuna helper, prepared	Meat/Fish/Poultry	1/2 cup	2.5
Tuna noodle casserole	Meat/Fish/Poultry	1 cup	3.5
Tuna Noodle Casserole, frozen, Stouffer's	Meat/Fish/Poultry	1/2 portion	0.0
Tuna salad	Meat/Fish/Poultry	1/2 cup	3.0
Tuna Salad, Nutripoint	Meat/Fish/Poultry	1/2 cup	5.0
Tuna, Albacore Solid White, in Oil, Chicken of the Sea	Meat/Fish/Poultry	1/2 cup	4.0
Tuna, canned in oil	Meat/Fish/Poultry	1/2 cup	2.0
Tuna, canned in water	Meat/Fish/Poultry	3/4 cup	7.5
Tuna, Chunk Light, in Oil, Chicken of the Sea	Meat/Fish/Poultry	1/2 cup	3.5
Tuna, Chunk Light, in Oil, Star-Kist	Meat/Fish/Poultry	1/2 cup	1.5
Tuna, Chunk Light, in Water, Chicken of the Sea	Meat/Fish/Poultry	3/4 cup	6.5
Tuna, Chunk Light, in Water, Low-Sodium, Chicken of the Sea	Meat/Fish/Poultry	1/2 cup	8.0
Tuna, Diet Albacore, Chunk White, in Water, Low-Sodium, Chicken of the Sea	Meat/Fish/Poultry	1/2 cup	5.0

Food Name	Nutrigroup	Serving Size	Nutripoints
Tuna, fresh, broiled	Meat/Fish/Poultry	3 ounces	6.5
Tuna, Light Chunk, in Water, Bumble Bee	Meat/Fish/Poultry	½ cup	7.0
Tuna, Lite Chunk Light, in Water and Oil, Chicken of the Sea	Meat/Fish/Poultry	½ cup	6.0
Tuna, Solid White, in Water, Star-Kist	Meat/Fish/Poultry	½ cup	5.5
Tuna, Tonno, Solid Light, in Oil, Chicken of the Sea	Meat/Fish/Poultry	½ cup	4.0
Tuna, White Solid, in Water, Bumble Bee	Meat/Fish/Poultry	½ cup	6.5
Turkey a la King, w/Rice, frozen, Budget Gourmet	Meat/Fish/Poultry	½ portion	−0.5
Turkey Breast Slices, Louis Rich	Meat/Fish/Poultry	3 pieces	3.5
Turkey Breast, frozen, Healthy Choice	Meat/Fish/Poultry	1 portion	2.0
Turkey Breast, Roasted, No Salt Added, Mr. Turkey	Meat/Fish/Poultry	4 ounces	1.0
Turkey Breast, Sliced, frozen, Budget Gourmet	Meat/Fish/Poultry	½ portion	0.5
Turkey Breast, Sliced, Mr. Turkey	Meat/Fish/Poultry	3 ounces	1.0
Turkey Breast, Sliced, w/Mushroom Sauce, frozen, Stouffer's	Meat/Fish/Poultry	1 portion	1.0
Turkey Breast, Stuffed, frozen, Weight Watchers	Meat/Fish/Poultry	½ piece	−1.0
Turkey Dinner, frozen, Morton	Meat/Fish/Poultry	1 portion	4.0
Turkey Ham, Louis Rich	Meat/Fish/Poultry	4 pieces	1.0

Food Name	Nutrigroup	Serving Size	Nutripoints
Turkey Pie, frozen, Stouffer's	Meat/Fish/Poultry	½ piece	−1.0
Turkey pot pie	Meat/Fish/Poultry	½ piece	0.5
Turkey Pot Pie, Swanson	Meat/Fish/Poultry	½ pie	−1.0
Turkey roll, light and dark meat	Meat/Fish/Poultry	4 ounces	1.0
Turkey roll, light meat	Meat/Fish/Poultry	3 ounces	3.0
Turkey Roll, White, Cooked, Mr. Turkey	Meat/Fish/Poultry	4 ounces	−0.5
Turkey, dark meat and skin, baked	Meat/Fish/Poultry	3½ ounces	1.0
Turkey, dark meat, baked, w/o skin	Meat/Fish/Poultry	3 ounces	3.0
Turkey, Divan, frozen, Le Menu	Meat/Fish/Poultry	1 portion	0.5
Turkey, frozen dinner	Meat/Fish/Poultry	½ portion	3.5
Turkey, Glazed, Slim, frozen, Budget Gourmet	Meat/Fish/Poultry	1 portion	0.5
Turkey, light meat and skin, baked	Meat/Fish/Poultry	3½ ounces	2.5
Turkey, light and dark meat, w/o skin, baked	Meat/Fish/Poultry	3 ounces	3.5
Turkey, light meat, baked, w/o skin	Meat/Fish/Poultry	3 ounces	4.5
Turkey, Luncheon Loaf, Louis Rich	Meat/Fish/Poultry	4 pieces	−1.0
Turkey, Pie, frozen, Morton	Meat/Fish/Poultry	½ piece	−0.5
Turkey, Sliced, frozen, Stouffer's Right Course	Meat/Fish/Poultry	1 portion	1.0
Turkey, Slices, frozen, Loma Linda	Legume/Nut/Seed	2 ounces	6.5
Turkey, w/Dressing and Potatoes, frozen, Swanson	Meat/Fish/Poultry	1 piece	−1.0

Food Name	Nutrigroup	Serving Size	Nutripoints
Turkey, w/Dressing, frozen, Morton	Meat/Fish/Poultry	1 portion	4.0
Turkey, White and Dark Meat, canned, Premium Chunk, Swanson	Meat/Fish/Poultry	4 ounces	0.0
Turkey, White, canned, Premium Chunk, Swanson	Meat/Fish/Poultry	4 ounces	3.5
Turmeric	Condiment	1 teaspoon	0.5
Turnip greens, chopped, cooked	Vegetable	1 cup	79.0
Turnip Greens, Seasoned, Nutripoint	Vegetable	1 cup	67.0
Turnips, cooked	Vegetable	1 cup	19.5
Turnips, raw	Vegetable	½ cup	18.0
Turnover, Blueberry, frozen, Pepperidge Farm	Grain	½ turnover	−2.0
Turnover, fruit	Grain	1 turnover	−1.5
Twinkies, Hostess	Grain	1 piece	−3.0
Vanilla extract	Condiment	1 teaspoon	0.0
Veal chop, medium fat, fried	Meat/Fish/Poultry	3 ounces	−0.5
Veal cutlet, medium fat, braised	Meat/Fish/Poultry	3 ounces	1.0
Veal cutlet/steak, lean, braised	Meat/Fish/Poultry	3 ounces	3.5
Veal Marsala, frozen, Le Menu	Meat/Fish/Poultry	1 portion	−0.5
Veal Parmigiana Patty, frozen, Weight Watchers	Meat/Fish/Poultry	1 portion	1.0
Veal Parmigiana	Meat/Fish/Poultry	½ piece	−1.5
Veal Parmigiana, frozen, Budget Gourmet	Meat/Fish/Poultry	½ portion	0.0
Veal Parmigiana, frozen, Morton	Meat/Fish/Poultry	1 portion	2.0

Food Name	Nutrigroup	Serving Size	Nutripoints
Veal patty, fried	Meat/Fish/Poultry	2 ounces	1.0
Veal Primavera, frozen, Stouffer's	Meat/Fish/Poultry	1 portion	−0.5
Veal roast, lean, braised	Meat/Fish/Poultry	3 ounces	2.0
Veal roast, medium fat, braised	Meat/Fish/Poultry	3 ounces	0.5
Vegeburger, Loma Linda	Legume/Nut/Seed	4 ounces	8.5
Vegetable Medley, Nutripoint	Vegetable	1 cup	48.5
Vegetable Stir-Fry, Nutripoint	Vegetable	½ cup	13.5
Vegetables, Custom Cuisine, w/Dijon Mustard, frozen, Birds Eye	Vegetable	½ cup	18.0
Vegetables, Italian Style, frozen, Birds Eye	Vegetable	½ cup	3.0
Vegetables, Japanese Style, frozen, Birds Eye	Vegetable	½ cup	2.5
Vegetables, mixed, canned	Vegetable	½ cup	22.0
Vegetables, Mixed, frozen, Birds Eye	Vegetable	½ cup	18.0
Vegetables, mixed, frozen, cooked	Vegetable	½ cup	18.0
Vegetables, Pasta Primavera Style, frozen, Birds Eye	Vegetable	½ cup	7.0
Vegetables, San Francisco Style, frozen, Birds Eye	Vegetable	½ cup	0.5
Vegetables, Spring, w/Cheese Sauce, frozen, Budget Gourmet	Vegetable	½ portion	4.5

Food Name	Nutrigroup	Serving Size	Nutripoints
Vegi-Patties, frozen, Lifestream	Legume/Nut/Seed	1 piece	1.5
Venison, baked	Meat/Fish/Poultry	4 ounces	8.5
Venison, w/Juniper Berry Sauce, Nutripoint	Meat/Fish/Poultry	6 ounces	6.5
Vinegar	Condiment	1 tablespoon	0.0
Vodka	Alcohol	2 fluid ounces	−16.5
Waffles	Grain	1 whole	4.0
Waffles, Blueberry, Aunt Jemima	Grain	2 waffles	2.0
Waffles, Buttermilk, Jumbo, DownyFlake	Grain	2 waffles	0.0
Waffles, Common Sense Oat Bran, Eggo	Grain	1½ waffles	3.5
Waffles, Homestyle, frozen, Eggo	Grain	1½ waffles	1.0
Waffles, Nutri-Grain, frozen, Eggo	Grain	1½ waffles	1.5
Waffles, Original, Aunt Jemima	Grain	2 waffles	1.0
Walnuts, Baking, Blue Diamond	Legume/Nut/Seed	1 ounce	−0.5
Walnuts, black	Legume/Nut/Seed	12 pieces	0.5
Walnuts, English or Persian	Legume/Nut/Seed	12 pieces	0.0
Water chestnuts, canned	Vegetable	1 cup	5.5
Watercress	Vegetable	20 pieces	52.5
Watermelon	Fruit	1 cup	10.5
Wendy's Apple Danish	Grain	½ Danish	−1.0
Wendy's Bacon Swiss Hamburger	Meat/Fish/Poultry	¼ piece	−0.5
Wendy's Big Classic Hamburger	Meat/Fish/Poultry	⅓ piece	0.0
Wendy's Big Classic Hamburger w/Cheese	Meat/Fish/Poultry	⅓ piece	−0.5

Food Name	Nutrigroup	Serving Size	Nutripoints
Wendy's Breakfast Sandwich	Milk/Dairy	½ piece	−2.5
Wendy's Buttermilk Biscuit	Grain	½ biscuit	−1.5
Wendy's Butterscotch Pudding	Milk/Dairy	¼ cup	−2.5
Wendy's California Coleslaw	Vegetable	¼ cup	1.0
Wendy's Cheddar Chips	Grain	1 ounce	−1.5
Wendy's Cheese Danish	Grain	½ Danish	−1.5
Wendy's Chef Salad (take-out)	Vegetable	¼ serving	6.0
Wendy's Chicken Fried Steak	Meat/Fish/Poultry	⅓ piece	−2.0
Wendy's Chicken Sandwich	Meat/Fish/Poultry	½ piece	2.0
Wendy's Chocolate Chip Cookie	Grain	½ cookie	−3.0
Wendy's Chocolate Pudding	Milk/Dairy	¼ cup	−2.0
Wendy's Cinnamon w/Raisin Danish	Grain	½ Danish	−1.5
Wendy's Creamy Peppercorn Dressing	Fat/Oil	1 tablespoon	−6.0
Wendy's Crispy Chicken Nuggets (fried in animal oil)	Meat/Fish/Poultry	4 pieces	−2.0
Wendy's Crispy Chicken Nuggets (fried in vegetable oil)	Meat/Fish/Poultry	4 pieces	−1.5
Wendy's Crushed Red Peppers	Vegetable	1 tablespoon	13.5
Wendy's Deluxe Three-Bean Salad	Vegetable	¼ cup	2.0
Wendy's Fish Fillet	Meat/Fish/Poultry	1 piece	−1.0
Wendy's French Toast	Grain	1 slice	−2.0

Food Name	Nutrigroup	Serving Size	Nutripoints
Wendy's Frosty Dairy Dessert	Milk/Dairy	½ piece	−3.5
Wendy's Garden Salad (take-out)	Vegetable	½ serving	16.5
Wendy's Hot Stuffed Potato	Vegetable	¼ serving	4.5
Wendy's Hot Stuffed Potato w/Bacon and Cheese	Vegetable	¼ piece	−0.5
Wendy's Hot Stuffed Potato w/Broccoli and Cheese	Vegetable	¼ piece	1.5
Wendy's Hot Stuffed Potato w/Cheese	Vegetable	¼ serving	−2.0
Wendy's Hot Stuffed Potato w/Sour Cream and Chives	Vegetable	¼ serving	0.0
Wendy's Imitation Cheese, Salad Bar	Milk/Dairy	1 ounce	1.5
Wendy's Imitation Parmesan Cheese	Milk/Dairy	1 ounce	4.5
Wendy's Imitation Sour Topping	Fat/Oil	2 ounces	−3.5
Wendy's Kids' Meal Cheeseburger	Meat/Fish/Poultry	½ piece	1.0
Wendy's Kids' Meal Hamburger	Meat/Fish/Poultry	½ piece	1.0
Wendy's New Beef Chili	Meat/Fish/Poultry	½ serving	1.5
Wendy's Old-Fashioned Corn Relish	Vegetable	¼ cup	−0.5
Wendy's Omelet #1 (eggs, ham, cheese)	Milk/Dairy	½ serving	−7.0
Wendy's Omelet #2 (eggs, ham, cheese, mushrooms)	Milk/Dairy	½ serving	−10.0
Wendy's Omelet #3 (eggs, ham, cheese, onions)	Milk/Dairy	½ serving	−10.0

Food Name	Nutrigroup	Serving Size	Nutripoints
Wendy's Omelet #4 (eggs, mushrooms, green peppers, onions)	Milk/Dairy	1 serving	−11.5
Wendy's Pasta Deli Salad	Grain	1 cup	1.5
Wendy's Philly Swiss Hamburger	Meat/Fish/Poultry	½ piece	0.0
Wendy's Picante Sauce	Condiment	2 ounces	3.0
Wendy's Plain Single Hamburger	Meat/Fish/Poultry	½ piece	0.5
Wendy's Plain Single Hamburger w/Cheese	Meat/Fish/Poultry	½ piece	0.0
Wendy's Potato Chili Cheese	Milk/Dairy	1 ounce	−1.0
Wendy's Red Bliss Potato Salad	Vegetable	¼ cup	−1.5
Wendy's Sausage Gravy	Fat/Oil	3 ounces	−3.0
Wendy's Sausage Patty	Meat/Fish/Poultry	1 piece	−3.0
Wendy's Single Cheese Hamburger w/Everything	Meat/Fish/Poultry	½ piece	0.5
Wendy's Single Hamburger w/Everything	Meat/Fish/Poultry	½ piece	0.5
Wendy's Sliced Pepperoni	Meat/Fish/Poultry	1 ounce	0.0
Wendy's Small Cheeseburger	Meat/Fish/Poultry	½ piece	1.0
Wendy's Small Hamburger	Meat/Fish/Poultry	½ piece	1.0
Wendy's Taco Beef Salad	Meat/Fish/Poultry	1 cup	2.0
Wendy's Taco Chips	Grain	1 ounce	0.0
Western Dinner, frozen, Morton	Meat/Fish/Poultry	1 portion	0.0

Food Name	Nutrigroup	Serving Size	Nutripoints
Wheat germ	Grain	1/4 cup	10.5
Wheat Germ, Kretschmer	Grain	1/4 cup	12.0
Wheat Germ, Honey Crunch, Kretschmer	Grain	1 ounce	8.0
Wheat, Whole Grain, Dry, Arrowhead Mills	Grain	2 ounces	4.5
Whiskey	Alcohol	2 fluid ounces	−16.5
Whiskey sour	Alcohol	3 fluid ounces	−19.0
White Russian	Alcohol	2 fluid ounces	−13.0
Whiting, baked/broiled	Meat/Fish/Poultry	4 ounces	2.0
Wine cooler	Alcohol	8 fluid ounces	−9.0
Wine spritzer	Alcohol	6 fluid ounces	−14.5
Wine, Chinese	Alcohol	6 fluid ounces	−14.5
Wine, light	Alcohol	6 fluid ounces	−14.0
Wine, sweet	Alcohol	4 fluid ounces	−13.0
Wine, table	Alcohol	6 fluid ounces	−14.0
Yeast, active dry	Miscellaneous	1 package	0.0
Yeast, Active Dry, Fleischmann's	Miscellaneous	1/4 ounce	0.5
Yeast, brewer's	Miscellaneous	1 tablespoon	3.5
Yellowtail, raw	Meat/Fish/Poultry	4 ounces	−0.5
Yogurt Drink, Low-Fat, Dan'Up, all flavors, Dannon	Milk/Dairy	1 cup	0.5
Yogurt, Banana Custard Style, Yoplait	Milk/Dairy	4 ounces	−1.0
Yogurt, Extra Smooth Fruit, all flavors, Dannon	Milk/Dairy	4 1/2 ounces	2.0
Yogurt, frozen, Almond Amaretto, Brice's	Milk/Dairy	1/2 cup	−0.5
Yogurt, frozen	Milk/Dairy	4 ounces	1.5
Yogurt, frozen, Low-Fat, Chocolate, Tuscan Pop	Milk/Dairy	1 piece	−2.0

Food Name	Nutrigroup	Serving Size	Nutripoints
Yogurt, frozen, Low-Fat, Fruit, Blue Bell	Milk/Dairy	½ cup	2.0
Yogurt, frozen, Low-Fat, Peaches 'n Cream, Blue Bell	Milk/Dairy	½ cup	2.0
Yogurt, Frozen, 90% Fat Free, Peanut Butter Cup, Columbo	Milk/Dairy	3 fluid ounces	−1.5
Yogurt, Frozen, 94% Fat Free, Bavarian Chocolate Crunch, Columbo	Milk/Dairy	3 fluid ounces	−1.0
Yogurt, Frozen, 94% Fat Free, Caramel Pecan Chunk, Columbo	Milk/Dairy	3 fluid ounces	−0.5
Yogurt, Frozen, 97% Fat Free, Strawberry Passion, Columbo	Milk/Dairy	4 fluid ounces	0.0
Yogurt, Frozen, 96% Fat Free, Vanilla Dream, Columbo	Milk/Dairy	4 fluid ounces	−0.5
Yogurt, Frozen, 92% Fat Free, Mocha Swiss Almond, Columbo	Milk/Dairy	3 fluid ounces	−1.5
Yogurt Frozen, TCBY	Milk/Dairy	5 fluid ounces	9.0
Yogurt, fruit	Milk/Dairy	6 ounces	2.0
Yogurt, Low-Fat, Boysenberry, Yoplait	Milk/Dairy	4 ounces	−0.5
Yogurt, Low-Fat, Cherry Vanilla, Borden	Milk/Dairy	4 ounces	−0.5
Yogurt, Low-Fat, Fresh Flavors, all flavors, Dannon	Milk/Dairy	6 ounces	2.0

Food Name	Nutrigroup	Serving Size	Nutripoints
Yogurt, Low-Fat, Fruit on Bottom, all flavors, Dannon	Milk/Dairy	4 ounces	1.0
Yogurt, Low-Fat, Nuts/Raisins/Fruit, Dannon	Milk/Dairy	4 ounces	0.5
Yogurt, Low-Fat, Nuts/Raisins/ Vanilla, Dannon	Milk/Dairy	4 ounces	0.0
Yogurt, Low-Fat, Peach, Borden	Milk/Dairy	4 ounces	−0.5
Yogurt, low-fat, plain	Milk/Dairy	8 ounces	7.0
Yogurt, Low-fat, Plain, Dannon	Milk/Dairy	8 ounces	5.5
Yogurt, Low-Fat, Strawberry, Borden	Milk/Dairy	4 ounces	−0.5
Yogurt, Low-Fat, Strawberry, Light n'Lively	Milk/Dairy	½ cup	−3.5
Yogurt, Low-Fat, Strawberry, Yoplait	Milk/Dairy	4 ounces	−0.5
Yogurt, Low-Fat, Swiss Style Plain, Lite-Line, Borden	Milk/Dairy	1 cup	1.5
Yogurt, Nonfat, Light, all flavors, Dannon	Milk/Dairy	1 cup	10.5
Yogurt, Nonfat, Light, all flavors, Yoplait	Milk/Dairy	1 cup	4.0
Yogurt, Nonfat, Lite, Plain, Columbo	Milk/Dairy	8 fluid ounces	4.0
Yogurt, Nonfat, Lite, Vanilla, Columbo	Milk/Dairy	8 fluid ounces	2.5
Yogurt, Nonfat, Peach, Weight Watchers	Milk/Dairy	1 cup	4.5
Yogurt, Nonfat, Plain, Dannon	Milk/Dairy	1 cup	9.0

Food Name	Nutrigroup	Serving Size	Nutripoints
Yogurt, Nonfat, Ultimate, all flavors, Weight Watchers	Milk/Dairy	1 cup	8.0
Yogurt, Nonfat, Yoplait 150	Milk/Dairy	6 fluid ounces	2.0
Yogurt, Pineapple, All Natural, Breyer's	Milk/Dairy	4 ounces	−2.0
Yogurt, Plain, Columbo	Milk/Dairy	8 fluid ounces	0.5
Yogurt, Soft Frozen Peach, Yoplait	Milk/Dairy	½ cup	−2.0
Yogurt, Strawberry, All Natural, Breyer's	Milk/Dairy	4 ounces	−2.0
Yogurt, whole milk, plain	Milk/Dairy	8 ounces	2.5
Zucchini, cooked	Vegetable	1 cup	15.0
Zucchini, raw	Vegetable	1 cup	16.0

POSTSCRIPT

"If your life-style does not control your body, eventually your body will control your life-style. The choice is yours."

Ern Baxter
Author of *I Almost Died*

WE ALL PAY LIP SERVICE TO THE VALUE OF GOOD HEALTH HABITS. We hear retired people say things such as, "As long as you've got your health . . . ," and we agree, even if we're years from thinking that anything could go wrong with our health. But as the years go by, and we begin to see how things *can* go wrong—how friends and family members can be stricken by chronic illness—we begin to appreciate the notion that good health is a very valuable commodity. Unfortunately, for many people, it can be too late.

Ern Baxter had a heart attack in middle age that frightened him more than he ever thought he could be frightened. Suddenly, he faced the possibility of his life ending much sooner than he'd thought. After a sea change in his attitudes about health and fitness, he rehabilitated himself to the point where he feels better than he had ever felt before his brush with death. I've quoted above from his book because I think his comment crystallizes everything you need to know about respecting your body and doing your best to keep it in optimum condition.

Good nutrition is a major component of a healthy life. I think that Nutripoints will help you achieve the best level of nutrition you've ever experienced. I would like to point out that to achieve an optimum sense of well-being, you must make both exercise and stress control part of your regimen. I strongly suggest that you investigate these areas and adopt some form of exercise, as well as techniques for stress control, so that you can enjoy the maximum benefits of Nutripoints.

Some excellent books on exercise include Dr. Kenneth

Cooper's *Aerobics Program for Total Well-Being* (M. Evans, 1982) and Casey Meyer's *Walking: A Complete Guide to the Exercise* (Random House, 1992).

For a good introduction to stress management I recommend Dr. Robert Eliot's *Is it Worth Dying For?* (Bantam, 1984); Drs. Kreigel and Kriegel's *The C Zone: Peak Performance Under Pressure* (Fawcett, Columbine, 1984); Dr. Herbert Bensen's *Beyond the Relaxation Response* (Berkeley, 1984); and Alan Lakein's *How to Get Control of Your Time and Your Life* (Signet, New American Library, 1974).

As a final note, I'd like to say that I don't think nutrition, exercise, and stress control are the most important things in life. I think eating should be pleasurable. I think exercise should be fun. I think time spent with loved ones and devotion to spiritual goals are at the core of a happy life. But I've seen that optimum health can affect life for the better, and I know that good health is achievable. So I want to convince you that it's a gift you can give yourself. It can enhance every other aspect of your life. I hope that *Nutripoints* will make your ultimate life goals easier to achieve.

For More Nutripoint Information

If you would like your name to be placed on a mailing list to learn about Nutripoint related products, you may do so by writing Dr. Vartabedian at Nutripoint Research, P.O. Box 1450, Loma Linda, CA 92354. A convenient order form for Nutripoints books and products is located in the back of this book.

REFERENCES

Association of Vitamin Chemists, The. *Methods of Vitamin Assay.* New York: Interscience Publishers, 1966.

Bland, Dr. Jeffrey. *Nutraerobics.* San Francisco: Harper & Row, 1983.

Brody, Jane. *Jane Brody's Nutrition Book.* New York: Norton, 1981.

Carper, Jean. *Jean Carper's Total Nutrition Guide.* New York: Bantam, 1987.

Connor, Sonja L., and William Connor. *The New American Diet.* New York: Simon & Schuster, 1986.

Hendler, Sheldon Saul, MD. *The Complete Guide to Anti-Aging Nutrients.* New York: Simon & Schuster, 1984.

Katch, Frank I., and William D. McArdle. *Nutrition, Weight Control, and Exercise.* Boston: Houghton Mifflin, 1988.

Last, John M., MD, ed. *Maxcy-Rosenau: Public Health and Preventive Medicine,* 11th ed. New York: Appleton-Century-Crofts, 1980.

Mayer, Jean. *A Diet for Living.* New York: David McKay, 1975.

National Research Council. *Diet and Health: Implications for Reducing Chronic Disease.* Washington, DC: National Academy Press, 1989.

National Research Council. *Recommended Dietary Allowances,* 9th revised ed. Washington, DC: National Academy of Sciences, 1980.

Paige, David M., MD, ed. *Manual of Clinical Nutrition.* Pleasantville, NJ: Nutrition Publications, 1983.

Pennington, Jean A. T., and Helen Nichols-Church. *Food Values of Portions Commonly Used,* 14th ed. New York: Harper & Row, 1985.

Saltman, Paul, Joel Gurin, and Ira Mothner. *California Nutrition Book.* Boston: Little Brown, 1987.

Schmid, Dr. Ronald F. *Traditional Foods Are Your Best Medicine.* New York: Ballantine, 1987.

Stunkard, Albert J., MD, ed. *Obesity.* Philadelphia: W. B. Saunders, 1980.

United States Department of Agriculture. *Composition of Foods.* Agriculture Handbooks 8-1 through 8-17 and 8-21, Washington, DC: USDA, 1978–1989.

United States Department of Agriculture. *Nutritive Value of Foods.* Home and Garden Bulletin No. 72, Washington, DC: U.S. Government Printing Office, 1988.

United States Department of Health and Human Services, Public Health Service, Centers for Disease Control. *Foodborne Disease Surveillance.* Annual Summary, 1982. Atlanta: U.S. Department of Health and Human Services, issued September 1985.

Walford, Roy L., MD. *The 120-Year Diet.* New York: Simon & Schuster, 1986.

Weiner, Michael A. *The Way of the Skeptical Nutritionist.* New York: Macmillan, 1981.

Whalen, Dr. Elizabeth, and Dr. Frederic J. Stare. *The 100% Natural, Purely Organic, Cholesterol-Free, Megavitamin, Low-Carbohydrate Nutrition Hoax.* New York: Atheneum, 1983.

INDEX

A, vitamin, 53, 81–82,
132, 172
alcohol and, 107
cancer-prevention diet,
174
in fruit, 19
storage in body, 53
Absorption of nutrients:
alcohol and, 107
calcium, 88
combinations, 158
interference with, 52,
171
iron, 88
phosphorus, 90
Acid stomach, calcium and,
88
Active women, calorie
levels, 139
Addictive drugs:
alcohol, 106–7
caffeine, 105–6
Additives to foods, 59–61,
177
Advanced Formula
Centrum, 57
Aerobics, Cooper, 546

Aerobics Burger, recipe,
250–51
Aerobics Program for Total
Well-Being, Cooper
Center, 33–34
*Aerobics Program for Total
Well-Being*, Evans,
546
Aerobic Walking, Meyers,
546
Air travel, 155
Alar (apple pesticide), 60
Alcohol, 106–7, 154, 158
American Cancer Society
Recommendations,
173–74
calcium and, 88
calories per serving, 74
guidelines, 70
Nutripoint ratings,
72–73, 378–79
portion sizes, 114
Allbee C-800 + Iron, 58
All Bran, 89, 91, 201
Extra Fiber, 201
Allergies, Nutripoints and,
181–82

553

Alphabetical lists,
Nutripoint ratings,
384–542
Aluminum, in antacids, 90
American Cancer Society,
40, 132, 173–74
American Dietetic
Association, 173
American Heart
Association, 173–74
cholesterol
recommendations,
96
Amino acids, 69, 145
in milk, 135
Anemia, iron-deficiency, 45,
88, 158
Angel Hair Pasta with
Sunshine Sauce,
recipe, 255
Animal protein, 69, 145
Anorexia nervosa, zinc
deficiency, 91
Antacids, 70
phosphorus and, 90
Antibiotics, 159
Antibodies:
pantothenic acid and, 85
vitamin B$_6$ and, 84
Anxiety:
caffeine and, 105
about diet, 8
Appetite, thiamin and, 83
Apple juice, 142
Apple pie, 133
Apples, 19, 70
Applesauce, recipe, 263

Apricots, 201
Arrowhead Mills dry
soybeans, 201
Arsenic, 59
Arteries, cholesterol and,
97
Arteriosclerosis, 40
Artificial sweetners, 104–5
Asada, beef, recipe, 251
Ascorbic acid. See Vitamin
C
Asparagus, 132
marinated, recipe, 244
Aspirin, folacin and, 86
Asthma, vitamin deficiency
and, 45
vitamin B$_6$, 84
Athletes:
diet for, 182
potassium deficiencies,
89–90
Avocado, 17

B
Bacon, 136
Baked beans, canned, 177
with tomato sauce, 202
Baking soda, 101, 159
and thiamin, 83
Balance in diet, 11–12,
118, 127, 165, 169
Nutripoint system, 21–22
Balsamic vinegar, salad
greens with, recipe,
238
Balsamic Vinegar Dressing,
recipe, 269

Banana cream pie, 133
Banana Gladje, 207
   recipe, 263
Banana Mint Sauce, recipe,
   278
Bananas, 85, 90
Bananas Flambé, recipe,
   262
Basic foods, 282
Bass, freshwater, 189
Baxter, Ern, 545
B-Complex vitamins, 80
   alcohol and, 107
   B_6, 45, 84–85
   B_{12}, 52, 85
      alcohol and, 158
      antibiotics and, 159
      vitamin C and, 158
   B_{15}, 58
   folic acid, 52, 80
      alcohol and, 107
   folacin, 86–87
      alcohol and, 107
   food combinations,
      158–59
   in fruit, 19
   in milk, 135
   niacin (B_3), 80, 83–84
   pantothenic acid, 80,
      85–86
   riboflavin (B_2), 80, 83
      alcohol and, 107
      baking soda and, 159
      in fruit, 19
   thiamin (B_1), 80, 82–83
      alcohol and, 107, 158
      in fruit, 19

Beans, 134
   baked, canned, 177
      with tomato sauce,
         202
   complementary protein
      relationships, 146
   dietary fiber, 80
   dried, 78
      to cook, 147
   protein, 78
Bean sprouts, 134, 188
Bed-wetting in children,
      vitamin B_6 and, 85
Beef, 74–75, 136
   Nutripoint values, 19
   recipes, 250–51
   shopping list, 197–98
Beef heart, cholesterol per
      calorie, 97
Beef liver, cholesterol per
      calorie, 96
Beer, alcohol-free, 107
Beet greens, 187
   and sodium in diet, 159
Beets, and sodium in diet,
      159
Benson, Herbert, *Beyond
      the Relaxation
      Response*, 546
Berries, 132
Beta-carotene, 81, 172
Beverages:
   alcohol-free, 107
   alcoholic, Nutripoint
      ratings, 378–79
   decaffeinated, 106
   fruit juice, 142

Beverages (*cont.*)
  Nutripoint ratings,
    382–83
  portion sizes, 114
  recipes, 278
  in restaurants, 154
Beyond the Relaxation
    Response, Benson,
    546
Bingeing, 150
Biotin, 80
Birds Eye broccoli, carrots
    and red peppers,
    200
Birds Eye frozen peas, 202
Birth control pills, 159
Birth defects, caffeine and,
    105
Black Bean Dip, recipe,
    238
Blackberries, 132
Blackberry Freeze, 207
  recipe, 262
Black currants, 187
Black-eyed peas, 147, 188,
    202
Blood:
  calcium and, 87
  iron and, 88
  vitamin B$_6$ and, 84
  vitamin B$_{12}$ and, 85
Blood cholesterol, 94–95,
    97
  See also Cholesterol
Blood pressure:
  caffeine and, 105
  potassium and, 89

Blood sugar, 76
  and brain function, 77
  NutraSweet and, 104–5
Blueberries, hot topping for
    pancakes, recipe,
    267
Blueberry soup, chilled,
    recipe, 234
Blue Cheese Dressing,
    recipe, 269
Bok choy, 87, 187, 200
  and sodium in diet, 159
Bones, phosphorus and, 90
Bowel movements, in
    vegetarian diet, 147
Brain function, 77
Bran Buds, 89, 91, 201
Bran cereals, 89, 91
Bran Chex, 89
Brand-name foods, 282
  information, 68, 178–79
  ratings, 177
Bran Flakes, 89, 91
Bran muffins, recipes, 229,
    264
  oat bran, recipe, 265
Breads, 133–34
  complementary protein
    relationships, 146
  in restaurants, 154
  shopping list, 192–94
Breakfast:
  fast-food, 137
  recipes, 264–68
Breast cancer, 41
  dietary fat and, 92,
    174

Breast disease, caffeine and, 105
Brine, 101
Broccoli, 87, 132, 187, 200
  Nutripoint values, 19
Brussels sprouts, 132, 200
Bulimia, zinc deficiencies, 91
Butter, 92
  cooking substitutions, 128
  in restaurants, 154
Buttermilk, skim, 189

C
C, vitamin, 17, 52, 80, 82, 132, 172
  alcohol and, 107
  cancer-prevention diet, 174
  diagnostic tests and, 55
  food combinations, 158
  in fruit, 15, 19
  iron and, 88
Cabbage, 200
Cadmium, 59
Caffeine, 105–6
  calcium and, 88
  guidelines, 70
Cajun Chicken Sandwich, recipe, 235
Calcium, 40, 45, 52–53, 80, 87–88, 171
  alcohol and, 107, 158
  in dairy foods, 13
  excess consumption, 54

magnesium and, 89
  in milk, 135
  protein and, 78
  in shellfish, 180
  in vegetables, 132
Calories, 93–94
  cholesterol and, 96–97
  daily needs, 137–42
  in fruit, 19
  nutrient analysis, low-calorie menu, 211
  nutrients and, 17, 25
  Nutripoint program and, 118, 159–61
  nutrition and, 41–45, 46
  serving size and, 74
  vegetarian diet, 147–48
Campbell's soups, Nutripoint ratings, 15
Cancer, 40
  calcium deficiency and, 45
  dietary fiber and, 78
  dietary recommendations, 173–74
  fat and, 92
  folacin and, 86
  vegetarian diet and, 143, 147
  vitamins and, 45, 132
    A, 81
    B₆, 84–85
Canned foods:
  evaporated skim milk, 189

Canned foods (cont.)
 fruits, 15
 to remove sodium, 102
 tuna, 14, 84, 136, 189
  Nutripoints per dollar, 202
  salad recipe, 240
  shopping list, 198
 vegetables, 190
Cantaloupe, 19, 132, 187, 200
 and sodium in diet, 159
Caper dressing, recipe, 271
Can'N Crunchberries, 179
Carbohydrates:
 alcohol, 106
 complex, 70, 76–77, 102
  fruits and vegetables, 176
  legumes, 134, 176
  milk, 135
  vegetarian diet, 143
 magnesium and, 89
 niacin and, 84
 pantothenic acid and, 85–86
 riboflavin and, 83
 sugar, 102–3
 thiamin and, 82
 vitamin B_6 and, 84
 vitamin B_{12} and, 85
Carcinogens, vegetarian diet and, 147
Cardiovascular disease:
 vitamin B_6 and, 84
 vitamin deficiency and, 45

Carnation Instant Breakfast, 202
 low-fat milk, no-sugar, 188
Carnation instant nonfat dry milk, 188, 202
Carnitine, 59
Carpal tunnel syndrome, vitamin B_6 and, 84
Carrots, 132
 dietary fiber, 79
Casaba melon, 201
Casserole, five-cheese, recipe, 228–29
Cauliflower, 132, 200
Caviar, cholesterol per calorie, 96
Cell replication, vitamin B_{12} and, 85
Center for Science in the Public Interest, 101
Cereals, 91
 bran, 89
 complementary protein relationships, 146
 cooked, Fruited Cinnamon Cereal, recipe, 266
 fortified, 133, 179–80
  Nutripoint ratings, 11
  top-ten, 188
 Nutripoints per dollar, 201
 sugar in, 103
Cervical dysplasia, folacin and, 86
Change of diet, 126–30

Cheese, 74, 135
  portion sizes, 113
  shopping list, 195–96
Cheese sauce, cholesterol
    per calorie, 97
Chemical additives, 59–61
Chemical fertilizers, 61–62
Chicken, 136
  in Chinese restaurants,
    155
  recipes, 252–55
    Cajun sandwich, 235
    marinades for, 274,
      275
    salad, 240
Chick-peas, 147
Children:
  diet for, 182
  iron deficiencies, 88
  vitamin supplements, 56
Chili, vegetarian, recipe,
    242
Chinese restaurants, 154,
    155
Chloride, 59
Chlorine, 81
Chocolate-chip cookies, 47
Choice of foods, 111, 149
  alteration of, 129
Cholera, 180
Cholesterol, 40–41, 94–99,
    170–71, 283, 284
  daily limit, 173
  guidelines, 70, 71
  niacin and, 83
  Nutripoint rating, 72

  in organ meats, 136
  soluble fiber and, 79
  in vegetables, 134
  vegetarian diet and, 143,
    147
  vitamin C and, 52
Choline, 59
Chromium, 81
Cioppino, 157
Cirrhosis of liver, 40
Citrus fruits, 132, 172
Clams, 180
  canned, 189
  raw, 136, 189, 202
Clear Spinach Soup, recipe,
    234
Cobalt, 59
Coenzyme Q, 59
Coffee, 130
  iron and, 88
  Nutripoint ratings, 382,
    383
  substitutes for, 106, 128
  See also Caffeine
Cold medications, caffeine
    in, 105
Cold Mixed-Vegetable
    Salad, recipe, 241
Coleslaw, recipe, 239
Collagen, Vitamin C and,
    82
Colon cancer, 40
  calcium deficiency, 45
  dietary fat and, 92, 174
  dietary fiber and, 78
  vegetarian diet and, 147

Combination dishes, 177
Combinations of foods,
    158–59
  for complete protein, 145
Complementary protein
    relationships, 146
Complete protein, 145
Complex carbohydrates, 70,
    76–77, 102
  in fruits and vegetables,
    176
  in legumes, 134, 176
  in milk, 135
  vegetarian diet, 143
Compote, fruit, recipe,
    259
Computer programs, 183
Condiments, 175
  calories per serving, 74
  Nutripoint ratings,
    379–82
Constipation, calcium and,
    88
Consumer Reports, 100
Contaminants, 177
  in meat, 143
  in shellfish, 136
Contraceptive pills, folacin
    and, 86
Convenience foods, 153
Cooking of foods:
  nutrient changes, 175
  substitutions, 128
Cooper, Kenneth, Aerobics,
    546
Cooper Aerobics Center, 8,
    27, 31–35
  Data Base, 177–78

In-Residence Program,
    137, 182
  Nutripoints program, 66,
    182–83
Copper, 52, 59, 81
Coronary heart disease:
  cholesterol and, 95, 96
  dietary fat and, 173–74
Costs of food, and
    nutritional value,
    200–202
Cottage cheese, 136
Crabs, cholesterol per
    calorie, 97
Crackers, shopping list,
    193
Cranberries, 132
Cream, heavy, cooking
    substitution, 128
Cream cheese, cooking
    substitution, 128
Croissants, 156
Cruciferous vegetables,
    132, 174
Crunchy Fish, recipe, 250
Current eating habits,
    evaluation, 112–25
The C-Zone: Peak
    Performance Under
    Pressure, Kreigel
    and Kreigel, 546

D
D, vitamin, alcohol and,
    107, 158
D$_2$, vitamin, 51
Daily calorie requirements,
    94

Daily Nutripoint scores, 20–22
Daily Stress Natural Vitamins, 57
Dairy foods, 13, 83, 135–36
  calcium in, 87
  calories per serving, 74
  Nutripoint ratings, 336–47
    top-ten, 188–89
  Nutripoints per dollar, 202
  protein, vegetarian diet, 144–45
  shopping list, 195–96
Dandelion greens, 187
Dannon nonfat light yogurt, 188
Data gathering, 177–78
Decaffeinated drinks, 106, 128
Dental caries, sugar and, 102
Depression, folacin and, 86
Desserts:
  in French restaurants, 156
  fruit recipes, 258–63
  fiber, 79
  magnesium, 89
  niacin, 83–84
  potassium, 90
  vitamin B_6, 85
  vitamin B_{12}, 85
  vitamin C, 158
Diet Sego, 202

Digestive diseases:
  caffeine and, 105
  potassium and, 89
Digestive system, niacin and, 84
Dining out, 153–57, 163
Dinner entrees, shopping list, 196, 198–99
Dip recipes:
  black bean, 238
  guacamole, 239
Diseases, from shellfish, 180
Diuretics, 130
  caffeine, 105
  potassium and, 89
Diverticulosis, 78
Diabetes, 40
  potassium and, 89
  sugar and, 102
  vitamin B_6 and, 84
  vitamin deficiency and, 45
Diagnostic tests, dietary supplements and, 55
Diary of eating habits, 112–26, 129, 131
Diet:
  change of, 126–30
  health and, 40–41
  Nutripoints and, 11–12
  unhealthy, 20–21, 25, 27–29, 51–53
Diet anxiety, 8
Dietary cholesterol, 97
Dietary fiber, 70, 76, 77, 78–80

Dietary fiber (*cont.*)
  daily recommendations,
    173, 174
  in fruits, 15, 132
  in legumes, 134, 176
  Nutripoint rating, 72
  in vegetables, 132
  in vegetarian diet, 143,
    147
Dietary supplements:
  calcium, 87–88
  evaluations, 56–58
Dressings:
  in French restaurants,
    156
  recipes, 268–73
  shopping list, 199
  Wendy's Creamy
    Peppercorn,
    cholesterol per
    calorie, 97
Dried beans, to cook, 80
Dried fruits, 192
Duran, Kathleen S., 205

E
Eating disorders, zinc
  deficiency and, 91
Eating habits:
  evaluation of, 111–26
  unhealthy, 20–21, 25,
    27–29, 51–53
Eating out, 153–57, 163
Eggs, 74
  cholesterol per calorie,
    96, 97

cooking substitutions,
  128, 129
salmonella
  contamination, 61
scrambled:
  garden scrambled,
    recipe, 266
  McDonald's, 136
shopping list, 196
substitutes, 15, 135,
  188, 202
Wendy's omelets, 96, 97,
  137
Egg white, 129, 202
Eliot, Robert, *Is It Worth
  Dying For?*, 546
Enchiladas, chicken, recipe,
  252
Energy sources, 76–77
  sugar, 102
Equal (NutraSweet), 104,
  128
Essential dietary elements,
  68–70, 75–91
Evaluation of food, 13
Evans, M., *Aerobics
  Program for Total
  Well-Being*, 546
Evaporated skim milk, 128,
  202
Excesses of calcium, 87–88
Excessive dietary elements,
  75–76, 91–92
  alcohol, 106–7
  caffeine, 105–6
  calories, 93–94

cholesterol, 94–99
fat, 91–93
limitation of, 162–63,
    164–65, 172–73,
    181
sodium, 99–102
standards, 70
sugar, 102–5
Exercise, 39, 546
and water, 130
weight-bearing, calcium
    and, 88

F

Fast foods, 17, 136–37,
    283
information, 68, 178
Fats, dietary, 14, 40–41,
    47, 91–93
calcium and, 87
label information, 43
magnesium and, 89
negative ratings, 167
niacin and, 84
Nutripoint ratings, 73,
    370–74
pantothenic acid and,
    85–86
portion sizes, 114
protein and, 77–78
recommendations, 70,
    173
riboflavin and, 83
shopping list, 199
vegetarian diet, 142
vitamin B$_6$ and, 84
vitamin B$_{12}$ and, 85

Fat-soluble vitamins, 55,
    80
A, 81–82
megadoses, 55
Fatigue:
from anemia, 45
caffeine and, 106
FDA (Food and Drug
    Administration), 42
Fertilizers, chemical, 61–62
Fetal problems, zinc
    deficiency and, 91
Fiber, dietary, 40, 70, 76,
    77, 78–80
daily recommendations,
    173, 174
in fruits, 15, 132
in legumes, 134, 176
Nutripoint rating, 72
in vegetables, 132
in vegetarian diet, 143,
    147
Fiber One, 201
Fish, 78, 136
calories per serving, 74
in Chinese restaurants,
    155
marinade for, recipe,
    275
Nutripoint ratings, 19,
    347–69
top-ten, 189
Nutripoints per dollar,
    202
portion sizes, 113
recipes, 246–50
shopping list, 197

Fish (cont.)
  See also Shellfish; Tuna,
    canned
Five-Cheese Casserole,
    recipe, 228–29
Flank steak, 202
Fleischmann's Egg Beaters,
    15, 128, 129, 135,
    188, 202
  with Cheeze, 135, 202
Flounder, Nutripoint
    values, 19
Fluoride, 59
Fluorine, 81
Folacin, 86–87
  alcohol and, 107, 158
  in fruit, 19
Folic acid, 52, 80
  alcohol and, 107
Food additives, 177
Food allergies, 181–82
Food and Drug
    Administration
    (FDA), 42
Food and Nutrition Board,
    National Academy
    of Sciences, 42
Food fads, 79
Food groups. See
    Nutrigroups
Foods:
  choice of, 111, 149
    alteration of, 129
  high in cholesterol,
    96–97
  nutritional value, 61–62
  safety of, 59–61

shopping for, 150–53
  lists, 190–99
  See also Labeling of
    foods
Formagg Cheese Substitute,
    135, 188
Fortified foods, 177,
    179–80, 283–84
  cereals, 133
Fortune cookies, 155
40% Bran Flakes, 91, 201
French Bread Pizza, recipe,
    236
French Market Soup,
    recipe, 231
French restaurants, 155–56
French Toast, recipe, 265
Fresh Fruit Platter, recipe,
    259
Fresh Fruit Slices, recipe,
    258
Fresh Pasta Salad, recipe,
    258
Fried chicken, low-fat,
    recipe, 254–55
Fried eggs, cholesterol per
    calorie, 96
Frozen foods:
  dinner entrees, 15, 196,
    198–99
  fruits, 191
  vegetables, 190
Fruited Cinnamon Cereal,
    recipe, 266
Fruitful Bran, 201
Fruits, 15, 132–33, 175,
    176

calories per serving, 74
dietary fiber, 79
juice, 142
Nutripoint ratings, 19, 296–304
top-ten, 187–88
Nutripoints per dollar, 200–201
recipes, 258–63
shopping list, 191–92
sodium and, 159
sugar from, 105

G
Garbanzo beans, 202
Garden Scrambled Eggs, recipe, 266
Garlic salt, 101
Gas, intestinal, vegetarian diet, 147
Generic foods, 282
Geritol, 56, 58
Getting Physical, Turock, 546
Ghee, Indian restaurants, 156
Glucose, 102
Goldbeck, David and Nikki, The Goldbeck's Guide to Good Food, 60
The Gradual Vegetarian, Tracy, 143
Grains, 133–34
calories per serving, 74
complementary protein relationships, 146
in menus, 206

Nutripoint ratings, 304–29
top-ten, 188
Nutripoints per dollar, 201
recipes, 255–58
shopping list, 192–94
Granola, 133
Grapefruit, 132, 201
Grapefruit juice, 17
Grape Nuts, 201
Grapes, 105
Green leafy vegetables, 132, 172
folacin in, 86
Grilled Salmon with Yellow Bell Pepper Sauce, recipe, 249
Groups of foods. See Nutrigroups
Growth:
pantothenic acid and, 85
thiamin and, 82
Guacamole, 157
dip recipe, 239
Guava, 132, 187, 201
Gum disease:
calcium deficiency, 45
zinc deficiency, 91

H
Hair, vitamin A for, 81
Halibut, 189, 202
Ham, Nutripoint values, 19
Hamburger, Nutripoint values, 19
Hawaiian Marinade, recipe, 275

Headache, caffeine and, 105, 106

Health problems:
  calcium excess, 87–88
  diet and, 40–41, 45–49
  niacin excess, 84
  Nutripoints program and, 34–35
  sodium excess, 99
  sugar and, 102–3
  vitamin B$_6$ and, 84–85

Health Valley black bean soup, 202

Health Valley minestrone soup, 202

Health Valley No Salt Chunky peanut butter, 135

Health Valley split pea soup, 188, 202

Health Valley vegetarian amaranth pilaf, 188

Heart:
  oxygen supply, 97–98
  potassium and, 89

Heart disease, 40
  cholesterol and, 95
  dietary fiber and, 78
  fat and, 92
  sodium and, 99
  sugar and, 103
  vegetarian diet and, 143

Heart rate:
  caffeine and, 105
  calcium and, 87

Hemorrhoids, 78

Hepatitis A, 180

Herbed Lentils and Wild Rice, recipe, 257

Herb Sauce, for fish, recipe, 247

Hiatal hernia, 78

High blood pressure, 40
  calcium and, 45, 88
  sodium and, 99

High-fiber Ryvita snackbread, 188

Home recipes, 282

Home-Style Potatoes, recipe, 245

Honey Buc Wheat Crisp, 201

Honey Cream Cheese, recipe, 268

Honeydew melons, 188, 201

Honey Yogurt Dressing, recipe, 270

Hot and Sour Soup, recipe, 232

Hot Blueberry Topping, recipe, 267

Hot Peach Topping, recipe, 267

Hot Red Raspberry Topping, recipe, 268

How to Get Control of Your Time and Your Life, Lakein, 546

Human Nutrition Information Service, 47

Hypercalcemia, 52

Hypertension, 40

I
Immune disorders, from
      anemia, 45
Immune system:
   vitamin A and, 81
   zinc and, 91
Imported foods, 60
Indian restaurants, 154,
      156
Infections:
   folacin and, 86
   Vitamin C and, 82
Information about diet,
      from Nutripoints
      program, 9–11
Information sources,
      177–78
   for Nutripoints program,
      68
In-Residence Program,
      Cooper Clinic, 137,
      182
Insoluble fiber, 78–79
Insomnia:
   caffeine and, 106
   vitamin B6 and 85
Integrated Pest
      Management
      System, 60
Interchangeable
      Nutrigroups, 165
Iodine, 59, 81
Iron, 81, 88
   alcohol and, 107
   deficiency of, 45, 48
   excess consumption, 54
   food combinations, 158
   in shellfish, 180

Irradiated ergosterol, 51
Is It Worth Dying For?,
      Eliot, 546
Italian restaurants, 157

J
Jambalaya, recipe, 248
Jams, 133
Japanese restaurants, 154,
      156–57
Jaundice, vitamin A and,
      81
*Jean Carper's Total
      Nutrition Guide*,
      158
Jellies, 133
Juices:
   fruit, 142
   Nutripoint ratings, 10
   shopping list, 191
   vegetable, 148
Juniper Berry Marinade
      and Sauce, recipe,
      274
Junk foods, 17, 153, 176
Just Right (cereal), 201
   with Fruit and Nuts, 201

K
K, vitamin, 159
Kabobs, scallop, recipe,
      245
Kellogg's Corn Flakes, 100,
      201
Ketchup, sugar in, 103
Key Lime Mousse, recipe,
      260
Kidney beans, 188, 202

Kidneys:
  disease of, sodium and, 99
  protein and, 78
  stones, calcium and, 88
Kiwi, 132, 187, 200
Koop, Surgeon General, 40
Kreigel, Drs., *The C Zone: Peak Performance Under Pressure*, 546
Kretschmer Toasted Wheat Bran, 201

L
Labeling of foods, 42–44
  cholesterol, 98
  sodium, 100–101
  sugar, 103
Lactovegetarians, 144
Lakein, Alan, *How to Get Control of Your Time and Your Life*, 546
Lasagna, 177
  spinach, recipe, 256
Laughing Cow Reduced Calorie Cheese, 15, 136
Lay's potato chips, 100
Leafy vegetables, 132, 172
  folacin in, 86
Learning problems in children, anemia and, 45
Lecithin, 58, 59
Legumes, 78, 86, 134–35, 176

calories per serving, 74
complementary protein relationships, 146
in menus, 206
Nutripoint ratings, 330–35
  top-ten, 188
Nutripoints per dollar, 201–2
shopping list, 194–95
substitutions, 163, 165
Lemon Chicken, recipe, 254
Lemons, 175
Lentils, 147, 202
  complementary protein relationships, 146
  herbed, with wild rice, recipe, 257
Lentil Soup, recipe, 230
Lettuce, 19
  Romaine, 187
Lettuce-Wrapped Salmon, recipe, 247
Life-style diseases:
  avoidance of, 176
  diet and, 40
Lima beans, 147, 188
Lists, 281–84
  alphabetical, 384–542
  Nutrigroup ratings, 285–369
  other groups of foods, 370–83
  for shopping, 151–52, 189–99
Litchi, 187

Lite Caper Dressing, recipe, 271
Lite Mayonnaise Mix, recipe, 270
Lite Orange Vinaigrette Dressing, recipe, 272
Lite Ranch Dressing, recipe, 273
Lite 16-Island Dressing, recipe, 270
Lite Spicy Mustard Dressing, recipe, 268
Lite Vinaigrette, recipe, 272
Lite Zero Salad Dressing, recipe, 269
Liver:
  cholesterol and, 170
  cirrhosis of, 40
  damage to:
    alcohol and, 106
    vitamin A and, 81
  protein and, 78
  vitamin A storage, 53
Loma Linda vegeburger, 134, 188
Low birth weight, zinc deficiencies, 91
Low-calorie diets:
  and vitamin supplements, 56
  zinc deficiencies, 90–91
Low-Fat Fried chicken, recipe, 254–55
Lunch meats, 136

M
McDonald's scrambled eggs, 136
McGovern, George, 40
Macrominerals, 80–81
Magnesium, 53, 80, 89, 171
  potassium and, 89
Mandarin oranges, 132, 188
  canned, 15
Manganese, 81
Mango, 132, 187, 201
Mango Sauce, recipe, 276–77
Margarine, 92
  low-calorie, 128
Marinades, recipes, 274–75
Marinated Asparagus, recipe, 244
Mayer, Jean, 51
Mayonnaise, lite mix, recipe, 270
Meal plans, Nutripoints and, 11–12
Meat, 136
  calories per serving, 74
  in Japanese restaurants, 156–57
  in Mexican restaurants, 157
  Nutripoint ratings, 19, 347–69
  top-ten, 189
  Nutripoints per dollar, 202
  portion sizes, 113

Meat (cont.)
  protein from, 145
  recipes, 250–51
  shopping list, 197–99
  toxic substances in, 143
  substitutes, 165
Medications, nutrients and, 159
Melons, 188, 200, 201
Men, weight-loss calorie levels, 139
Menus, 205–24
Metabolism:
  of carbohydrates, thiamin and, 82
  niacin and, 84
  pantothenic acid and, 85–86
  phosphorus and, 90
  riboflavin and, 83
  vitamin B$_6$ and, 84
  vitamin B$_{12}$ and, 85
  zinc and, 90
Mexican restaurants, 157
Meyers, Casey, Aerobic Walking, 546
Microminerals, 81
Milk, 135
  calcium in, 87
  calories per serving, 74
  cholesterol in, 71
  complementary protein relationships, 146
  in menus, 207
  nonfat dry, 83, 87, 135, 188, 202

Nutripoint ratings, 336–47
  top-ten, 188–89
Nutripoints per dollar, 202
  portion sizes, 114
  shopping list, 195–96
Minerals, 76n, 80–81
  calcium, 87–88
  deficiencies, 48–49
  iron, 88
  magnesium, 89
  phosphorus, 90
  potassium, 89–90
  sodium, 99–102
  zinc, 90–91
Minestrone, 157
Miscellaneous foods, Nutripoint ratings, 382–83
Miso soup, 156
Modifications:
  of Nutripoint program, 164–65
  of recipes, 226–27
Molybdenum, 59, 81
Monosodium glutamate (MSG), 101
  in Chinese restaurants, 155
Mousse, key lime, recipe, 260
Mucous membranes, vitamin A for, 81
Muffins, 193–94
  bran, recipes, 229, 264
  oat bran, recipe, 265

Mung bean sprouts, 201
Muscle action, calcium and,
   87
Muscle tone, thiamin and,
   82–83
Muscle weakness, from
   anemia, 45
Mussels, steamed, 157
Mustard dressing, recipe,
   268
Mustard greens, 187, 200
Myadec, 57

N
National Cancer Institute,
   174
National Centers for
   Disease Control,
   180
National Research Council,
   calcium report, 88
Natural nutrition, 50–55
Nature Valley Oats 'n
   Honey Granola Bar,
   133
Nausea, calcium and, 88
Navy beans, 134, 188, 202
Nectarines, 201
Negative Nutripoint foods,
   18, 164–65, 167,
   168
Nerve function:
   calcium and, 87
   potassium and, 89
   thiamin and, 82
Nervous system:
   niacin and, 84
   vitamin B$_{12}$ and, 85

New Way Sour Cream, 128
   recipe, 271
Niacin (vitamin B$_3$), 80,
   83–84
Nickel, 59
Nitrite-cured foods, 174
Nonfat dry milk, 83, 87,
   135, 188, 202
Nonfat yogurt, 128, 135,
   188, 202
Nonrecommended foods,
   19, 164, 172–73
NutraSweet, 104–5, 128
Nutrient analysis, diet
   record, 120, 122,
   124–25
Nutrients, 166
   alcohol and, 107
   per calorie, 17, 25,
      160
   in fruits and vegetables,
      176
   in legumes, 134
   in meats, 136
Nutri-Grain, 91
Nutrigroups, 21–22
   calories per serving,
      74
   daily recommendations,
      117
   ratings, 285–369
      differences, 166
      fruits, 296–304
      grains, 304–29
      legume/nut/seed,
         330–35
      meat/fish/poultry,
         347–69

Nutrigroups (*cont.*)
milk/dairy, 336–37
top-ten Nutripoints, 187–89
vegetables, 285–96
trends, 130–37
Nutripoint program, 46, 50, 111
balance in diet, 11–12
calories, 94, 138–39
development of, 65–71
information, 9–11
life changes, 31–35
questions, 159–83
real-life applications, 26–35
Nutripoints, 9–18
calculation of ratings, 70–71
daily scores, 20–22
food values and, 44–45
recovery, 23–26, 149–50
values, 18–19
See also Nutrigroups, ratings
Nutritional information, 9–11
Nutritional labeling, 42–44
Nutritional needs, individual differences, 137–38
Nutritional value of foods, 61–62
and cost, 200–202
Nuts, 134–35
Nutripoint ratings, 330–35

O
Oat bran, 79
Oat Bran Muffins, recipe, 265
Oatmeal, 133
fruited cinnamon, recipe, 266
Obesity, 40, 92
avoidance of, 174
sugar and, 103
Oils:
calories per serving, 74
in Indian restaurants, 156
Nutripoint ratings, 370–74
shopping list, 199
Okra, 132
Old people, vitamin supplements, 56
Omelets, Wendy's, 137
cholesterol per calorie, 96, 97
One-A-Day Maximum Formula, 56
One-A-Day Stressgard, 57
100% Bran, 201
Onion soup, 156
Open-Face Pita Sandwich, recipe, 236
Optimum diet, 17–18, 49, 162
balance, 165
Orange juice, 88, 90, 142, 200
iron absorption and, 158
Orange-pineapple juice, 142

Oranges, 70–71, 132, 200
Orange Vinaigrette, recipe,
    272
Organically grown foods,
    60
Organ meats, 83, 136, 170
Osteoporosis, 45, 52, 87
    zinc deficiency, 91
Overdoses of calcium,
    87–88
Ovolactovegetarians, 144
Oxalic acid, 171
Oysters, 180
    raw, 91, 136, 189, 202

P
PABA, 59
Pancakes, 194
    whole grain, recipe,
        266–67
Pantothenic acid, 80,
    85–86
Papaya, 132, 187, 201
Parasites, to avoid, 61
Parsley, 187, 200
Pasta, 133
    recipes, 255–58
    in restaurants, 157
    shopping list, 193
Paté, chicken liver,
        cholesterol per
        calorie, 97
Peaches, 201
    hot topping for pancakes,
        recipe, 267
Peanut butter, 74, 134–35
Pears, 15
    poached, recipe, 261

Peas, 134, 188, 202
    complementary protein
        relationships, 146
    dried, 78
Pepperidge Farm bread,
    100
Peppers:
    sweet red, 82, 200
    Yellow Bell Pepper
        Sauce, recipe, 249
Pesticides, 59–60
Phenylketonouria, 104n
Phosphorus, 59, 80, 90
    in shellfish, 180
Pie, fruit-yogurt, recipe,
    260
Pike, baked, 189
Pinto beans, 202
Pita sandwich, open-face,
    recipe, 236
Pizza, 134, 137
    French bread recipe, 236
Pizza Hut:
    Hand-Tossed Supreme
        Pizza, 134
    Thin and Crispy Pizza,
        137
Planters Cocktail Peanuts,
    100
Plums, canned, 200
PMS (pre-menstrual
        syndrome):
    vitamin B_6 and, 84
    vitamin deficiency and,
        45
Poached Pears, recipe, 261
Portion size:
    adjustments, 115

Portion size (*cont.*)
  calories and, 73–74
  ratings and, 161
  typical, 113–14
Post Natural Bran, 201
Postum, 106, 128
Potassium, 59, 70, 80, 89–90
  in shellfish, 180
  sodium and, 159
Potatoes:
  home-style recipe, 245
  Nutripoint ratings, 13, 19
  portion sizes, 114
  salad recipe, 241
Pot roast, 91
Poultry, 136
  calories per serving, 74
  Nutripoint ratings, 347–69
  portion sizes, 113
  salmonella contamination, 61
  shopping list, 197
Pregnancy:
  diet for, 182
  nutritional imbalances, 52
  vitamins during, 55, 56
Preparation for shopping, 151–52
Preserves, 133
Preventive diets, 181
Pritikin, Nathan, 95
Processed foods:
  grains, 133
  legumes, 134–35
  meats, 136
  Nutripoint ratings, 13
  sodium and, 100–101
  vegetables, 132
Product 19, 201
Protein, 69, 77–78
  complementary relationships, 146
  in legumes, 134, 176
  magnesium and, 89
  meats, 136
  in milk, 135
  niacin and, 84
  riboflavin and, 83
  sources, 142–43
  in vegetarian diet, 144–45
  vitamin B_6 and, 84
  vitamin B_{12} and, 85

Q
Quail, marinade for, recipe, 274
Quaker Oat Bran cereal, 188
Questions:
  about diet, 5–9
  about Nutripoints, 72–75, 159–83
Quotas, Nutripoints, 19–21

R
Rainbow compote, recipe, 259
Ralston hot, high-fiber cereal, 188
Ranch dressing, lite, recipe, 273

Raspberries, 132
  red, hot topping for
      pancakes, recipe,
      268
Ratings, Nutripoints, 160,
      166–67
  calculation of, 167–68
Raw seafood, 61
  Shellfish, 180, 189
    clams, 136, 202
    oysters, 91, 136, 189,
      202
RDAs (Recommended Daily
      Allowances), 12, 42,
      68–69, 169, 173
  Nutripoint program and,
      20, 111
  shortcomings, 47
Rebound scurvy, 55
Recipes, 205, 225–78
  identification, 282
Recommended Daily
      Allowances. See
      RDAs
Recommended level,
      dividing line, 167
Record of eating, 112–26,
      129, 131
  calorie consumption,
      140–41
Rectum cancer, dietary
      fiber and, 78
Red blood cells, vitamin B6
      and, 84
Red meat, 136
  avoidance of, 144
  See also Meat

Red snapper, 189, 202
Red Snapper Veracruz, 206
  recipe, 246
Red wine, iron absorption
      and, 158
Remoulade dishes, 156
Reproduction, vitamin A
      and, 81
Respiration, caffeine and,
      105
Restaurants, 153–57
Rheumatoid arthritis, 52
Riboflavin (vitamin B2), 80,
      83
  alcohol and, 107
  baking soda and, 159
  in fruit, 19
Rice, 133, 194
  in Chinese restaurants,
      155
  to cook, 83
Rice bran, 79
Romaine lettuce, 187, 200
Roughage. See Dietary
      fiber

S
Saccharin, 104
Safety of foods, 59–61
Safflower Oil, 128
Salad dressings, 154–55
  fat in, 92
  recipes, 268–73
  shopping list, 199
  sugar in, 103
Salads:
  portion sizes, 113

Salads (*cont.*)
recipes, 237–41
fruit, 258
pasta, 258
in restaurants, 154–55
Salmon, 202
grilled, recipe, 249
lettuce-wrapped, recipe, 247
steamed/poached, 189
Salmonella contamination, to avoid, 61
Salt, 100
substitutes, 101–2
See also Sodium
Salt-cured foods, 174
Saltman, Paul, 49–50
Sandwiches, recipes, 234–36
Saturated fats, 73, 98, 99
guidelines, 70
limitations, 93
Sauces:
cheese, cholesterol per calorie, 97
in Chinese restaurants, 155
in French restaurants, 156
in Indian restaurants, 156
in Italian restaurants, 157
recipes, 276–78
herb, for fish, 247
yellow bell pepper, for salmon, 249
Scallop Kabobs, recipe, 245

Scallop Sauce, recipe, 277
Scrambled eggs:
cholesterol per calorie, 96
garden scrambled, recipe, 266
McDonald's, 136
Scramblers egg substitute, 188
Seafood:
Nutripoints per dollar, 202
raw, 61, 91, 136, 189, 202
recipes, 245–50
shopping list, 197
shrimp, 14
cholesterol per calorie, 97
See also Fish; Shellfish
Seasoned Turnip Greens, recipe, 244
Sedatives, alcohol, 106
Sedentary women, calorie levels, 138
Seeds, 134
complementary protein relationships, 146
Nutripoint ratings, 330–35
Sego Diet Lite milk drink, 188
Selenium, 81
Serum cholesterol, 97, 99
dietary fiber and, 96
See also Cholesterol
Servings:
limitations, 21–22

recommended number, 161
size of:
  calories and, 73–74
  list information, 283
  ratings and, 161
Sesame seeds, complementary protein relationships, 146
Shellfish, 284
  clams, 180
    canned, 189
  oysters, 136, 180
  raw, 61, 91, 136, 189, 202
  See also Fish; Seafood
Shopping for Nutripoints, 150–53
  lists, 189–99
Shredded Wheat, 179–80
Shrimp, 14
  cholesterol per calorie, 97
Silicon, 59
Skim milk, 189
  nonfat dry, 83, 87, 135, 188, 202
Skin:
  niacin and, 84
  pantothenic acid and, 85
  vitamin A and, 81
Smoked foods, 174
Smoking, calcium and, 88
Smucker's Concord Grape Jelly, 133
Snack foods, 153
Soda, diet, 130

Sodium, 59, 80, 99–102
  guidelines, 70, 173
  potassium and, 89, 159
Sodium bicarbonate, 101
Sodium citrate, 101
Soil conditions, and food value, 62
Soluble fiber, 79
Soups:
  canned, 15
  in French restaurants, 156
  in Italian restaurants, 157
  in Japanese restaurants, 156
  recipes, 230–34
  shopping list, 190–91, 198
Sour cream:
  cooking substitutions, 128
  new way, recipe, 271
South-of-the-Border Vegetarian Chili, recipe, 242
Soy-based foods, 78, 134
Spaghetti sauces, shopping list, 190
Special K, 91
Sperm count, low, zinc deficiency, 91
Spinach, 19, 86, 89, 187, 200
  recipes:
    Clear Spinach Soup, 234
    lasagna recipe, 256
    salad recipe, 237

Spinach (*cont.*)
  salad, cholesterol per
    calorie, 97
  and sodium in diet, 159
Split peas, 201
Spreads, shopping list, 199
Squash, 132
Squid, cholesterol per
    calorie, 96, 97
Standards, Nutripoint
    ratings, 68–71
Stir-fried foods, 155
  chicken recipe, 253
  vegetables, 86
    recipe, 243
Storage of foods, and
    nutritional value,
    62
Strawberries, 187, 201
Strawberry Smoothie,
    recipe, 278
Stress management, 546
Stroke, 40
  sodium and, 99
Styles in foods, 16
Substitutes:
  for coffee, 106
  for salt, 101–2
  for sugar, 104–5
Substitutions in diet
    program:
  Nutrigroups, 163–64,
    165
  upgrade, 128–29
  vegetarian diet, 148
  for water, 130
Sugar, 76–77, 102–5
  calories per serving, 74

guidelines, 70
  Nutripoint ratings,
    375–77
  substitutes, 104–5,
    128
Sulfur, 80
Sunflower seeds,
    complementary
    protein
    relationships, 146
Sunrise Cooler, recipe,
    278
Supplemental minerals:
  calcium, 87–88
  iron, 88
  magnesium, 89
  potassium, 90
Supplemental vitamins,
    50–55
  B_6, 84, 85
  B_{12}, 85
  C, 158
  niacin, 84
Supplemented foods,
    179–80
Sushi, 157
Sussman, Vic, *The
    Vegetarian
    Alternative*, 143
Sweetbreads, 170
  cholesterol per calorie,
    96
Sweeteners, artificial,
    104–5
Sweet potatoes, 82
Swordfish, 202
Systemic conditioning, to
    vitamins, 55

T
Table salt, 100
  See also Sodium
Taco Bell, 136–37
Tacos, 157
Tangerines, 132
Tea, 130
  and iron, 88, 158
  Nutripoint ratings, 382,
    383
  substitutes, 128
Tension headaches, caffeine
    and, 106
Theragran-M, 57
Theragran-M Stresstabs,
    58
Thiamin (Vitamin B$_1$), 80,
    82–83
  alcohol and, 107, 158
  in fruit, 19
3 Minute Brand instant oat
    bran cereal, 188
Time frame of Nutripoint
    diet, 16, 23–26,
    149–50
Timing of shopping trips,
    152–53
Tin, 59
Tobacco, calcium and,
    88
Tofu, 44, 78, 134
  Nutripoints per dollar,
    202
Tofutti Egg Watchers egg
    substitute, 188
Tomatoes, 132
  and sodium in diet, 159
Tomato Sauce, recipe, 276

Tongue, health of, niacin
    and, 84
Tooth decay, sugar and,
    102
Topping recipes:
  hot blueberry, 267
  hot peach, 267
  hot red raspberry, 268
Top-ten Nutripoint Foods,
    187–89
Tortillas, 157
Tossed Salad, recipe, 237
Total Corn Flakes, 201
Total Oatmeal, 201
Total Raisin Bran, 201
Toxicity of vitamins, 53–54
  vitamin A, 81
Toxic substances:
  alcohol, 106–7
  in liver, 170
  vegetarian diet and, 143
Trace elements, 48–49, 81
Tracy, Lisa, *The Gradual
    Vegetarian*, 143
Travel, airline food, 155
Tuna:
  canned, 14, 84, 136,
    189
    Nutripoints per dollar,
      202
    salad recipe, 240
    shopping list, 198
    to remove sodium, 102
  fresh, 202
Turkey, 136
  sandwich, recipe, 234–35
Turnip greens, 187, 200
  recipe, 244

Turock, Arthur, *Getting Physical*, 546
Typhoid fever, 180

U

Unhealthful diets, 20–21, 25, 27–29, 40–41
United States, dietary shortcomings, 47
U.S. Department of Agriculture, Human Nutrition Information Service, 47
U.S. Department of Health and Human Services, cholesterol recommendations, 98
Unsaturated fat, 98
Urination, frequent, vitamin B_6 and, 85

V

Values, Nutripoint ratings, 18–19, 68–71
Vanadium, 59
Varicose veins, 78
Variety in diet, 118, 127–28, 160
Vegans, 144
Vegetable Medley, recipe, 243
Vegetables, 132, 175–76
    calories per serving, 74
    canned, to remove sodium, 102
    in Chinese restaurants, 155
    to cook, 83, 86
    dietary fiber in, 79
    folacin in, 86
    green leafy, 86, 132, 172
    Nutripoint ratings, 19, 21, 22, 285–96
    top-ten, 187
    Nutripoints per dollar, 200
    portion sizes, 114
    recipes, 242–45
    salad, 241
    shopping list, 190–91
    sodium and, 159
The Vegetarian Alternative, Sussman, 143
Vegetarian diet, 142–48
    vitamin B_{12} deficiency, 85
    vitamin supplements, 56
Venison:
    baked, 189
    marinade for, recipe, 274
Vichyssoise, 156
Vinaigrettes, recipes, 272
Virgin Mary (beverage), 107
Viruses, from shellfish, 180
Vision, vitamin A for, 81
Vitamins, 76n, 80
    A, 53–54, 81–82, 132, 172
        alcohol and, 107
        cancer-prevention diet, 174

B-complex, 80
    alcohol and, 107
    B₆, 45, 84–85
    B₁₂, 52, 85
        alcohol and, 158
        antibiotics and, 159
        vitamin C and, 158
    B₁₅, 58
    folacin, 86–87
        alcohol and, 107
    folic acid, 52, 80
    food combinations,
        158–59
    in fruit, 19
    in milk, 135
    niacin (B₃), 80, 83–84
    pantothenic acid, 80,
        85–86
    riboflavin (B₂), 80, 83
        alcohol and, 107
        baking soda and,
            159
        in fruit, 19
    thiamin (B₁), 80,
        82–83
        alcohol and, 107,
            158
        in fruit, 19
C, 17, 52, 80, 82, 132,
    172
    alcohol and, 107
    cancer-prevention diet,
        174
    diagnostic tests and,
        55
    food combinations,
        158

in fruit, 15, 19
    iron and, 88
cancer prevention diet,
    174
in combinations, 158–59
D, alcohol and, 107, 158
    D₂, 51
deficiencies, 45, 47
dietary supplements,
    50–55
in fruits, 132
in milk, 135
P, 59
Q, 59
in vegetables, 132

W
Waffles, 194
Wall street Journal, 60
Walton, Bill, 48–49
Wasa Fiber-Plus
        Crispbread, 188
Washing of fresh foods, 60
Water, 130
Watercress, 187, 200
Watermelon, 105, 200
Water-soluble vitamins, 80
    B₆, 84–85
    B₁₂, 85
    C, 82
    systemic conditioning to,
        55
    thiamin (B₁), 82–83
Waxed foods, 60
Weight loss diets, 42, 46,
    49
    calorie levels, 138–39

Wendy's Creamy
    Peppercorn
    dressing, cholesterol
    per calorie, 97
Wendy's omelets, 137
    cholesterol per calorie,
        96, 97
Wheat bran, 133, 188
Wheat germ, 133, 188
White beans, 147
White wine, iron absorption
    and, 158
Whole Grain Pancakes,
    recipe, 266–67
Whole milk, 207
    cooking substitution,
        128
    See also Milk
Whole wheat bread/English
    muffin, 188
Whole Wheat Total, 133,
    179–80, 201
Wild rice:
    herbed lentils with,
        recipe, 257
    soup, recipe, 233
Wine, iron absorption and,
    158
Women:
    calcium deficiency, 87

calorie levels, 138–39
    dietary needs, 45
    folacin deficiency,
        86
    high-calorie diet, 41
    iron deficiency, 88
    zinc deficiency, 91
Wonder Hi-Fiber bread,
    133, 188

Y

Yeast, Nutripoint ratings,
    382
Yellow/orange vegetables,
    172
Yogurt, 46
    fruit pie, recipe, 260
    Honey Yogurt Dressing,
        recipe, 270
    nonfat, 87, 128, 135,
        188, 202
    Nutripoint ratings,
        14
    shopping list, 195

Z

Zinc, 52, 81, 90–91
    alcohol and, 107
    in shellfish, 180

Nutripoints	Food Name	Serving size	Nutrigroup
46.5	*Juice, Vitamin Supreme, Snapple	10 oz	Fruit
41.0	*Milk Drink, Spiru-Tein (w/skim milk)	8 oz	Milk/Dairy
29.0	*Sports Drink, Splash	8 oz	Fruit
21.5	*Snack Bar, Tiger's Sports Bar	1 bar	Grain
21.0	*Snack Bar, Power Bar	1 bar	Grain
16.5	*Sports Drink, Power Burst (all flavors)	8 oz	Fruit
14.5	Chlorella (powder or w/water)	3 oz powder	Misc.
13.0	*Cereal, Cheerios, Multi-Grain, General Mills	1 cup	Grain
10.5	Waffles, Wholegrain Wheat/Oatbran, Aunt Jemima	2 waffles	Grain
8.5	Pancakes, Whole Wheat, Aunt Jemima (from mix)	3 small	Grain
8.5	Cereal, Multi-Grains/Raisins/Oats, Healthy Choice	1 cup	Grain
8.0	Pancakes, Lite Buttermilk, Aunt Jemima (from mix)	3 small	Grain
7.5	Hamburger, (Vege) Harvest Burger, Green Giant	1 burger	Legume
7.0	Soup, Healthy Request, Vegetable, Campbell's	1 cup	Vegetable
6.5	Turkey, Ground Breast Meat, Turkey Store	4 oz	M/F/P
6.5	Turkey, Breast Slices, Turkey Store	4 oz	M/F/P
6.5	Turkey, Breast Tenderloins, Turkey Store	4 oz	M/F/P
6.0	Soup, Healthy Classics, Chicken Noodle, Progresso	1 cup	M/F/P
6.0	Pancakes, Buckwheat, Aunt Jemima (from mix)	3 small	Grain
6.0	Snack Bar, FIBAR (all flavors)	1 bar	Grain
5.5	Soup, Healthy Request, Vegetable Beef, Campbell's	1 cup	M/F/P
5.0	Soup, Minestrone, Healthy Choice	1 cup	Legume
5.0	Broc/Caul/Car/97% fat-free sauce, fzn, Green Giant	2/3 cup	Vegetable
4.5	Wheat Cakes, Quaker	3 cakes	Grain
4.5	Rye Cakes, Quaker	3 cakes	Grain
4.5	Milk Drink, Nutrament	6 oz (1/2 can)	Milk/Dairy

* Fortified: 50% or greater of total nutritional value added.

Nutripoints	Food Name	Serving size	Nutrigroup
4.5	Soup, Healthy Classics, Garlic & Pasta, Progresso	1 cup	Grain
4.5	Soup, Garden Vegetable, Healthy Choice	1 cup	Vegetable
4.5	Soup, Healthy Classics, Beef Vegetable, Progresso	1 cup	M/F/P
4.0	Milk Substitute, Non-Dairy, Vitamite	1 cup	Milk or Legume
4.0	Sports Drink, Bodyfuel	8 oz	Fruit
4.0	Cheese, Non-Fat, Processed American or Swiss	2 slices	Milk/Dairy
3.5	Juice, Mango Nectar, Kern's	8 oz	Fruit
3.5	Snack Bar, Nutri-Grain, Kellogg's (all flavors)	1 bar	Grain
3.5	Chicken, (Vege) Chick Patties, Morningstar Farms	1 patty	Legume
3.5	Juice, Strawberry/Banana Nectar, Kern's	8 oz	Fruit
3.0	Rice Cakes, Plain, Salt-Free, Quaker	3 cakes	Grain
3.0	Rice Cakes, Plain, Lightly Salted, Quaker	3 cakes	Grain
3.0	Rice Cakes, Sesame, Lt. Salted, Quaker	3 cakes	Grain
3.0	Juice, Guava Nectar, Kern's	8 oz	Fruit
3.0	Soup, Chicken w/Rice, Healthy Choice	1 cup	Grain or M/F/P
2.5	Soup, Healthy Request, Chicken Noodle, Campbell's	1 cup	M/F/P
2.5	Cracker, Fat-Free, Premium Saltine, Nabisco	10 crackers	Grain
2.5	Corn Cakes, Quaker	3 cakes	Grain
2.5	Cookies, Fat-Free, Health Valley (all flavors)	3 cookies	Grain
2.5	Turkey, Burger Patties, Turkey Store	3.5 oz	M/F/P
2.0	Tarts, Fat-Free, Health Valley (all flavors)	1 tart	Grain
2.0	Cracker, 5-grain, Harvest Crisps, Nabisco	12 crackers	Grain
2.0	Fruit Drink Mix, Crystal Light (all flavors)	8 oz	Misc.
2.0	Frozen Dessert, Fudgesicle, Sugar-Free, Good Humor	2	Misc.
1.5	Cracker, Low Salt, Saltine, Nabisco	10 crackers	Grain
1.5	Pretzel, Fat-Free, Mr. Salty, Nabisco	1 oz	Grain
1.5	Sports Drink, Exceed	8 oz	Fruit
1.5	Cracker, Whole Wheat, Saltine, Nabisco	10 crackers	Grain
1.5	Cracker, Saltine, Nabisco	10 crackers	Grain

Nutripoints	Food Name	Serving size	Nutrigroup
1.5	Peanut Butter, 25% less fat, Laura Scudder's Natural	2 Tbls	Legume
1.0	Peanut Butter, 30% less fat, Peter Pan Smart Choice	2 Tbls	Legume
1.0	Peanut Butter, 25% less fat, Skippy	2 Tbls	Legume
1.0	Margarine, 20% Corn Oil, Smart Beat	1 oz	Fat/Oil
1.0	Peanut Butter, Reduced Fat, Jiff	2 Tbls	Legume
1.0	Cracker, Wheat 'n Bran, Triscuit, Nabisco	6 crackers	Grain
1.0	Cracker, Low Salt, Triscuit, Nabisco	6 crackers	Grain
.5	Frozen Dessert, Popsicle, Sugar-Free, Good Humor	2	Misc.
.5	Crackers, Teddy Grahams, Nabisco	22 pieces	Grain
.5	Cracker, Whole Wheat, Ritz	10 crackers	Grain
.5	Cracker, Low Salt, Ritz	10 crackers	Grain
.5	Creamer, Non-Dairy, Fat-Free, Mocha Mix	2 Tbls	Misc.
0.0	Dressing, Lite Red French, Wish-Bone	1 Tbls	Fat/Oil
0.0	Dressing, Non-Fat, Healthy Sensation (all flavors)	1 Tbls	Fat/Oil
0.0	Corn Chips, Pringles	11 chips	Grain
0.0	Mayonnaise, Non-Fat, Kraft Free	1 Tbls	Fat/Oil
-.5	Dressing, Non-Fat, Kraft Free (all flavors)	1 Tbls	Fat/Oil
-.5	Dressing, Lite Italian, Wish-Bone	1 Tbls	Fat/Oil
-.5	Dressing, Non-Fat, Take Heart, Hidden Valley (all flav)	1 Tbls	Fat/Oil
-1.5	Snack Cake, 97% Fat-Free, Hostess (all flavors)	1 cake	Grain
-1.5	Granola Bar, Chewy, Low-Fat, Quaker (all flavors)	1 bar	Grain
-2.0	Milk Drink Mix, Non-Fat, Hot Cocoa, Swiss Miss	1 cup	Milk/Dairy
-2.5	Mayonnaise, Canola Oil, Smart Beat	1 Tbls	Fat/Oil
-2.5	Pudding, Fat-Free, Swiss Miss (all flavors)	1/2 cup	Milk/Dairy
-3.0	Brownie/Blondie, Fat-Free, Pepperidge Farm	1 piece	Sugar
-4.5	Syrup, Lite, Aunt Jemima	1 fl oz	Sugar
-5.5	Syrup, Original, Aunt Jemima	1 fl oz	Sugar
-6.0	Syrup, Butterlite, Aunt Jemima	1 fl oz	Sugar

ABOUT THE AUTHOR

Roy E. Vartabedian, Dr.P.H., M.P.H., F.A.P.C.A. is a clinical preventive care specialist in private practice in Southern California, and President of Vartabedian & Associates/Designs for Wellness. A frequent lecturer and popular guest speaker, Dr. Vartabedian has appeared on the *Today Show*, *Live With Regis & Kathy Lee*, *Everyday With Joan Lunden* and a variety of other national and regional TV and radio programs. His breakthrough Nutripoint method has also been the subject of numerous articles in leading newspapers and magazines across the country such as *Ladie's Home Journal*, *The New York Daily News* and *The Dallas Morning News*.

Previously, he held the position of Executive Director of the Cooper Clinic Residential Wellness Programs in Dallas for 6 years. He received his Doctor of Public Health degree (clinical preventive care) and Master of Public Health degree (nutrition, health education) from Loma Linda University, Loma Linda, California. Prior to his work in Dallas he taught Preventive Medicine at the Florida Hospital Family Practice Residency in Orlando for 4 years.

Dr. Vartabedian is available for public speaking engagements to your group. He also works as a consultant in the development of nutrition, wellness, and preventive medicine programs. To contact Dr. Vartabedian, write to:

**VARTABEDIAN & ASSOCIATES
DESIGNS FOR WELLNESS**
PO Box 1671, Carlsbad CA 92018
(760) 804-5999